T0221201

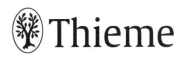

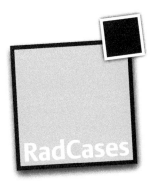

RadCases Plus Q&A Neuro Imaging
Second Edition

Edited by

Roy F. Riascos, MD
Professor of Radiology
Chief of Neuroradiology
Department of Diagnostic and Interventional
  Imaging
The University of Texas Health Science Center at
  Houston
Houston, Texas

Eliana Bonfante, MD
Associate Professor of Radiology
Department of Diagnostic and Interventional
  Imaging
The University of Texas Health Science Center at
  Houston
Houston, Texas

Susana Calle, MD
Staff Neuroradiologist
Department of Diagnostic and Interventional
  Imaging
The University of Texas Health Science Center at
  Houston
Houston, Texas

Series Editors

Jonathan M. Lorenz, MD, FSIR
Professor of Radiology
Section of Interventional Radiology
The University of Chicago
Chicago, Illinois

Hector Ferral, MD
Senior Medical Educator
NorthShore University HealthSystem
Evanston, Illinois

776 illustrations

Thieme
New York • Stuttgart • Delhi • Rio de Janeiro

Executive Editor: William Lamsback
Managing Editors: J. Owen Zurhellen IV and Kenneth Schubach
Director, Editorial Services: Mary Jo Casey
Production Editor: Teresa Exley, Absolute Service, Inc.
International Production Director: Andreas Schabert
Editorial Director: Sue Hodgson
International Marketing Director: Fiona Henderson
International Sales Director: Louisa Turrell
Director of Institutional Sales: Adam Bernacki
Senior Vice President and Chief Operating Officer: Sarah Vanderbilt
President: Brian D. Scanlan
Printer: King Printing

Library of Congress Cataloging-in-Publication Data

Names: Riascos, Roy, editor. | Bonfante, Eliana, editor. | Calle,
   Susana, editor.
Title: RadCases plus Q&A neuro imaging / edited by
   Roy F. Riascos, Eliana Bonfante, Susana Calle.
Other titles: Neuro imaging (Riascos) | Q&A neuro imaging |
   RadCases.
Description: Second edition. | New York : Thieme, 2018. | Series:
   RadCases | Preceded by Neuro imaging / edited by Roy Riascos,
   Eliana Bonfante. 2011. | Includes bibliographical references.
Identifiers: LCCN 2018035072| ISBN 9781626232372 | ISBN
   9781626232433 (e-book)
Subjects: | MESH: Central Nervous System Diseases--diagnostic
   imaging | Radiography | Central Nervous System--diagnostic
   imaging | Diagnostic Techniques, Neurological | Case Reports
Classification: LCC RC349.R3 | NLM WL 141.5.N47 | DDC
   616.8/047572–dc23
LC record available at https://lccn.loc.gov/2018035072

Copyright © 2019 by Thieme Medical Publishers, Inc.
Thieme Publishers New York
333 Seventh Avenue, New York, NY 10001 USA
+1 800 782 3488, customerservice@thieme.com

Thieme Publishers Stuttgart
Rüdigerstrasse 14, 70469 Stuttgart, Germany
+49 [0]711 8931 421, customerservice@thieme.de

Thieme Publishers Delhi
A-12, Second Floor, Sector-2, Noida-201301
Uttar Pradesh, India
+91 120 45 566 00, customerservice@thieme.in

Thieme Publishers Rio de Janeiro, Thieme Publicações Ltda.
Edifício Rodolpho de Paoli, 25º andar
Av. Nilo Peçanha, 50 – Sala 2508,
Rio de Janeiro 20020-906 Brasil
+55 21 3172-2297/+55 21 3172-1896

Cover design: Thieme Publishing Group
Typesetting by Absolute Service, Inc.
Printed in the United States by King Printing
5 4 3 2 1

ISBN 978-1-62623-237-2

Also available as an e-book:
eISBN 978-1-62623-243-3

Important note: Medicine is an ever-changing science undergoing continual development. Research and clinical experience are continually expanding our knowledge, in particular our knowledge of proper treatment and drug therapy. Insofar as this book mentions any dosage or application, readers may rest assured that the authors, editors, and publishers have made every effort to ensure that such references are in accordance with **the state of knowledge at the time of production of the book**.

Nevertheless, this does not involve, imply, or express any guarantee or responsibility on the part of the publishers in respect to any dosage instructions and forms of applications stated in the book. **Every user is requested to examine carefully** the manufacturers' leaflets accompanying each drug and to check, if necessary in consultation with a physician or specialist, whether the dosage schedules mentioned therein or the contraindications stated by the manufacturers differ from the statements made in the present book. Such examination is particularly important with drugs that are either rarely used or have been newly released on the market. Every dosage schedule or every form of application used is entirely at the user's own risk and responsibility. The authors and publishers request every user to report to the publishers any discrepancies or inaccuracies noticed. If errors in this work are found after publication, errata will be posted at www.thieme.com on the product description page.

Some of the product names, patents, and registered designs referred to in this book are in fact registered trademarks or proprietary names even though specific reference to this fact is not always made in the text. Therefore, the appearance of a name without designation as proprietary is not to be construed as a representation by the publisher that it is in the public domain.

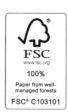

FSC
www.fsc.org
100%
Paper from well-
managed forests
FSC® C103101

Dedicated to the woman for whom my heart surrenders, Maria Claudia, and to our three sons, Camilo, Felipe, and Pablo, for making my life this wonderful experience.

—RFR

This book is dedicated to my loving and supporting soulmate, Darren, and to our two wonderful and inspiring children, Matthew and Zachary.

—EB

This book is dedicated to my incredible husband, Jaime, and to my beautiful baby daughter, Elena: you mean the world to me.

—SC

Series Preface

As enthusiastic partners in radiology education, we continue our mission to ease the exhaustion and frustration shared by residents and the families of residents engaged in radiology training! In launching the second edition of the RadCases series, our intent is to expand rather than replace this already rich study experience that has been tried, tested, and popularized by residents around the world. In each subspecialty edition, we serve up 100 carefully chosen new cases to raise the bar in our effort to assist residents in tackling the daunting task of assimilating massive amounts of information. RadCases second edition primes and expands on concepts found in the first edition with important variations on prior cases, updated diagnostic and management strategies, and new pathological entities. Our continuing goal is to combine the popularity and portability of printed books with the adaptability, exceptional quality, and interactive features of an electronic case–based format. The new cases will be added to the existing electronic database to enrich the interactive environment of high-quality images that allows residents to arrange study sessions, quickly extract and master information, and prepare for theme-based radiology conferences.

We owe a debt of gratitude to our own residents and to the many radiology trainees who have helped us create, adapt, and improve the format and content of RadCases by weighing in with suggestions for new cases, functions, and formatting. Back by popular demand is the concise point-by-point presentation of the Essential Facts of each case in an easy-to-read bulleted format, and a short critical differential starting with the actual diagnosis. This approach is easy on exhausted eyes and encourages repeated priming of important information during quick reviews, a process we believe is critical to radiology education. New since the previous edition is the addition of a question-and-answer section for each case to reinforce key concepts.

The intent of the printed books is to encourage repeated priming in the use of critical information by providing a portable group of exceptional core cases to master. Unlike the authors of other case-based radiology review books, we removed the guesswork by providing clear annotations and descriptions for all images. In our opinion, there is nothing worse than being unable to locate a subtle finding on a poorly reproduced image even after one knows the final diagnosis.

The electronic cases expand on the printed book and provide a comprehensive review of the entire specialty. Thousands of cases are strategically designed to increase the resident's knowledge by providing exposure to a spectrum of case examples—from basic to advanced—and by exploring "Aunt Minnies," unusual diagnoses, and variability within a single diagnosis. The search engine allows the resident to create individualized daily study lists that are not limited by factors such as radiology subsection. For example, tailor today's study list to cases involving tuberculosis and include cases in every subspecialty and every system of the body. Or study only thoracic cases, including those with links to cardiology, nuclear medicine, and pediatrics. Or study only musculoskeletal cases. The choice is yours.

As enthusiastic partners in this project, we started small and, with the encouragement, talent, and guidance of Timothy Hiscock and William Lamsback at Thieme Publishers, we have further raised the bar in our effort to assist residents in tackling the daunting task of assimilating massive amounts of information. We are passionate about continuing this journey and will continue to expand the series, adapt cases based on direct feedback from residents, and increase the features intended for board review and self-assessment. First and foremost, we thank our medical students, residents, and fellows for allowing us the privilege to participate in their educational journey.

Jonathan M. Lorenz, MD, FSIR
Hector Ferral, MD

Preface

It is a thrill for us to come together again and create this second edition. We have designed this book with great care to maximize the amount of retained material. Our advice is to truly analyze each case as if it were presented to you at your institution of practice. As always, our patients are our best teachers. Try to extract the greatest amount of information from each image, and resist the urge to quickly turn the page and read the provided material. The flow of the cases intends to mimic what is encountered at the reading station with the added benefit of a third party signaling which images are relevant to the diagnosis. A short and concise clinical presentation is provided. Readers are invited to test their knowledge by establishing differential diagnoses and determining which is the main consideration and why the other diagnoses are less probable. The exercise of developing a working diagnosis based on a presented case is the essence of learning in radiology and will truly enhance the review process.

New technologies including perfusion techniques, spectroscopy, nuclear medicine, and 3D reconstructions, among others, are included in this current edition. The purpose of this is to guide the reader to incorporate this additional information into the thought process as these modalities become more common in the workplace.

In contrast to the previous edition, questions and answers have now been added to each case in an attempt to better simulate how neuroradiology is currently taught. Our hope is that the interactive and dynamic nature of the book will serve to further strengthen the concepts presented.

Acknowledgments

There are not enough words of gratitude to thank everybody who allowed this second edition of our book to become a reality. I would like to acknowledge first of all the readers who have supported the material and have helped make this new edition. I must sincerely thank my amazing coauthors and friends, Eliana and Susana, for working with me on this project. A special thank you to all the medical students, residents, research assistants, and fellows at University of Texas Health Science Center and University of Texas Medical Branch for inspiring me to come to work every day. Appreciation to my team, to my colleagues, and to Susan John for the support. Special thanks to my beautiful wife Maria Claudia and my three wonderful kids, the true loves of my life, for being there for me and for sacrificing so much of their time to make a project like this come true. Gratitude to Lucy, Roy Sr., and Roberto for helping become who I am.
Thank you.

—RFR

With each one of my academic projects, the list of people I am grateful to keeps growing and growing. It has been an honor to be invited to collaborate on a second edition of this book. It has been a blessing to receive feedback from residents and colleagues to improve and update our cases. Roy and Susana are the best partners to have. They made this project seem like we were not working, we were just having fun. Thanks to my colleagues in the Neuroradiology section, to our amazing fellows, and to our inquisitive residents for enriching my world every day. The love and support of my husband Darren and our fantastic sons, Matthew and Zachary, are the fuel that keeps me here every day. And as always, I owe who I am to my beloved parents, Juan and Ester, who taught me what perseverance gives you at the end of the day.

—EB

First and foremost, I would like to thank my coauthors for inviting me to participate in this project. It has been an honor to collaborate with you both on this second edition, and I have learned so much throughout the process. To the groups of outstanding neuroradiologists at University of Texas at Houston and MD Anderson Cancer Center, I appreciate your role in transforming me into a neuroradiologist. I have learned so much from each of you. I am forever indebted to my teachers and coresidents at Pontificia Universidad Javeriana. You were the foundation of my training and I still hear your words of advice in my daily practice. Last but definitely not least, I would like to thank my parents and my brother and sister. You are behind everything I am and all that I do.

—SC

Case 1

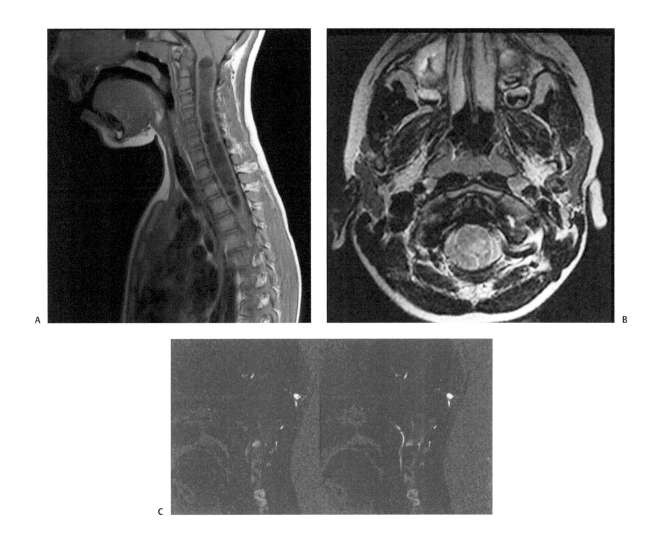

■ Clinical Presentation

A 6-year-old boy presents with headaches.

■ Imaging Findings

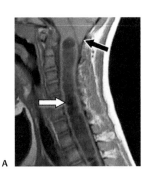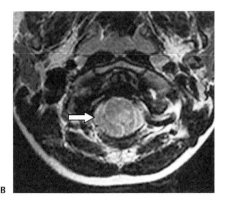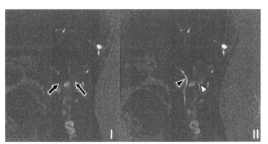

(A) Sagittal T1 image shows peg-shaped cerebellar tonsils lying > 5 mm below the level of the foramen magnum, at the level of the posterior arch of C1 (*black arrow*). There is associated dilatation of the central canal of the cervical cord (*white arrow*). **(B)** Axial T2-weighted image demonstrates crowding of the foramen magnum with effacement of the subarachnoid space at the craniocervical junction (*white arrow*). **(C)** Transverse gated phase-contrast MR images (cerebrospinal fluid flow study) during the systolic phase (*I*) and diastolic phase (*II*) demonstrate lack of flow-related signal at the foramen magnum during systole (*black arrows*). During the diastolic phase, there is patent flow ventrally at the foramen magnum (*black arrowhead*) with obstruction to flow dorsally due to the herniated tonsils (*white arrowhead*).

■ Differential Diagnosis

- *Chiari I malformation:* A malformation of the posterior fossa and cerebellum characterized by peg-shaped cerebellar tonsils positioned > 5 mm below the level of the foramen magnum. This condition is commonly associated with altered cerebrospinal fluid (CSF) flow dynamics at the craniocervical junction, which leads to syringohydromyelia.
- *Intracranial hypotension:* Acquired or spontaneous condition leading to decreased pressure typically resulting from CSF leaks secondary to trauma, surgery, or interventional spine procedures. Apart from the inferiorly displaced tonsils, intracranial hypotension also demonstrates chronic subdural collections, dilated dural sinuses, enlargement of the pituitary gland, and a "sagging" midbrain below the level of the dorsum sellae. There is no associated syringohydromyelia.
- *Tonsillar ectopia:* Position of the cerebellar tonsils below the level of the foramen magnum measuring < 5 mm. Generally, the morphology of the tonsils is preserved, no CSF flow alterations occur, and the posterior fossa has normal size.

■ Essential Facts

- Unclear pathogenesis, generally believed to be secondary to para-axial mesodermal insufficiency.
- The basion-opisthion line (BOL) marks the inferior margin of the foramen magnum. A perpendicular measurement of the inferior tip of the cerebellar tonsils to the BOL > 5 mm is generally considered diagnostic for Chiari I malformation.

- Tonsils typically herniate through the foramen magnum to the level of C1 or C2.
- The location of the brainstem is usually normal.
- The tonsils adopt a pointed or peg-shaped morphology.
- Cerebellar folia exhibit a vertical or oblique orientation sometimes referred to as "sergeant's stripes."

■ Other Imaging Findings

- Altered CSF dynamics ensue because of abnormal flow between spinal and intracranial CSF spaces, leading to syringohydromyelia in 40 to 80% of patients with symptomatic Chiari I.
- There is effacement of the subarachnoid spaces at the craniocervical junction with the appearance of "crowding" at the foramen magnum, which is better seen on axial T2 images.
- Hydrocephalus can be seen as a complication of Chiari I malformation in ~10% of cases.
- Other rare associations include callosal dysgenesis and absence of the septum pellucidum.

✓ Pearls and ✗ Pitfalls

- ✓ No association with spinal dysraphism.
- ✓ Cervical anomalies associated with Chiari I include Klippel–Feil syndrome.
- ✓ In axial images, visualization of the cerebellar tonsils at the level of the dens is indicative of ectopia.
- ✗ Borderline inferiorly displaced and normally shaped cerebellar tonsils are consistent with tonsillar ectopia and do not fit the criteria for Chiari I malformation.

Case 2

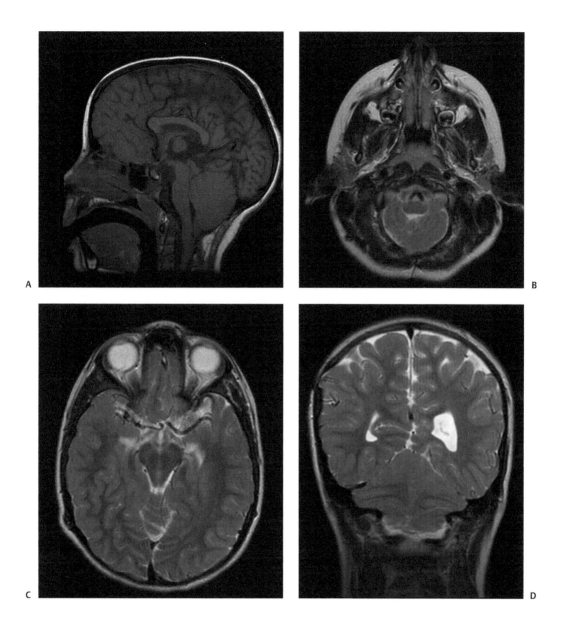

■ Clinical Presentation

A 7-year-old male patient with developmental delay.

■ Imaging Findings

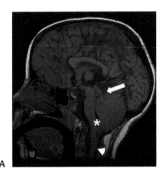 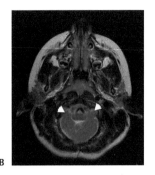 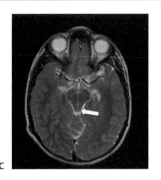 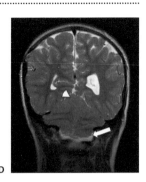

(A) Sagittal T1-weighted image (WI) demonstrates beaking of the tectum (*arrow*), effacement of the fourth ventricle (*asterisk*), small posterior fossa secondary to a low-riding torcula, and descent of the cerebellar tonsils down to the level of C2–C3 (*arrowhead*). **(B)** Axial T2WI demonstrates wrapping of the cerebellar tonsils around the medulla oblongata (*arrowheads*). **(C)** Axial T2WI at the level of the midbrain shows beaking of the tectum (*arrow*). **(D)** Coronal T2WI demonstrates descent of the cerebellar tonsils (*arrow*) below the level of the foramen magnum and towering of the cerebellum (*arrowhead*).

■ Differential Diagnosis

- ***Chiari II malformation:*** Hindbrain anomaly characterized by a small posterior fossa with crowding, deformity, and herniation of the cerebellum and brainstem. This condition is associated with lumbar myelomeningocele.
- *Chiari I malformation:*
  ○ Low-lying cerebellar tonsils
  ○ Cervical cord syrinx
  ○ Hydrocephalus in up to 30% of cases
  ○ Associated with skeletal anomalies including: platybasia, basilar invagination, atlanto-occipital assimilation, Sprengel deformity, Klippel–Feil syndrome
- *Spinal hypotension:*
  ○ Most commonly results from cerebrospinal fluid (CSF) leaks in the cervical and thoracic spine.
  ○ Sagging brainstem
  ○ Subdural effusions
  ○ Increased fluid around the optic nerves
  ○ Venous sinus engorgement
  ○ Pachymeningeal enhancement

■ Essential Facts

- In Chiari II malformation, the posterior fossa is small with a low insertion of the tentorium. The cerebellum herniates superiorly (towering cerebellum) and the resultant mass effect on the tectum causes a characteristic beaking effect (tectal beaking). Furthermore, the inferior displacement of the brainstem leads to medullary kinking and herniation of the tonsils and/or vermis into the cervical spinal canal.
- Other anomalies are frequent in the cerebrum (obstructive hydrocephalus, dysgenesis of the corpus callosum, prominent masa intermedia, absent septum pellucidum), dura (fenestration of the falx with interdigitated gyri, heart-shaped incisura, hypoplastic tentorium), and cranial vault (enlarged foramen magnum, scalloping of petrous temporal bone, lacunar skull).

■ Other Imaging Findings

- CSF flow studies demonstrate abnormal CSF dynamics at the foramen magnum and may be used for decisions regarding therapy.
- Associated spinal malformations include syringohydromyelia, scoliosis, segmentation anomalies, and diastematomyelia.

✓ Pearls and ✗ Pitfalls

- ✓ If only axial images are available, search for wrapping of the cerebellar tonsils around the medulla oblongata, beaking of the tectum, and colpocephaly as clues for this diagnosis.
- ✓ If there is no basilar invagination, observing the cerebellar tonsils at the same level on axial imaging as the tip of the dens indicates tonsillar ectopia.
- ✗ The herniated cerebellar tonsils may undergo atrophy and can be difficult to detect in the cervical spinal canal.

Case 3

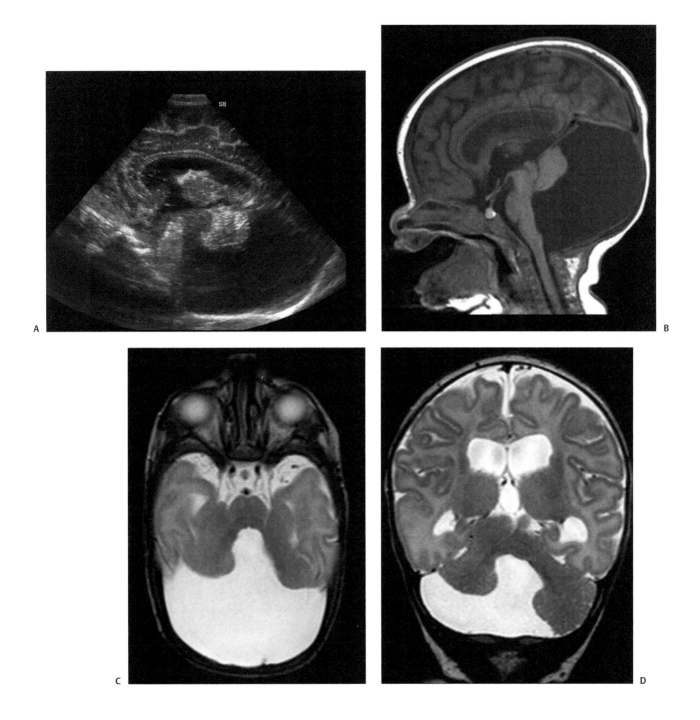

■ Clinical Presentation

A neonate presents with an abnormal obstetric ultrasound.

■ Imaging Findings

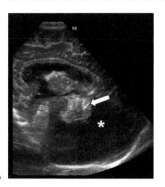 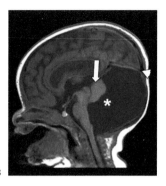 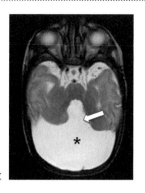 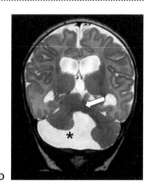

A   B   C   D

(A) Sagittal ultrasound shows a small cerebellar vermis that is tilted superiorly (*arrow*), with the presence of a large cyst in the posterior fossa (*asterisk*). **(B)** Sagittal T1-weighted image (WI) shows the hypoplastic vermis (*arrow*) with a superiorly inserted torcula (*arrowhead*) and a large posterior fossa cyst (*asterisk*). **(C)** Axial T2WI shows a large posterior fossa cyst (*asterisk*) with an abnormal connection with the fourth ventricle (*arrow*). **(D)** Coronal T2WI shows the hypoplastic cerebellar vermis (*arrow*) and the large posterior fossa cyst (*asterisk*).

■ Differential Diagnosis

- *Dandy–Walker malformation:*
  ○ Hypoplasia and elevation of the cerebellar vermis.
  ○ Large cyst in the posterior fossa that is a continuation of the fourth ventricle.
  ○ Enlargement of the posterior fossa with a high tentorium.
- *Blake pouch cyst:*
  ○ Not associated with vermian hypoplasia.
  ○ Cyst that extends through the foramen of Magendie and communicates with the fourth ventricle. In contrasted images, the choroid plexus will be seen extending through the cyst.
  ○ Typically will not have superior displacement of the tentorium.
  ○ No communication of the cyst with the subarachnoid space.
- *Posterior fossa arachnoid cyst:*
  ○ Variable locations within the posterior fossa.
  ○ The cerebellar vermis can either exhibit a normal configuration or can be deformed by mass effect from the cyst.
  ○ Large cysts may cause hydrocephalus.
  ○ The cerebellar falx may be displaced off the midline.
  ○ No communication of the cyst with the fourth ventricle.

■ Essential Facts

- Hydrocephalus is present in 90% of cases and is the most common manifestation in the first months of life.

- Thirty to 50% of cases can have additional malformations such as callosal dysgenesis, occipital encephalocele, polymicrogyria, and heterotopia.

■ Other Imaging Findings

- Dandy–Walker malformation can be identified in prenatal ultrasound.
- MRI is the best diagnostic tool.
- Contrast helps differentiate between a Blake pouch cyst and Dandy–Walker malformation by identifying enhancing choroid plexus extending through the cyst in Blake pouch cysts.

✓ Pearls and ✗ Pitfalls

✓ Fifty percent of cases are associated with chromosomal anomalies or Mendelian disorders.
✓ Most patients present with symptoms of increased intracranial pressure in the first year of life.
✗ Look for associated anomalies to identify different syndromes:
  • Meckel–Gruber syndrome: encephalocele, polydactyly
  • Walker–Warburg syndrome: encephalocele, lissencephaly, microphthalmia
✗ If axial scans are acquired with a steep angle, an abnormal communication between the fourth ventricle and the cisterna magna can be erroneously suggested.

Case 4

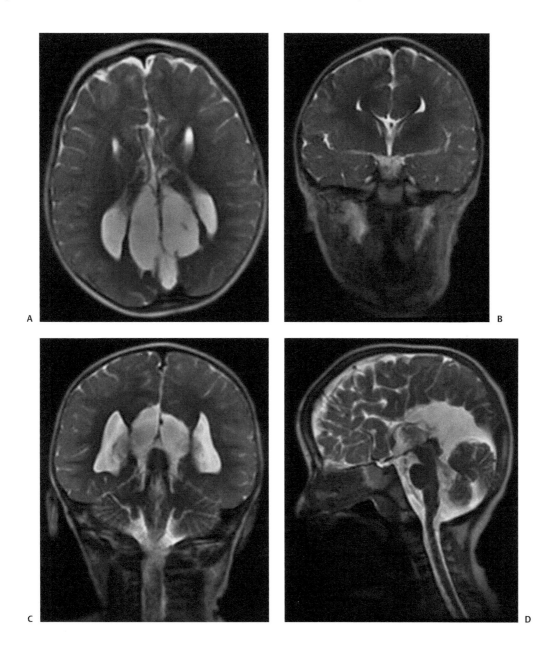

■ Clinical Presentation

A child presents with developmental delay.

■ Imaging Findings

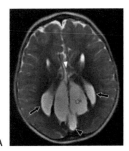 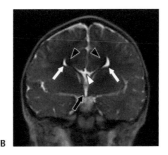 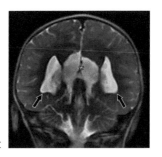 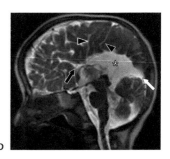

A   B   C   D

(A) Axial T2-weighted image (WI) demonstrates a parallel orientation of the lateral ventricles (*black arrows*), also termed the "race car sign." Between the widely spaced lateral ventricles there is a midline cyst (*asterisk*), with a vessel running through it, extending from the third ventricle (*white arrowhead*) to the subarachnoid space (*black arrowhead*). **(B)** Coronal T2WI shows a high-riding third ventricle due to absence of the corpus callosum (*white arrowhead*), with bundles of Probst indenting the superomedial bodies of the lateral ventricles (*black arrowheads*). The configuration of the ventricles mimics a "moose head" with the third ventricle representing the moose's head (*black arrow*) and the lateral ventricles being the antlers (*white arrows*). **(C)** Coronal T2WI shows the cystic structure (*asterisk*) at the midline between the posterior bodies of the lateral ventricles (*black arrows*). **(D)** Sagittal T2WI of the brain demonstrates agenesis of the corpus callosum with eversion of the cingulate gyrus. The vertically oriented paramedic gyri radiate toward the expected location of the corpus collosum and conform the so-called "sun ray appearance" (*black arrowheads*). The interhemispheric cyst (*asterisk*) communicates the ventricular system (*black arrow*) with the subarachnoid space (*white arrow*).

■ Differential Diagnosis

- **Callosal agenesis with interhemispheric cyst (CA with IHC):** CA with IHC is a distinct condition that is believed to vary in cause when compared to other forms of agenesis of the corpus callosum. This condition is characterized by a deficient formation of the corpus callosum associated with a midline cyst that can present with or without communication to the ventricular system.
- *Porencephaly:* Congenital or acquired condition secondary to a wide range of traumatic, ischemic, and/or infectious causes. The insult ultimately leads to a cerebrospinal fluid (CSF)–filled cyst or cleft, lined by white matter, that communicates with the subarachnoid space and/or the ventricular system.
- *Cystic encephalomalacia:* Irregular cystic cavity at the anatomic site of remote insult with surrounding gliosis and no communication with the adjacent ventricle. Cystic encephalomalacia has no specific association with dysgenesis of the corpus callosum.

■ Essential Facts

- Type 1:
  - Single cyst
  - Signal intensity follows CSF.
  - Thought to represent a diverticulum of the ventricle. Therefore, the cyst and the ventricle communicate.
  - More common in males.
  - Associated with macrocephaly and cranial malformations.

- Type 2:
  - Multiple cysts/multiloculated cyst
  - Does not communicate with the ventricle.
  - Signal intensity does not exactly follow CSF.
  - Associated with subcortical heterotopia and polymicrogyria.

■ Other Imaging Findings

- CA with IHC can also be associated with Dandy–Walker malformation.
- The cyst tends to grow proportionally to increasing ventricular size, which may indicate that cysts may develop as a consequence of elevated ventricular pressure.

✓ Pearls and ✗ Pitfalls

- ✓ The conditions associated with agenesis of the corpus callosum include anomalies of cortical development, lipomas, Dandy–Walker complex, Chiari II malformation, holoprosencephaly, and encephalocele.
- ✓ The communication of the IHC to the ventricle, the number of cysts, and their internal signal intensity allow for an accurate classification.
- ✗ Although the cyst is located at the midline, its morphology may be asymmetric and involve one side preferentially.
- ✗ In patients with an enlarged third ventricle secondary to hydrocephalus, the evaluation of the corpus callosum is limited because of the thinning and superior displacement of the fibers. Evaluation after decompression facilitates the diagnosis.

Case 5

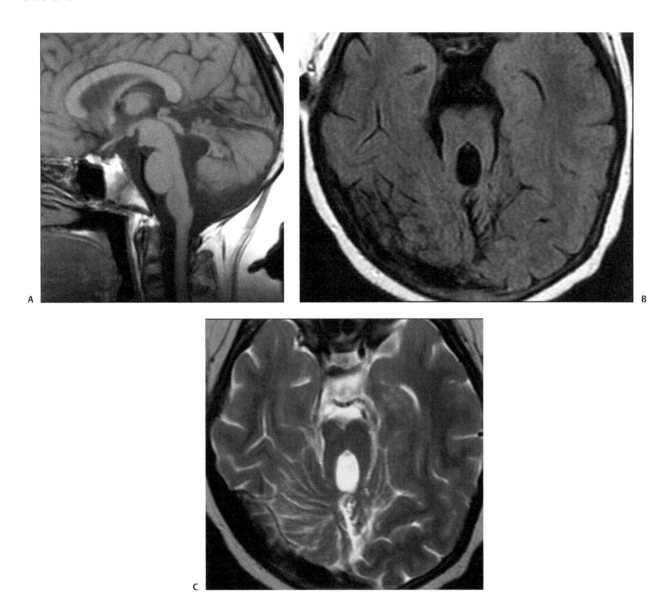

■ Clinical Presentation

Clinical history was withheld.

■ Imaging Findings

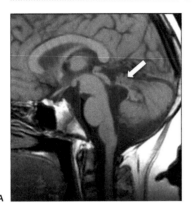 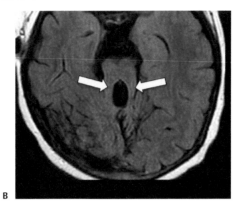 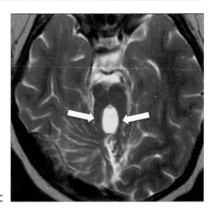

A   B   C

(A) Sagittal T1-weighted image (WI) without contrast shows cerebellar atrophy most prominent at the superior aspect (*arrow*). **(B)** Axial fluid-attenuated inversion recovery (FLAIR) image shows thickened superior cerebellar peduncles (*arrows*), which give the midbrain the characteristic "molar tooth appearance." **(C)** Axial T2WI shows thickened superior cerebellar peduncles (*arrows*) and the "molar tooth" configuration of the midbrain.

■ Differential Diagnosis

- **Joubert syndrome:** Agenesis or dysgenesis of the vermis, a deep interpeduncular fossa, and long thickened superior cerebellar peduncles give the midbrain the characteristic "molar tooth" appearance on axial MR images. There is absence of normal fiber tract decussation at the superior cerebellar peduncles. Axial MR images in the posterior fossa classically show the "bat wing" configuration of the fourth ventricle, reminiscent of a bat with outstretched wings.
- *Progressive supranuclear palsy:*
  ○ Neurodegenerative disorder
  ○ Decreased cognition, abnormal eye movements (supranuclear vertical gaze palsy), postural instability and falls, as well as parkinsonian features and speech disturbances
  ○ MRI: midbrain atrophy (Mickey Mouse appearance, morning glory sign, hummingbird sign). T2 hyperintense lesions involve the pontine tegmentum, the tectum, and the inferior olivary nuclei.
- *Walker–Warburg syndrome:*
  ○ A genetically heterogeneous disease presenting with congenital muscular dystrophy, type II lissencephaly, hydrocephalus, cerebellar malformations, and eye abnormalities.
  ○ Cerebellar/brainstem malformations include cerebellar hypoplasia, primitive Z-shaped configuration of the brainstem, and bifid pons/medulla oblongata.

■ Essential Facts

- Joubert syndrome represents a group of disorders that present clinically with ataxia, hypotonia, abnormal breathing, and mental retardation.

- Autosomal recessive inheritance.
- Several causal genes have been identified, all involved in the function of the primary cilia and basal body organelle, which are believed to play a role in signaling pathways during cerebellar development.

■ Other Imaging Findings

- Other associated central nervous system abnormalities include hydrocephalus, cystic enlargement of the posterior fossa, corpus callosum anomalies, white matter cysts, hypothalamic hamartomas, absence of the pituitary gland, migration anomalies, and occipital encephalocele.
- Associated multiorgan involvement such as retinal dystrophy, nephrolithiasis, hepatic fibrosis, and polydactyly may be present.

✓ Pearls and ✗ Pitfalls

- ✓ In Joubert syndrome, diffusion tensor imaging and fiber tractography reveal absence of decussation of both the superior cerebellar peduncles and corticospinal tracts.
- ✗ Vermian hypoplasia is best assessed on sagittal views. Thin slices help prevent volume averaging with the hemispheres.
- ✗ The size of the vermis must also be assessed on axial and coronal views, paying particular attention to whether cerebrospinal fluid is present at the midline between the hemispheres.

Case 6

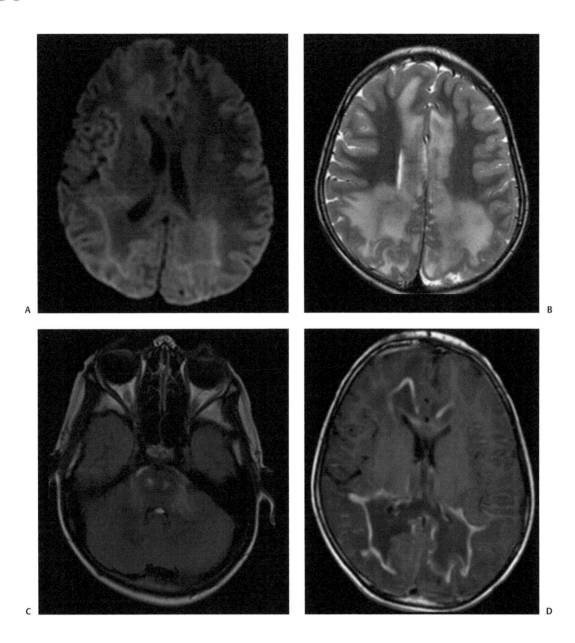

■ Clinical Presentation

A 7-year-old boy presents with seizures.

■ Imaging Findings

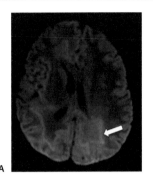 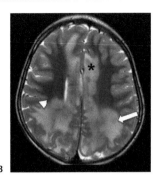 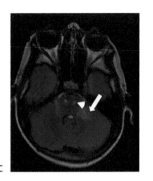 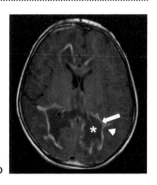

(A) Diffusion-weighted image (WI) shows a well-defined line of increased signal that affects mostly the deep white matter of the parietal lobes (*arrow*). **(B)** Axial T2WI shows confluent symmetric areas of hyperintensity that affect mostly the periventricular and deep white matter in the parietal lobes (*arrow*). The signal abnormality extends anteriorly in the medial aspect of the frontal lobes (*asterisk*). The subcortical "U" fibers are spared in some areas (*arrowhead*). **(C)** Axial fluid-attenuated inversion recovery (FLAIR) T2 sequence shows increased signal in the corticospinal tracts (*arrowhead*) and in the middle cerebellar peduncles (*arrow*). **(D)** There are three concentric layers of signal abnormality in the periatrial region: central low signal (*asterisk*), surrounded by linear enhancement (*arrow*), and a peripheral nonenhancing area of low T1 signal (*arrowhead*). The areas of linear enhancement correspond to the areas of restricted diffusion.

■ Differential Diagnosis

- **X-linked adrenoleukodystrophy (ALD):**
  - Peroxisomal disorder affecting males.
  - Approximately 35% of the cases present in childhood.
  - The radiologic presentation precedes the clinical symptoms.
  - Symmetric periventricular and deep white matter hyperintensities with parietal and occipital predominance, sparing the subcortical "U" fibers in the initial stages.
  - Not associated with macrocephaly.
- *Alexander disease (fibrinoid leukodystrophy):*
  - This leukodystrophy typically presents with symmetric bifrontal subcortical U-fiber involvement early in the disease.
  - The brainstem involvement of the long fibers is frequent. Contrast enhancement is not characteristic.
  - The patients are typically macrocephalic.
- *Canavan disease (spongiform degeneration of the white matter):*
  - Presents with macrocephaly, extensive white matter changes with frontal predominance, and abnormalities of the thalamus and globus pallidus, sparing the striatum.
  - This disease typically begins in the subcortical white matter and progresses to the deep white matter.
  - The cerebellum is a common site of involvement.
  - No enhancement is seen.
  - Increased *N*-acetylaspartate (NAA) and NAA:creatinine ratio on MR spectroscopy.

■ Essential Facts

- ALD presents with white matter changes, hypoadrenalism, and/or primary hypogonadism. It has been described in the parieto-occipital lobes (typical), the anterior frontal lobe, and the temporal lobes. The visual and auditory tracts, the corpus callosum, and the corticospinal projection fibers can also be involved. Lastly, involvement of the middle cerebellar peduncles has recently been described.
- MRI shows three zones: a central zone of irreversible gliosis, an intermediate enhancing zone that represents active inflammation and breakdown of the blood–brain barrier, and a third peripheral zone of active demyelination.

■ Other Imaging Findings

- MR is important for the diagnosis and the follow-up of therapy with hematopoietic stem cell transplantation.
- Diffusion-weighted imaging (DWI) shows a decrease in the fraction of anisotropy in the demyelinating zone and increased DWI signal on the intermediate zone.

✓ Pearls and ✗ Pitfalls

- ✓ Consider ALD if white matter changes involve the posterior brain.
- ✓ Pontomedullary junction and corticospinal tract involvement is rarely seen in any other form of leukodystrophy.
- ✓ ALD is not associated with macrocephaly.
- ✗ Not all patients with ALD present with the typical posterior cerebral pattern.
- ✗ Spectroscopy findings are not specific in ALD.

Case 7

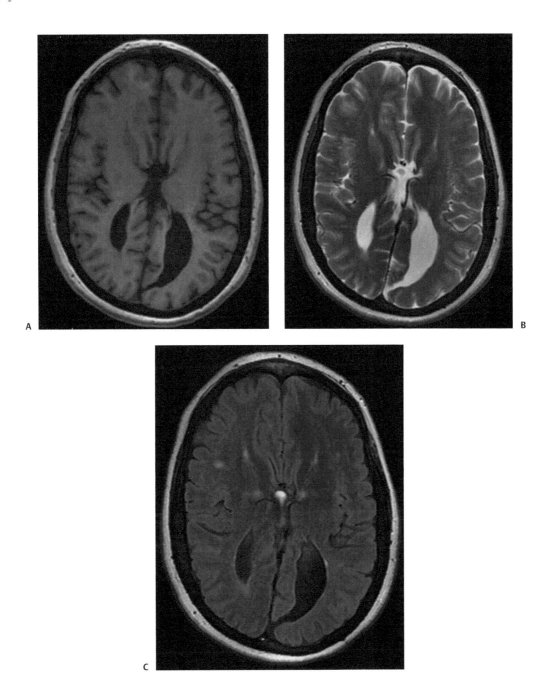

■ Clinical Presentation

A 40-year-old woman presents with known agenesis of the corpus callosum with an additional abnormal finding.

■ Imaging Findings

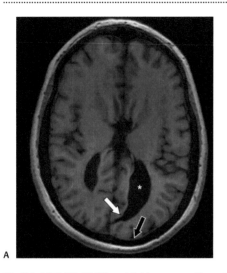
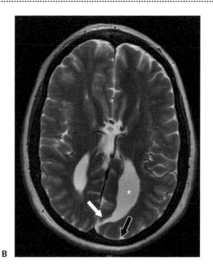
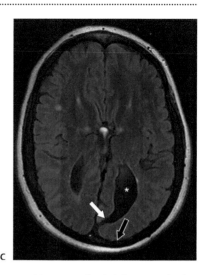

A   B   C

(A–C) Axial T1 (A), T2 (B), and fluid-attenuated inversion recovery (FLAIR) (C) images of the brain demonstrate a white matter–lined cleft communicating the occipital horn of the left lateral ventricle with the subarachnoid space (*white arrows*). The left lateral ventricle is enlarged (*asterisk*) due to associated parenchymal volume loss. The adjacent skull shows subtle thinning and remodeling (*black arrows*).

■ Differential Diagnosis

- **Porencephaly:** Congenital or acquired condition secondary to a wide range of traumatic, ischemic, and/or infectious causes that ultimately lead to a cerebrospinal fluid (CSF)-filled cyst or cleft, lined by white matter, that communicates with the subarachnoid space and/or the ventricular system.
- *Open lip schizencephaly:* Early brain malformation characterized by a cleft lined by dysplastic gray matter extending from the ventricle to the pial cortical surface. The cleft can show intervening CSF space (open lip), or the sides of the cleft can closely appose each other (closed lip).
- *Cystic encephalomalacia:* Irregular cystic cavity at the anatomic site of remote insult, with surrounding gliosis and no communication with the adjacent ventricle.

■ Essential Facts

- Smooth, well-demarcated CSF-filled cavities resulting from a wide range of damaging processes including trauma, ischemia, infection, or surgery.
- The cysts vary widely in size and can be small or involve almost entire hemispheres.
- Characteristically, porencephaly or porencephalic cysts extend from the ventricle to the cortex.
- CSF pulsation caused by the communication between the ventricle and the subarachnoid space may secondarily remodel the adjacent skull.
- Parenchymal volume loss adjacent to the involved region of brain causes a focally enlarged ventricle.
- The contents of the cyst or cleft follow CSF on all sequences and completely suppress on fluid-attenuated inversion recovery (FLAIR) image.

■ Other Imaging Findings

- Can be unilateral or bilateral.
- Often follows an arterial territory distribution.
- Heterogeneous internal signal intensity can be seen in large porencephalic cysts due to CSF flow turbulence.
- White matter lining the cleft may be gliotic or spongiotic.

✓ Pearls and ✗ Pitfalls

✓ The porencephalic cyst may communicate with the subarachnoid space while schizencephaly communicates with the subpial space. This feature is not appreciable on imaging.

✓ Porencephaly is not a static process. Adhesions within the defect may create valve effects that gradually enlarge the CSF-filled space or ventricle over time.

✗ Gliotic or spongiotic white matter along the cleft surface may simulate dysplastic gray matter, making differentiation between porencephaly and schizencephaly difficult.

Case 8

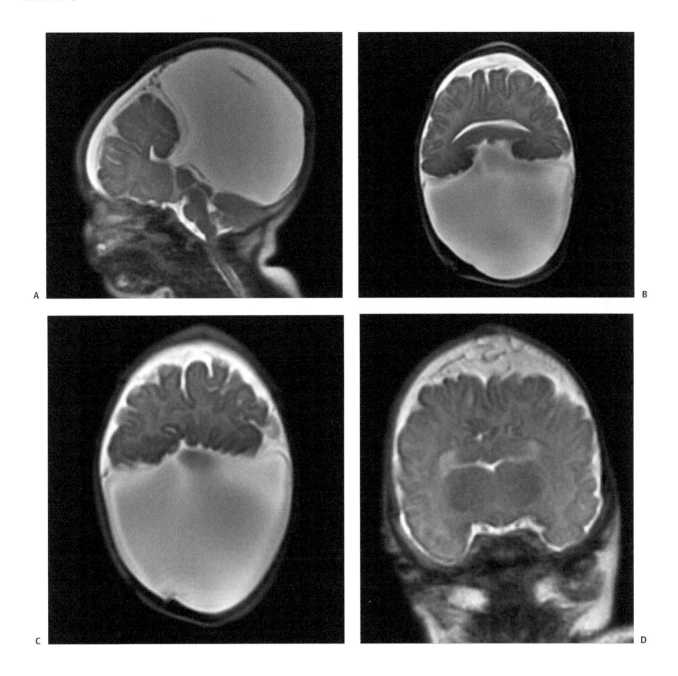

A

B

C

D

■ Clinical Presentation

A newborn presents with increased head circumference and a history of abnormal fetal ultrasound.

■ Imaging Findings

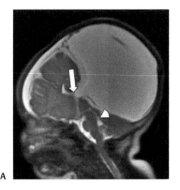 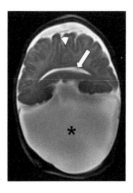 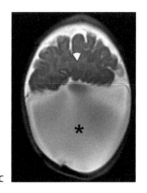 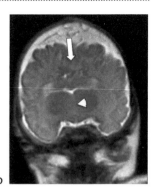

(A) Sagittal T2-weighted image (WI) demonstrates a large supratentorial cystic structure communicating with the ventricular system (*arrow*). The aqueduct and fourth ventricle are small (*arrowhead*). **(B)** Axial T2WI shows fusion of the frontal lobes (*arrowhead*), a monoventricle (*arrow*), and absence of the falx. A large cystic structure (*asterisk*) replaces the posterior temporal, occipital, and parietal lobes. **(C)** Axial T2WI shows fusion of the frontal lobes (*arrowhead*), absence of the interhemispheric fissure, and a large cystic structure (*asterisk*) replacing the posterior temporal, occipital, and parietal lobes. **(D)** Coronal T2WI shows continuity of the frontal lobes at the midline (*arrow*) and fusion of the thalami (*arrowhead*).

■ Differential Diagnosis

- ***Alobar holoprosencephaly:***
  - The most severe form of holoprosencephaly.
  - Prosencephalic cleavage fails, resulting in a single midline forebrain with a primitive monoventricle often associated with a large dorsal cyst.
- *Hydranencephaly:*
  - In utero destruction of the cerebral hemispheres.
  - Absent cortical tissue with preserved thalami and posterior fossa.
  - Islands of residual tissue can be seen at the occipital poles and orbitofrontal regions.
  - The falx is usually present.
  - Choroid can often be identified within the fluid-filled sac.
- *Dandy–Walker malformation:*
  - Posterior fossa cyst that communicates with the fourth ventricle.
  - Abnormal development of the cerebellar vermis.
  - Cystic dilatation of the fourth ventricle extending posteriorly.
  - Enlarged posterior fossa with torcular-lambdoid inversion.

■ Essential Facts

- Holoprosencephaly is the result of failed or incomplete separation of the forebrain early in gestation.
- Types:
  - Alobar holoprosencephaly: Small single forebrain ventricle, no interhemispheric division, absent olfactory bulbs and tracts, absent corpus callosum, no separation of the deep gray nuclei.
  - Semilobar: Rudimentary cerebral lobes with incomplete interhemispheric division, varying separation of the deep gray nuclei.

- Lobar: Fully developed cerebral lobes, except for continuous midline frontal neocortex; distinct interhemispheric division; absent, hypoplastic, or normal corpus callosum; separation of deep gray nuclei.
- Middle interhemispheric variant (also known as syntelencephaly): Failure of separation of the posterior frontal and parietal lobes. The body of the corpus callosum is absent, whereas the genu and splenium are normally formed. The hypothalamus and lentiform nuclei are normally separated.

■ Other Imaging Findings

- Other anomalies include cyclopia, proboscis, median or bilateral cleft lip/palate in severe forms, ocular hypotelorism, or solitary median maxillary central incisor.
- "The face predicts the brain": If facial malformations are present, the brain must be studied.

✓ Pearls and ✗ Pitfalls

- ✓ Semilobar holoprosencephaly is one of the few pathologies where the rostrum and splenium of the corpus callosum are well formed in the absence of a callosal body.
- ✓ In the sagittal images, the large cyst is in the supratentorial compartment, unlike the infratentorial location and communication with the fourth ventricle seen in Dandy–Walker malformation.
- ✗ Prominence of the masa intermedia seen in Chiari II malformation should not be confused with fused thalami.

Case 9

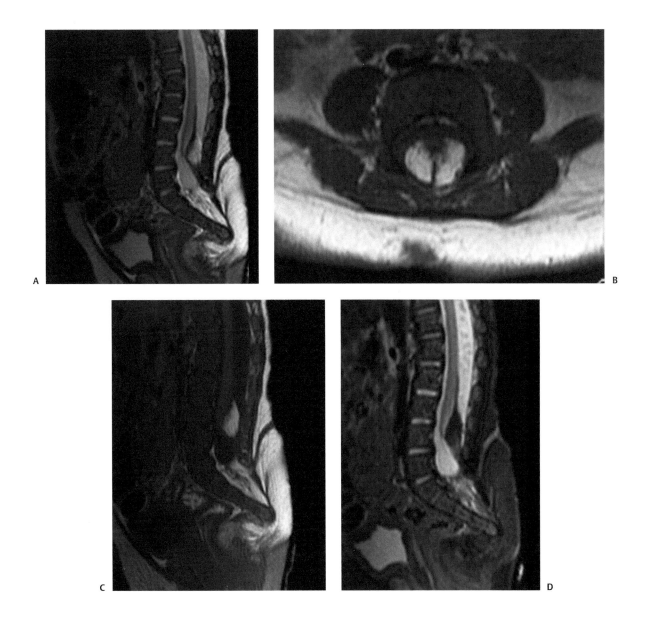

■ Clinical Presentation

....

A newborn boy presents with a hairy patch on his lower back.

■ Imaging Findings

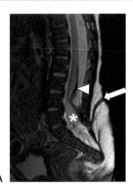
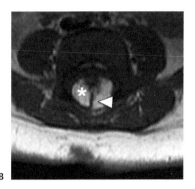
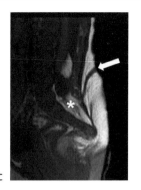
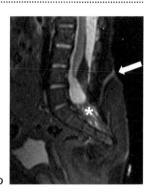

A   B   C   D

(A) Sagittal T2-weighted image (WI) of the lumbosacral region shows a superficial lipoma and a dermal sinus (*arrow*). The lipoma extends into the spinal canal through a sacral dysraphism (*asterisk*). The patient has a tethered cord, and the placode–lipoma interface is inside of the spinal canal (*arrowhead*). **(B)** Axial T1WI of the lower lumbar spine shows a lipoma in the spinal canal (*asterisk*) and a linear hypointensity corresponding to a dermal sinus (*arrowhead*). **(C, D)** Sagittal T1WI **(C)** and sagittal short tau inversion recovery (STIR) images **(D)** of the lumbosacral region show a superficial lipoma and a dermal sinus (*arrow*). The lipoma extends into the spinal canal through a sacral dysraphism (*asterisk*).

■ Differential Diagnosis

- **Lipomyelocele and lipomyelomeningoceles:** These correspond to closed spinal dysraphisms with subcutaneous lumbosacral lipomas and dural defects. The subcutaneous lipoma is located above the intergluteal crease. The lipoma tends to be excentric and extends into the spinal canal through a large sacral dorsal dysraphism. All cases are associated with tethered cord. No abnormal enhancement is seen.
- *Sacrococcygeal teratoma:* Unlike lipomyelocele and lipomyelomeningoceles, sacrococcygeal teratomas are located below the intergluteal crease. These are complex masses that may present with calcifications (60%), debris, and skin appendages. The solid components of the teratoma typically enhance.
- *Terminal myelocystocele:* Terminal hydromyelia associated with expansion of the central canal of the caudal spinal cord and surrounding distension of the dural sac. Typically associated with a dural lipoma.

■ Essential Facts

- Lipomyelocele and lipomeningocele are types of closed spinal dysraphism that feature a lipoma and a dural defect.
- They are considered abnormalities of primary neurulation, disjunction between the neuroectoderm and cutaneous ectoderm.
- If the lipoma–placode interface is inside of the canal, is it called lipomyelocele or lipomyeloschisis (75%).
- If the lipoma–placode interface is outside of the canal, the condition is termed lipomyelomeningocele (25%), and the dural defect is typically located laterally toward the lipoma.

■ Other Imaging Findings

- Prenatal ultrasound can detect the fat in the spinal canal.
- MRI shows the defect, and the lipoma–placode interface is seen as hypointense on both T1- and T2-weighted images.
- The size of the canal can increase depending on the size of the lipoma, but the subarachnoid space ventral to the spinal cord is always normal.

✓ Pearls and ✗ Pitfalls

- ✓ If treatment is not established before 6 months of age, irreversible neurologic sequelae will likely occur.
- ✓ In half of the cases, skin abnormalities such as hypertrichosis, sacral dimple, dermal sinus tract, and capillary hemangioma are present.
- ✗ Look closely for the location of the lipoma–placode interface to differentiate lipomyelocele from lipomyelomeningocele.

Case 10

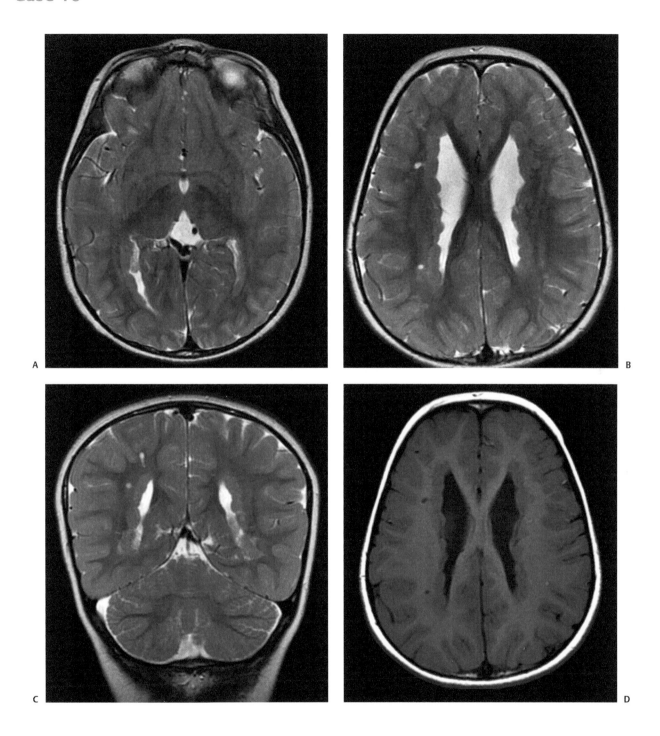

A

B

C

D

■ Clinical Presentation

A child presents with seizures.

■ Imaging Findings

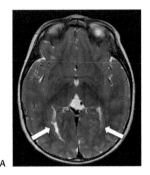
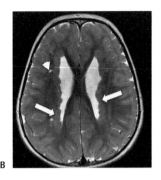
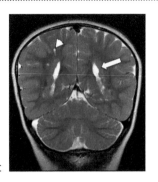
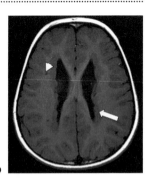

A   B   C   D

(A) Axial T2-weighted image (WI) demonstrates gray matter signal intensity along the lateral walls of the lateral ventricles, causing a wavy appearance of the lumen (*arrows*). **(B)** Axial T2WI demonstrates gray matter signal intensity along the lateral walls of the lateral ventricles, causing a wavy appearance of the lumen (*arrows*). Small cysts in the deep white matter are also noted (*arrowhead*). **(C)** Coronal T2WI demonstrates gray matter signal intensity along the lateral walls of the lateral ventricles, causing a wavy appearance of the lumen (*arrow*). Small cysts in the deep white matter are also noted (*arrowhead*). **(D)** Axial T1WI demonstrates gray matter signal intensity along the lateral walls of the lateral ventricles, causing a wavy appearance of the lumen (*arrow*). Small cysts in the deep white matter are also noted (*arrowhead*).

■ Differential Diagnosis

- **Heterotopia:** Heterotopias are a group of malformations of cortical development secondary to abnormal neuronal migration. Malformations of cortical development are a major cause of developmental delay, refractory epilepsy, and cerebral palsy.
- *Closed lip schizencephaly:* Neuronal migration anomaly characterized by a cerebrospinal fluid–filled cleft, lined by gray matter. The cleft extends from the ventricular surface (ependyma) to the periphery (pial surface) of the brain, with apposition of the cleft walls.
- *Tuberous sclerosis:* Tuberous sclerosis is a neurocutaneous syndrome characterized by hamartoma formation in almost every organ. In the central nervous system, it features cortical tubers (disorganized cerebral and cerebellar brain cortex, usually multiple, appearing as enlarged misshapen gyri with a core of water signal intensity replacing the myelinated white matter signal) and subependymal nodules (along the lateral margins of the lateral ventricles, most common near the caudothalamic grove).

■ Essential Facts

- Malformations of cortical development are currently classified according to their development in three categories:
  ○ Malformations secondary to abnormal neuronal and glial proliferation or apoptosis.
    ▪ Reduced proliferation or accelerated apoptosis (congenital microcephalies).
    ▪ Increased proliferation or decreased apoptosis (megalencephalies).
    ▪ Cortical dysgeneses with abnormal cell proliferation: focal and diffuse dysgenesis and dysplasia.
  ○ Malformations due to abnormal neuronal migration.
    ▪ Heterotopia.
    ▪ Lissencephaly.
    ▪ Subcortical heterotopia and sublobar dysplasia.
    ▪ Cobblestone malformations.
  ○ Malformations secondary to abnormal postmigrational development.
    ▪ Polymicrogyria and schizencephaly.
    ▪ Cortical dysgenesis secondary to inborn errors of metabolism.
    ▪ Focal cortical dysplasias.
    ▪ Postmigrational microcephaly.

■ Other Imaging Findings

- Advanced MR imaging such as diffusion tensor imaging (DTI) and MR spectroscopy can be used to aid in lesion localization and identification of eloquent cortex and white matter tracts for epilepsy surgery work-up.
- Functional MR imaging is used to map the sensorimotor cortex and lateralize language.
- DTI tractography can be used to map the corticospinal tracts and the optic radiations.
- Magnetoencephalography and nuclear medicine studies such as positron emission tomography (PET) and single-photon emission CT (SPECT) may be used to lateralize seizure focus when clinical, electrophysiologic, and structural MR imaging findings are discordant.

✓ Pearls and ✗ Pitfalls

- ✓ In patients who have not completed white matter myelination, the poor gray–white matter distinction may limit the ability to identify migration anomalies.
- ✗ The caudate nucleus features a wide head that tapers into a body and a thin tail. The tail of the caudate nucleus should not be confused with ectopic gray matter along the wall of the lateral ventricle.

Case 11

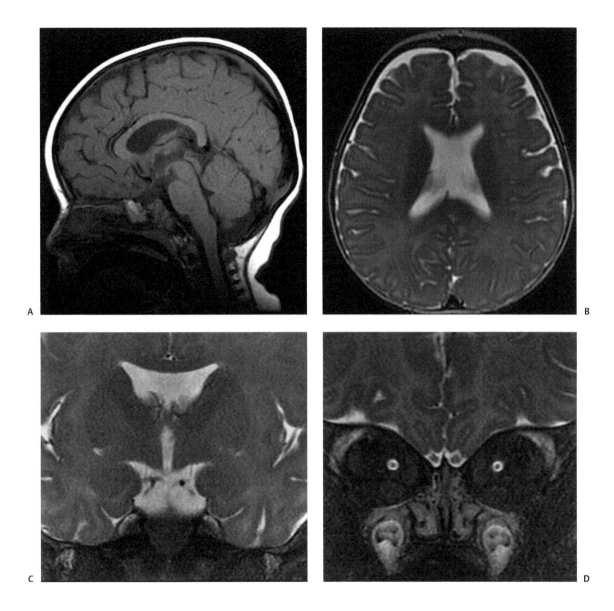

A

B

C

D

■ Clinical Presentation

A 24-year-old presents with hypopituitarism and visual defects.

■ Imaging Findings

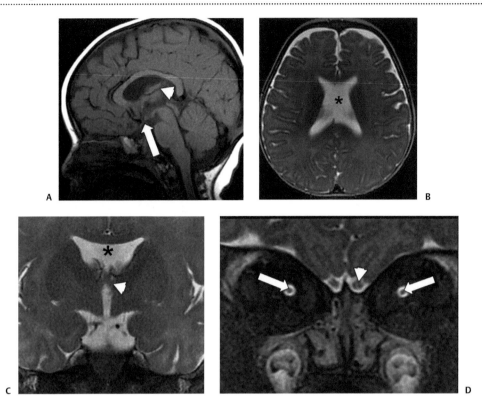

(A) Sagittal T1-weighted image (WI) shows a diminutive optic chiasm (*arrow*) and a thick body of the fornix (*arrowhead*). **(B)** Axial T2WI of the brain shows absence of the septum pellucidum (*asterisk*). **(C)** Coronal T2WI shows absence of the septum pellucidum (*asterisk*) with a thick central fused fornix (*arrowhead*). **(D)** Coronal T2WI at the level of the posterior orbits shows small optic nerves bilaterally (*arrows*) surrounded by cerebrospinal fluid within the optic nerve sheaths. The olfactory nerves (*arrowhead*) have a normal size in this patient.

■ Differential Diagnosis

- **Septo-optic dysplasia:** The classic triad of optic nerve hypoplasia, pituitary hormone abnormalities, and midline brain defects is present in only 33% of these patients. The midline abnormalities consist of complete or partial absence of the septum pellucidum with fusion of the fornix at the midline (60%) and callosal abnormalities. The olfactory bulbs may also be absent. Around half of the patients show mid-hindbrain abnormalities, which include hypoplasia of the pons.
- *Lobar holoprosencephaly:* This is the milder form of the holoprosencephaly spectrum. It presents with absence of the septum pellucidum and fusion of the mid fornix but has normal-sized optic nerves and chiasm. The most inferior portions of the frontal lobes are fused. Pituitary anomalies are uncommon.
- *Isolated agenesis of the septum pellucidum:* Not associated with cleavage anomalies. The fornix is not fused.

■ Essential Facts

- Previously known as de Morsier syndrome. Two distinct forms of septo-optic dysplasia (SOD) have been

described: (1) The classic form features two of the three findings of the triad. This form is also associated with hypoplasia of the white matter, including the optic radiations. (2) A second form, known as SOD-plus, presents with unilateral migration anomalies including schizencephaly and callosal dysgenesis.

■ Other Imaging Findings

- Prenatal diagnosis is difficult. Fusion of the fornix may be seen on ultrasound.
- MR is the diagnostic modality of choice.

✓ Pearls and ✗ Pitfalls

- ✓ SOD is a heterogeneous condition, with only a third of the patients demonstrating the classic triad.
- ✓ SOD-plus is an asymmetric variant associated with schizencephaly, which typically does not present with pituitary symptoms.
- ✗ Fusion of the fornix was considered a unique finding in lobar holoprosencephaly; a variety of conditions, including SOD, are now associated with this finding.

Case 12

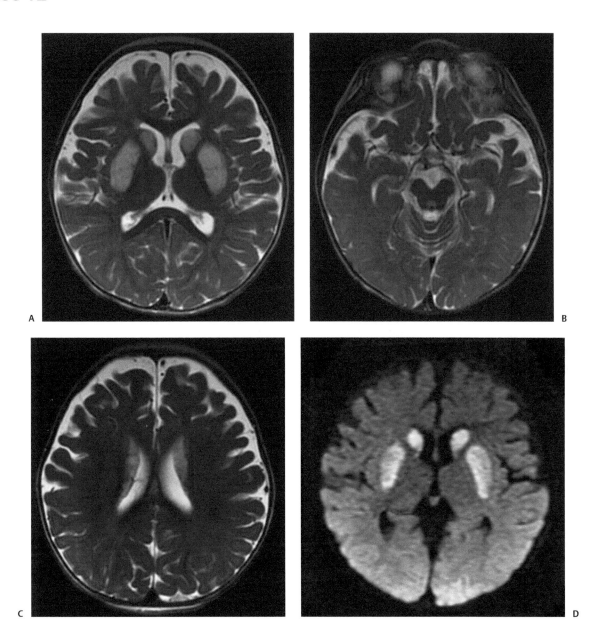

■ Clinical Presentation

A 9-month-old girl presents with dystonia.

■ Imaging Findings

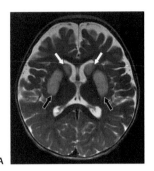 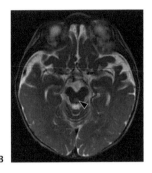 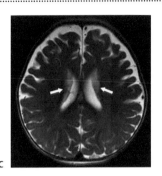 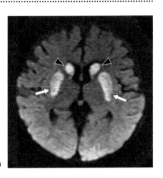

A   B   C   D

(A) Axial T2 image demonstrates increased T2 signal and hypertrophy in the caudate heads (*white arrows*) and the bilateral putamina (*black arrows*). **(B)** Axial T2 image shows increased signal intensity involving the periaqueductal gray matter (*arrowhead*). **(C)** Axial T2-weighted image shows increased signal intensity involving the caudate bodies bilaterally, right slightly greater than left (*arrows*). **(D)** Diffusion-weighted image demonstrates increased signal consistent with restricted diffusion within the putamina (*arrows*) and caudate heads (*arrowheads*).

■ Differential Diagnosis

- **Leigh syndrome:** Subacute necrotizing encephalopathy with a special predilection for the putamina and caudate heads, which are consistently affected, showing increased T2 signal intensity. Other frequently affected sites include the periaqueductal gray matter and the brainstem.
- *Myoclonic epilepsy with ragged red fibers (MERRF):* MERRF is a multisystem mitochondrial disorder that causes degeneration of the basal ganglia, particularly the globus pallidus, unlike our case in which the putamina are predominantly affected. Furthermore, the cortex is more commonly involved than the cerebral white matter.
- *Kearns–Sayre syndrome (KSS):* KSS is a mitochondrial DNA disorder characterized by increased T2 signal intensity in the basal ganglia, white matter, and cerebellum. However, unlike this particular case, KSS shows early involvement of the subcortical arcuate fibers with relative sparing of the periventricular white matter.

■ Essential Facts

- Progressive disorder leading to spongiform degeneration predominantly affecting watershed regions, the basal ganglia, and the brainstem.
- T2/fluid-attenuated inversion recovery (FLAIR) hyperintensity is typically bilateral and symmetric.
- The putamina, in particular their posterior segments, and the heads of the caudate nuclei are consistently involved.
- Lesions involving the inferior and middle portion of the brainstem are common and can even be the sole finding.

- If detected in the acute stage, lesions may demonstrate associated restricted diffusion.
- Lesions are typically nonenhancing regardless of the stage of imaging.

■ Other Imaging Findings

- MR spectroscopy generally shows an elevated lactate peak at 1.3 parts per million.
- Abnormally increased T2 signal can also commonly be seen in the cerebellar peduncles, dorsomedial thalami, and periaqueductal gray matter.
- Occasionally, cerebral white matter may demonstrate extensive gliosis and even cystic degeneration.
- Global volume loss may occur at later stages of the disease.

✓ Pearls and ✗ Pitfalls

✓ Bilateral and symmetric involvement of deep gray structures in the absence of hypoxic or ischemic etiologies.

✓ Mitochondrial diseases involve multiple organ systems, especially the central nervous system, cardiac system, and musculoskeletal system.

✗ Mitochondrial disorders can exhibit multiple overlapping features.

✗ Many times, earlier imaging studies can be the best method to detect characteristic patterns of disease.

✗ In the later stages of evolution of mitochondrial conditions, the extensive involvement of multiple structures makes the imaging appearance less specific.

Case 13

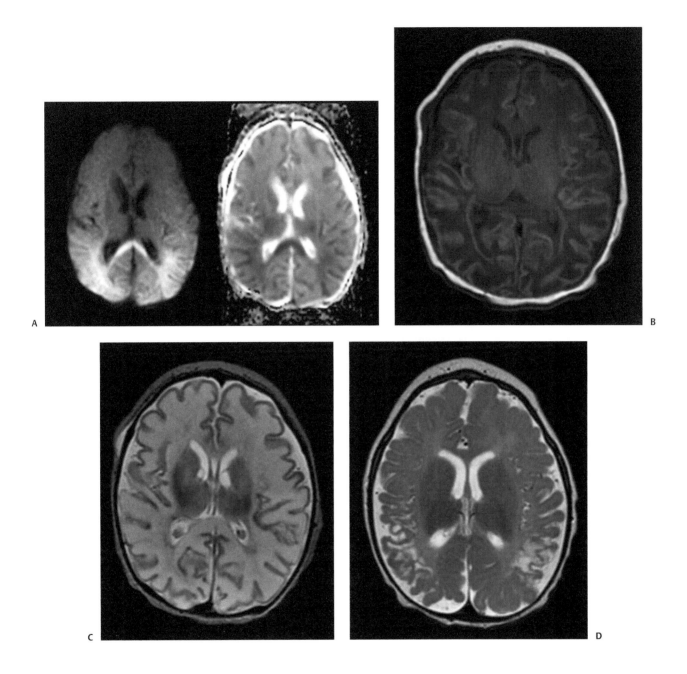

A

B

C

D

An 11-day-old neonate presents with a history of placental abruption.

■ Imaging Findings

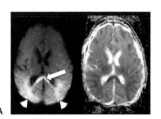 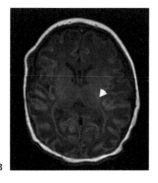 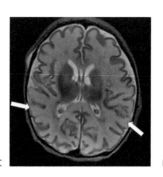 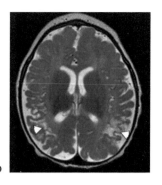

(A) Diffusion-weighted image (WI) and corresponding apparent diffusion coefficients map (*right*) demonstrate restricted diffusion in the splenium of the corpus callosum (*arrow*) and in the white matter of both temporal and occipital lobes (*arrowheads*). **(B)** Axial T1WI demonstrates T1 shortening of the cerebral cortex bilaterally. Note the higher signal intensity of the cortex in relation to the posterior limb of the internal capsule (*arrowhead*). **(C)** Axial T2WI demonstrates generalized edema in the white matter and in the temporal and occipital cortex bilaterally. Note the lack of anatomic detail in the cerebral cortex posteriorly (*arrows*). **(D)** Follow-up T2WI at 6 months of age demonstrates extensive areas of cystic encephalomalacia in the white matter of the temporal lobes (*arrowheads*), with generalized volume loss.

■ Differential Diagnosis

- ***Hypoxic-ischemic injury (HII):*** HII refers to the imaging pattern of injury due to acquired global arterial hypoperfusion. Not all the patients with HII meet clinical criteria for hypoxic-ischemic encephalopathy (HIE).
- *Herpes encephalitis:*
  ○ Neonatal herpes simplex encephalitis caused by herpes simplex virus type 2 (HSV-2).
  ○ In early stages, MRI shows variable diffusion-weighted image (DWI) signal. In later stages, it shows atrophy, cysts, ventriculomegaly, and calcifications.
  ○ Involves white matter, cortex, basal ganglia, and brainstem.
  ○ Unlike HSV encephalitis in adults and older children, neonates do not have a temporal lobe predilection.
- *Neonatal hypoglycemia:*
  ○ Low glucose values are often seen in term infants with neonatal encephalopathy, including those with HII.
  ○ Both entities may demonstrate overlapping features.
  ○ Features most commonly seen in hypoglycemia include bilateral, symmetric selective posterior white matter edema, associated edema in the pulvinar and anterior medial thalamic nuclei, and restricted diffusion in the optic radiations.

■ Essential Facts

- Diffuse hypoxic-ischemic brain injury in neonates results in neonatal HIE. Because of differences in brain maturity at the time of insult, in the severity of hypotension, and in the duration of the insult, there are four distinct patterns of brain injury.
- Preterm neonates:
  ○ Mild hypotension causes periventricular injury.
  ○ Severe hypotension results in infarction of the deep gray matter, brainstem, and cerebellum.

- Term neonates:
  ○ Mild hypotension causes parasagittal cortical and subcortical injury.
  ○ Severe hypotension causes characteristic injury of the lateral thalami, posterior putamina, hippocampi, corticospinal tracts, and sensorimotor cortex.

■ Other Imaging Findings

- Cranial ultrasonography is sensitive for the detection of hemorrhage, periventricular leukomalacia, and hydrocephalus. Doppler interrogation and the assessment of resistive index provide additional information on cerebral perfusion.
- CT is the least sensitive modality for evaluation of HIE because of the high water content in the neonatal brain and high protein content of the cerebrospinal fluid, which result in poor parenchymal contrast resolution. However, this modality provides a quick method of screening for intracranial hemorrhage in a sick neonate without the need for sedation.

✓ Pearls and ✗ Pitfalls

✓ Analysis of the myelination milestones at the corrected gestational age of the patient is essential to interpret brain MRI in newborns.

✓ The appearance of the DWI/apparent diffusion coefficients map varies with time.

✗ MR imaging changes due to hypoxic-ischemic cerebral damage can be subtle and difficult to distinguish from normal myelinated areas because both have similar increases in signal intensity on T1-weighted images. In HII, search for a higher T1 signal in the posterior putamen with respect to the posterior limb of the internal capsule.

Case 14

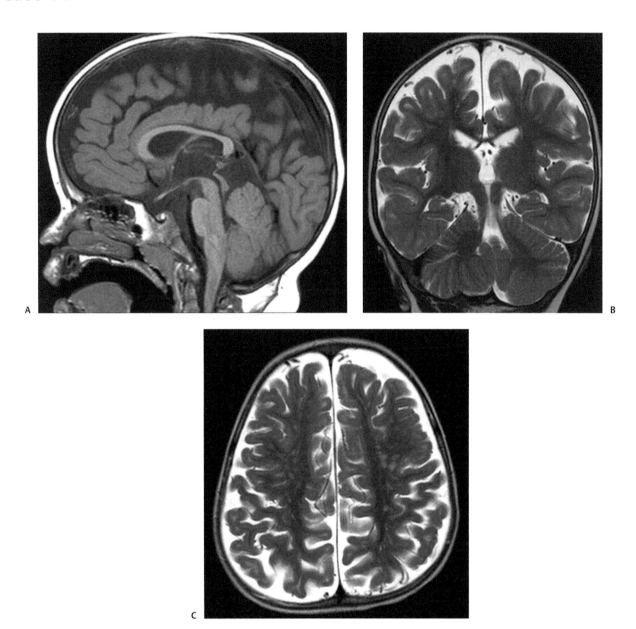

■ Clinical Presentation

A 2-year-old presents with macrocephaly.

■ Imaging Findings

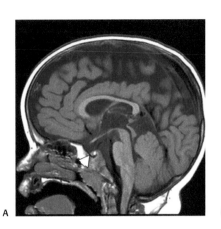
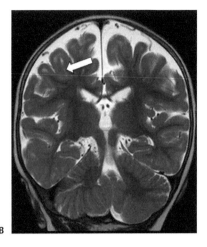
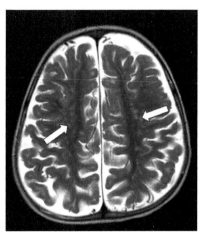

(A) Sagittal T1-weighted image (WI) shows a "J-shaped" sella (*arrowhead*). **(B, C)** Coronal **(B)** and axial **(C)** T2WI show prominent perivascular spaces (*arrows*).

■ Differential Diagnosis

- ***Mucopolysaccharidosis:***
  - Presents with white matter lesions, enlargement of the perivascular spaces, slowly progressive hydrocephalus, and brain atrophy. Spinal canal stenosis at the craniocervical junction, typically due to odontoid process dysplasia and laxity of the transverse ligament, can lead to myelopathy.
  - White matter lesions are nonspecific and present as symmetric focal or confluent increased T2 hyperintensities most common in the periventricular white matter.
  - Dysotosis multiplex refers to multiple abnormalities of the skeletal system, mainly seen as wedge-shaped vertebrae, platyspondyly, anterior beaking, and posterior scalloping (bullet-shaped vertebrae).
- *Metachromatic leukodystrophy:*
  - May have confluent periventricular T2 hyperintensities that spare the perivenular white matter, giving the "tigroid" appearance.
  - Late involvement of the subcortical "U" fibers.
  - Does not have spinal manifestations.
- *Achondroplasia:*
  - The most common skeletal dysplasia. Classically presents with a large cranial vault, frontal bossing, and a narrowed foramen magnum.
  - No brain parenchymal abnormalities.
  - Communicating hydrocephalus is common.
  - Bullet-shaped vertebrae are present, not to be confused with Hurler syndrome.
  - Spinal canal stenosis is due to short pedicles.
  - Rhizomelic dwarfism.

■ Essential Facts

- Mucopolysaccharidosis (MPS) is a group of lysosomal storage disorders with accumulation of partially degraded glycosaminoglycans in the lysosomes and extracellular space. Seven distinct types have been described.
- The posterior fossa shows a megacisterna magna in MPS type II.
- A "J-shaped" sella turcica conformation is described.
- Craniocervical junction: odontoid process dysplasia and atlantoaxial instability with thickening of the intrinsic ligaments.
- Cortical bone is thickened with premature closure of sagittal suture that leads to dolichocephaly.

■ Other Imaging Findings

- MR is the method of choice to diagnose and evaluate for treatment response in MPS. Patients with MPS should have an MR scan of the whole neuraxis because the disease is not limited to the brain.
- Broad ribs and trident hands are part of the imaging spectrum.

✓ Pearls and ✗ Pitfalls

✓ Always scan the whole neuraxis in patients with MPS; the findings are characteristic of these diseases.

✗ CNS involvement is more frequent in MPS I, II, III, and VII.

Case 15

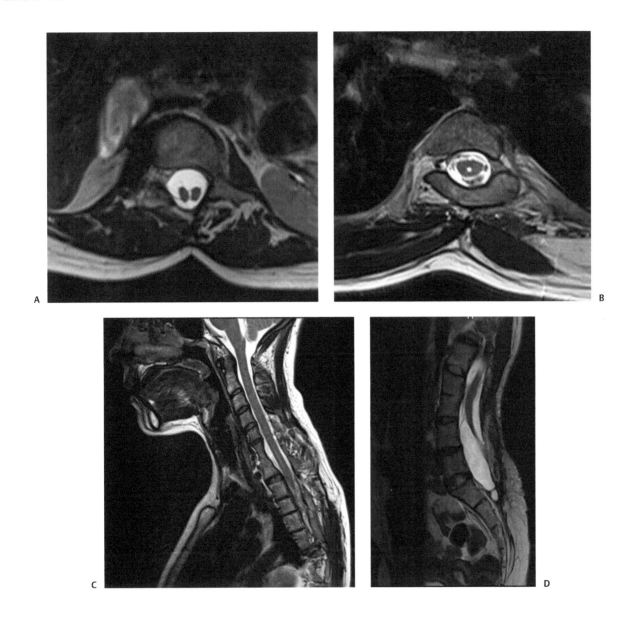

A

B

C

D

■ Clinical Presentation

An 8-year-old girl presents with leg weakness and back pain.

■ Imaging Findings

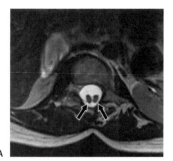 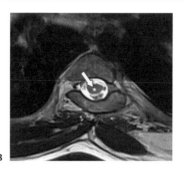 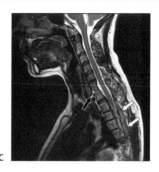 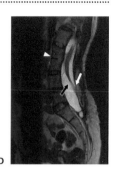

(A) Axial T2-weighted image (WI) through the lower thoracic spine shows two separate hemicords within a common thecal sac (*arrows*). **(B)** Axial T2WI through the midthoracic spine shows dilatation of the central ependymal canal consistent with mild syringohydromyelia (*arrow*). **(C)** Sagittal T2WI of the cervicothoracic spine shows vertebral body fusions (*black arrow*) and intersegmental laminar fusions (*white arrows*). The upper thoracic cord is off of midline due to scoliosis. **(D)** Sagittal T2WI through the lumbar spine shows partial vertebral interbody fusion (*white arrowhead*). The conus medullaris terminates at approximately the L4 level (*black arrow*) and shows abnormal adhesions to the dorsal thecal sac (*white arrow*).

■ Differential Diagnosis

- **Diastematomyelia:** Diastematomyelia is an abnormal sagittal split of the spinal cord into two distinct hemicords and is associated with numerous spinal malformations.
- *Tethered cord syndrome:* Tethered cord syndrome is classified under the spectrum of closed spinal dysraphisms and is characterized by a conus medullaris that lies below the level of L2–L3. Similar to this case, there can be scoliosis and syringohydromyelia. However, the presence of two distinct hemicords indicates diastematomyelia.
- *VACTERL association:* VACTERL is an acronym that summarizes the group of nonrandom anomalies of the following systems: vertebral, anorectal, cardiac, tracheoesophageal, renal, and musculoskeletal (limb). Within the spinal anomalies there is a predisposition for hemivertebrae, scoliosis, caudal regression, and spina bifida. However, split cord deformities are not characteristic of this association.

■ Essential Facts

- Also referred to as split cord malformation.
- Each hemicord contains an individual central canal, a single dorsal horn, and one ventral horn.
- The most common site of splitting is the lumbar region.
- The cord can either split in two and remain separate, with two individual coni medullaris and two fila terminale, or can split and meet again inferior to the cleft.
- Two types:
  ○ Type I—25%.
    ▪ Each hemicord has its own sac.
    ▪ A bony or cartilaginous spur separates the hemicords at the inferior part of the cleft.
    ▪ Cortical dysgeneses with abnormal cell proliferation: focal and diffuse dysgenesis and dysplasia.
  ○ Type II—75%.
    ▪ One single subarachnoid space/sac.
    ▪ A fibrous band separates the hemicords at the inferior part of the cleft.

■ Other Imaging Findings

- The sagittal division of the cord can lead to symmetric or asymmetric hemicords.
- The separation of the cord may be incomplete, involving only the ventral and dorsal portions of the cord and not its entire thickness.
- Approximately 85% of patients have associated spinal abnormalities, including:
  ○ Low-lying conus.
  ○ Thickened filum terminale.
  ○ Myeloceles/myelomeningoceles.
  ○ Tethering adhesions.
  ○ Dermal sinuses.
  ○ Syringohydromyelia (50%).
  ○ Intersegmental laminar fusion—essentially pathognomonic, seen in 60%.
  ○ Klippel–Feil anomaly.

✓ Pearls and ✗ Pitfalls

✓ Diastematomyelia is commonly one finding within a constellation of malformations.
✓ Occasionally imaging is insufficient in determining the type of tissue that separates the hemicords.
✓ Cutaneous stigmata are common in diastematomyelia.
✓ CT is helpful for the evaluation of a bony spur.
✗ Imaging of these patients is often difficult due to severe scoliosis.
✗ Diastematomyelia is a separate entity from diplomyelia which is duplication of the spinal cord, in which case each cord demonstrates two dorsal horns and two ventral cords as well as a central ependymal canal.

Case 16

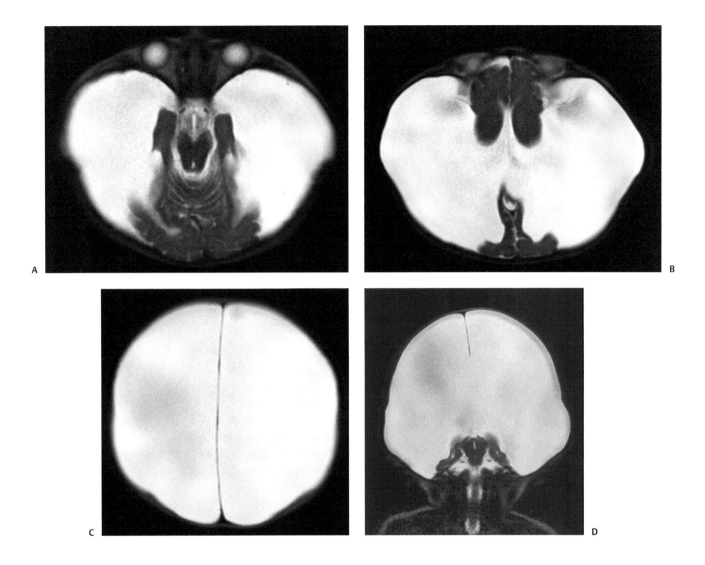

A

B

C

D

■ Clinical Presentation

A neonate presents with increased head circumference.

■ Imaging Findings

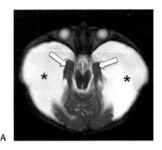 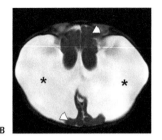 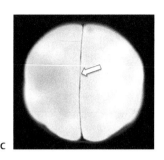 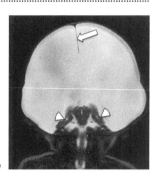

A   B   C   D

(A) Axial T2-weighted image (WI) demonstrates enlargement of the head with cystic spaces filling the middle cranial fossa bilaterally (*asterisks*). Notice the preservation of the medial temporal lobes (*arrows*). **(B)** Axial T2WI demonstrates enlargement of the head with cystic spaces filling the middle cranial fossae (*asterisks*), converging at the midline. Portions of the frontal lobes anteriorly and the occipital lobes posteriorly are preserved (*arrowheads*). **(C)** Axial T2WI demonstrates cystic spaces replacing the cerebrum. The falx is present (*arrow*). **(D)** Coronal T2WI demonstrates cystic spaces replacing the cerebrum, with preservation of the medial temporal lobes (*arrowheads*). The falx is present (*arrow*).

■ Differential Diagnosis

- **Hydranencephaly:** Acquired destructive process of the cerebral hemispheres in which (1) the major portions of both cerebral hemispheres are replaced by thin-walled, fluid-filled sacs; (2) the falx, tentorium, and other meninges remain intact, and (3) the thalami, brainstem, and cerebellum are usually intact.
- *Extreme hydrocephalus:* A cortical mantle is present, although in severe cases it may be difficult to discern. Posterior fossa abnormalities or aqueductal stenosis may be present.
- *Alobar holoprosencephaly:*
  - The most severe form of holoprosencephaly.
  - Prosencephalic cleavage fails, resulting in a single midline forebrain with a primitive monoventricle often associated with a large dorsal cyst.
    - No interhemispheric division, absent falx.
    - Absent olfactory bulbs and tracts, absent corpus callosum, no separation of deep gray nuclei.

■ Essential Facts

- Most authors believe that hydranencephaly is the result of intrauterine bilateral internal carotid artery (ICA) occlusion, likely occurring between the 8th and 12th weeks of gestation.
- The ICAs may be severely hypoplastic or absent. The carotid artery bony canals can be missing or hypoplastic.

■ Other Imaging Findings

- Findings on second trimester fetal ultrasound include absent cerebral hemispheres, which are replaced by homogeneous echogenic material filling the supratentorial space. The thalami, brainstem, and cerebellum are generally preserved.

✓ Pearls and ✗ Pitfalls

- ✓ Facial features are uniformly normal in hydranencephaly, which may help in the distinction from holoprosencephaly.
- ✗ In some cases of hydranencephaly, more distal occlusions of the vasculature likely explain cases with preservation of inferomedial strips of the inferior frontal lobes and preservation of postero-inferomedial crescents of temporal, parietal, and occipital lobes.

Case 17

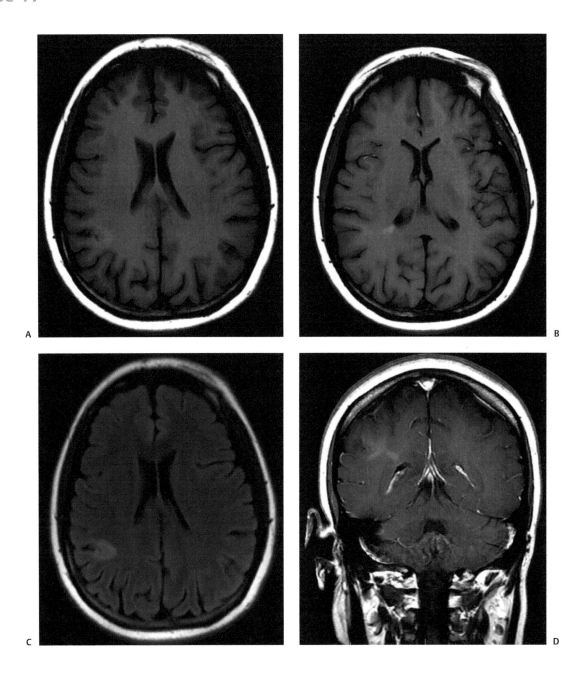

A

B

C

D

■ Clinical Presentation

A 22-year-old woman presents with seizure.

■ Imaging Findings

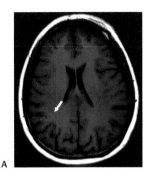 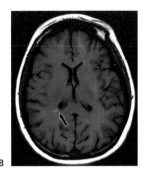 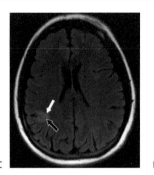 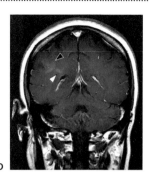

(A) Axial T1-weighted image (WI) shows a focal area of subtle increased signal intensity involving the subcortical white matter deep to a right parietal lobe sulcus (*arrow*). **(B)** Axial T1WI at a level below the previous image shows extension of the abnormal T1 hyperintense signal, in a slightly bandlike or linear fashion, to the periventricular white matter adjacent to the posterior body of the right lateral ventricle (*arrow*). **(C)** Fluid-attenuated inversion recovery (FLAIR) image shows increased signal intensity of the subcortical white matter at the same site, with blurring of the gray–white matter interface (*white arrow*) and mild thickening of the adjacent cortex (*black arrow*). **(D)** Coronal T1-weighted postcontrast image shows the entire extension of the hyperintense signal abnormality from the subcortical region of the right parietal lobe to the ventricular surface without significant associated enhancement. This morphology has occasionally been termed the "wine glass" sign, where the bowl of the glass is the U-shaped subcortical involvement (*black arrowhead*) and the stem of the glass is the linear extension to the ventricle (*white arrowhead*).

■ Differential Diagnosis

- ***Focal cortical dysplasia (type IIb):*** Focal cortical dysplasia (FCD) is a wide spectrum of congenitally malformed cerebral cortex. The subtype IIb of the Blümcke classification of FCD is characterized by the "transmantle sign." This sign is seen as white matter signal abnormality that extends from the bottom of a sulcus and tapers to the periventricular region. This appearance has been compared to the shape of a wine glass, predominantly on coronal images.
- *Low-grade glioma:* Low-grade gliomas can also present as focally ill-defined increased T2 signal. Typically, these tumors are hypointense on T1, hyperintense on T2, and do not enhance. The signal abnormality is generally associated with a greater degree of mass effect, a feature that is not present in this case. Lastly, the tapering radial extension to the ventricular surface is not a common feature in low-grade gliomas.
- *Subcortical tuber:* Subcortical tubers, seen in patients with tuberous sclerosis (TS), may have similar imaging features, including increased T2 signal in the subcortical white matter with blurring of the gray–white matter interface. Also, patients with TS may exhibit radial bands of white matter T2 hyperintensity that extend from the cortex to the ventricle, similar to the "transmantle sign." TS typically shows multiple subcortical lesions and numerous radial bands, as well as subependymal nodules.

■ Essential Facts

- FCDs occur secondary to errors in cortical lamination, cytoarchitecture, and white matter development.
- They are a common cause of intractable epilepsy in children and adults.
- The Blümcke classification was developed in 2011 as a revision to the prior classification systems created by Palmini and Barkovich, and describes three distinct types.

- Within the Blümcke classification, type II FCDs, also known as Taylor dysplasias, can be further classified into FCD with dysmorphic neurons (type IIa) and FCD with dysmorphic neurons and balloon cells (type IIb).
- FCD type IIb on imaging is seen as blurring of the gray–white matter interface with subcortical white matter T2 hyperintensity.
- The overlying cortex can appear to have normal or increased thickness.
- The "transmantle sign" was originally coined by Barkovich in 1997 and is thought to reflect the abnormality of the glioneural units in a radial distribution.

■ Other Imaging Findings

- The adjacent cortical segment may also have increased T2 signal.
- FCDs can be associated with abnormal sulcation patterns and lobar/segmental volume loss.
- FCD type II is slightly more likely to occur in the frontal lobes and less in the temporal lobes as compared to FCD type I.

✓ Pearls and ✗ Pitfalls

- ✓ Heavily T2-weighted and FLAIR sequences can be useful to better delineate focal white matter hyperintensities.
- ✓ Although the majority of FCDs have decreased T1 signal intensity, these abnormalities can occasionally show increased T1 signal.
- ✗ The T2 hyperintensity associated with low-grade gliomas has a more expansile appearance with greater mass effect.
- ✗ Solitary lesions are uncommon in TS and should orient the diagnosis to an FCD.
- ✗ Infants with incomplete myelination have high T2 signal in the subcortical U fibers, which can limit the assessment of FCD.

Case 18

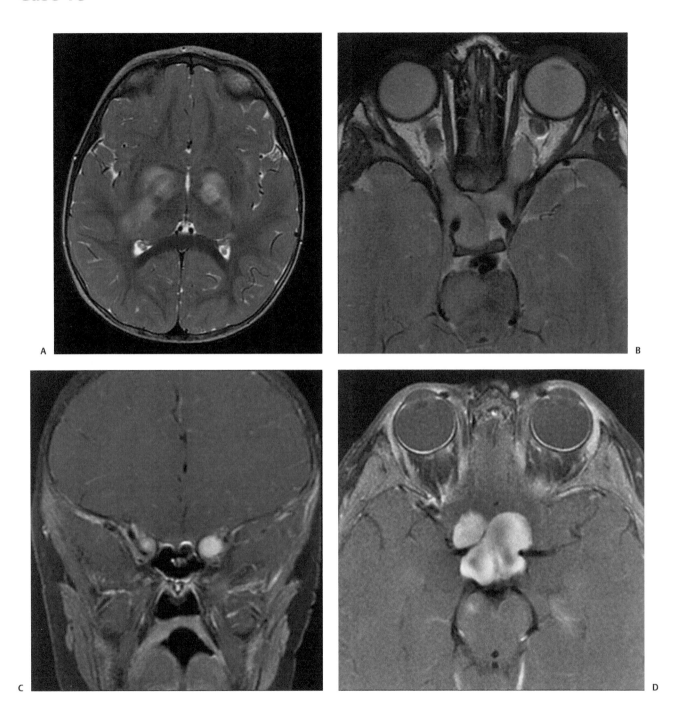

■ Clinical Presentation

History withheld.

■ Imaging Findings

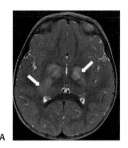 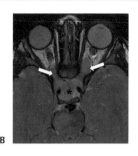 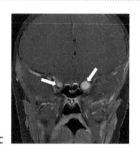 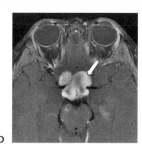

(A) Axial T2-weighted image (WI) demonstrates hyperintense lesions without mass effect in the lentiform nuclei and right internal capsule (*arrows*). **(B)** Axial T2WI demonstrates enlargement and increased signal intensity of the optic nerves (*arrows*) and chiasm (*asterisk*). **(C)** Coronal postcontrast T1WI shows marked homogeneous enhancement of the enlarged optic nerves (*arrows*). **(D)** Axial postcontrast T1WI shows significant enhancement of the enlarged optic chiasm (*arrow*).

■ Differential Diagnosis

- *Neurofibromatosis type I (NF1):*
  ○ Autosomal-dominant neurocutaneous disorder (phakomatosis).
  ○ Two or more of the following must be present:
    ▪ Six café au lait spots measuring ≥ 5 mm in prepubertal and ≥ 15 mm in postpubertal patients.
    ▪ ≥ 2 neurofibromas or one plexiform neurofibroma (PNF).
    ▪ Axillary/inguinal freckling.
    ▪ Visual pathway glioma.
    ▪ Two or more Lisch nodules (iris hamartomas).
    ▪ Distinctive bony lesion.
    ▪ Sphenoid wing dysplasia.
    ▪ Thinning of long bones ± pseudarthrosis.
    ▪ First-degree relative with NF1.
- *Hypothalamic hamartoma:*
  ○ Tumorlike masses located in the tuber cinereum of the hypothalamus.
  ○ May present with gelastic seizures and precocious puberty.
  ○ Contain nerve cells that resemble those of the normal hypothalamus, along with normal glial cells.
  ○ MRI: Well-defined pedunculated or sessile lesions at the tuber cinereum, which are isointense or mildly hypointense on T1-weighted images and iso- to hyperintense on T2-weighted images, with no contrast enhancement or calcification.
  ○ Stable in size, shape, and signal intensity over time.
- *ADEM:*
  ○ Monophasic demyelinating disease of the central nervous system (CNS).
  ○ Numerous T2 hyperintense lesions in gray and white matter, poorly marginated, and asymmetric. Contrast enhancement is infrequent.
  ○ Prior infectious episode or vaccination triggers the inflammatory response.
  ○ Young and adolescent children are most affected.

■ Essential Facts

- NF1 is an autosomal-dominant disorder with genetic locus on chromosome 17q11.2.
- White matter lesions: Hyperintense T2 abnormalities in the brainstem, middle cerebellar peduncles, cerebellar white matter, cerebral peduncles, basal ganglia (especially the globus pallidus), thalamus, and internal capsule. Most common in children younger than 7 years, and the lesions tend to improve with advancing age.
- Optic pathway glioma: Isolated to a single optic nerve or involving both optic nerves, chiasm, and optic tracts. Although tumors in the optic nerves and chiasm often enhance, parenchymal involvement (optic tracts and beyond), in the setting of optic pathway gliomas, does not typically enhance.
- Other associated tumors and tumorlike conditions include astrocytomas and hamartomatous enlargement of the brainstem and hypothalamus.

■ Other Imaging Findings

- MR angiography delineates the intracranial vasculopathy: Stenoses, occlusions, ectasia, moyamoya disease, and fusiform aneurysm formation.
- Fluorodeoxyglucose (FDG) positron emission tomography (PET) imaging helps differentiate benign from malignant nerve sheath tumors. A standardized uptake value with a maximum > 3 is indicative of malignant transformation in a PNF.

✓ Pearls and ✗ Pitfalls

✓ Astrocytomas are more common in children with NF1 than in the general population and can arise anywhere in the CNS. These are most commonly pilocytic astrocytomas, but other low-grade and higher-grade tumors also occur.

✓ The brainstem also is often involved, especially the tectum and the medulla.

✗ Differentiation between retrochiasmatic parenchymal tumor involvement and the characteristic hyperintense T2 lesions encountered in children with NF1 can be difficult. Features that favor optic pathway glioma infiltration include contiguity, mass effect, significant elevations of choline (at MR spectroscopy), low T1 signal on precontrast images, and enhancement after contrast agent administration.

Case 19

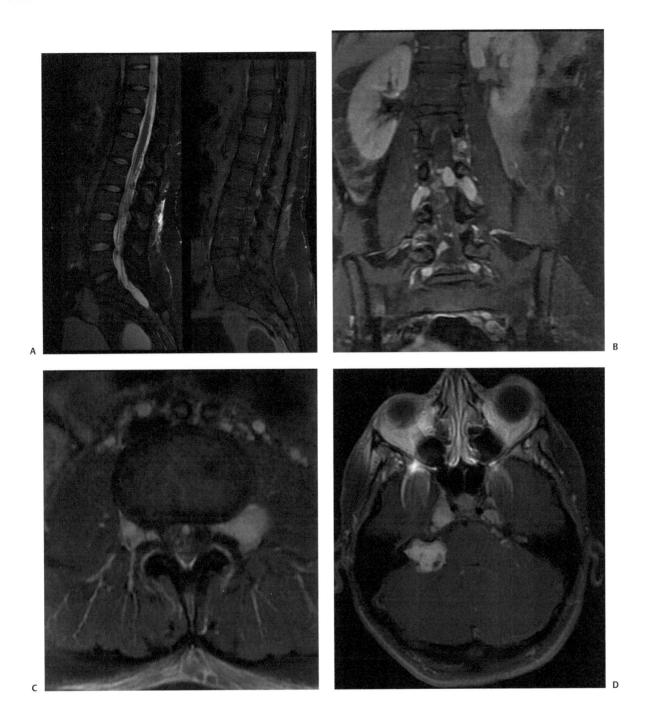

■ Clinical Presentation

A 36-year-old man presents with bilateral weakness in the lower extremities and hearing loss on the right side.

■ Imaging Findings

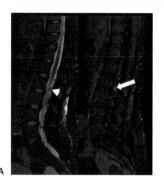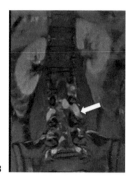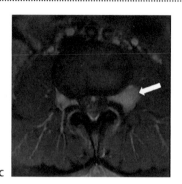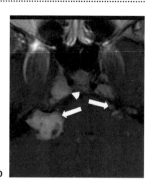

(A) Sagittal T2-weighted image (WI) without contrast and T1 fat-saturated image with contrast show multiple intrathecal extramedullary nodular lesions (*arrowhead*) that demonstrate avid enhancement (*arrow*). **(B, C)** Coronal **(B)** and axial **(C)** T1 fat-saturated images with contrast show multiple dumbbell-shaped lesions at multiple levels of the lumbar spine, exiting through the neural foramina (*arrow*). **(D)** Axial T1WI with contrast of the head shows bilateral enhancing lesions in the cerebellopontine angles that extend into the internal auditory canals (*arrows*). Other enhancing lesions are noted adjacent to the cavernous sinuses bilaterally (*arrowhead*).

■ Differential Diagnosis

- **_Neurofibromatosis type 2 (NF2):_**
  - Congenital syndrome that results in multiple intracranial schwannomas, meningiomas, and ependymomas ("MISME").
  - Lesions can be distributed throughout the intracranial compartment and spine.
  - Mutation on chromosome 22.
  - Mean age at presentation is 25 years old.
- *Neurofibromatosis type 1:*
  - Cutaneous café au lait spots.
  - Plexiform neurofibromas.
  - Intracranial hamartomas and gliomas.
  - Spinal scoliosis, posterior vertebral body scalloping, dural ectasia, and lateral meningoceles.
  - Mutation in chromosome 17.
  - Plexiform neurofibromas are imbedded in the nerve fibers.
- *Schwannomatosis:*
  - A third type of neurofibromatosis.
  - Adult patients in the third to sixth decades of life.
  - Presence of multiple peripheral schwannomas and/or meningiomas.
  - Absence of bilateral vestibular schwannomas.
  - Chronic pain.

■ Essential Facts

- Bilateral vestibular schwannomas are a characteristic finding.
- Generally, multiple meningiomas, ependymomas, and schwannomas are seen distributed throughout the neuroaxis.
- The schwannomas are not imbedded in the nerve fibers.
- The inheritance pattern is autosomal dominant.

■ Other Imaging Findings

- CT can demonstrate the widening of the internal auditory canals and calcifications within the nerve sheath tumors, if present.
- MR is the imaging modality of choice. Schwannomas show increased T2 intensity and enhancement. Mural cysts can also be seen.
- Small 3D thin-slice, heavy-weighted T2-weighted image of the posterior fossa can aid in the identification of nerve contour irregularities.

✓ Pearls and ✗ Pitfalls

- ✓ Whole-body MR imaging provides adequate data with which to accurately quantify tumor burden in patients with nerve sheath tumors.
- ✓ Not all the cerebellopontine angle schwannomas are from the vestibular nerve; these tumors can arise from the facial or acoustic nerves as well.
- ✗ When irregularities are seen in the cauda equina, contrast is needed to exclude enhancing masses.

Case 20

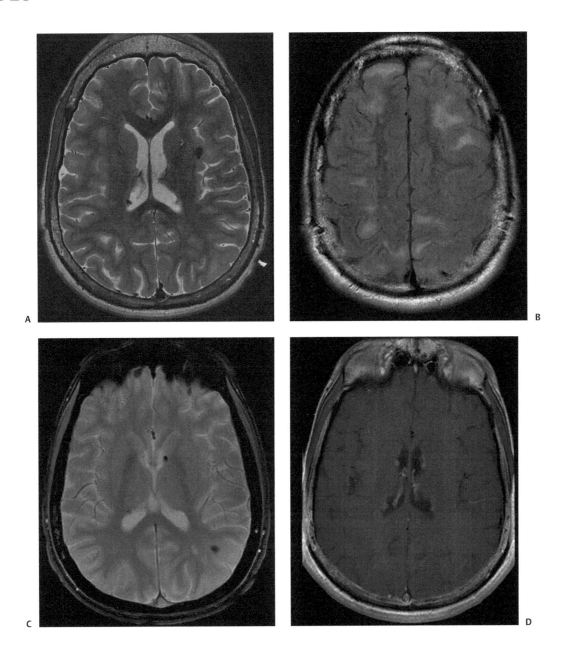

A

B

C

D

■ Clinical Presentation

A 12-year-old patient presents with recurrent seizures.

■ **Imaging Findings**

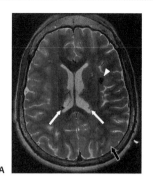 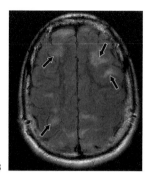 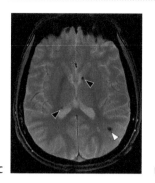 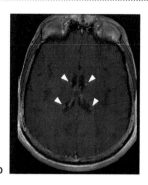

(A) Axial T2-weighted image shows multiple hypointense subependymal nodules lining the lateral ventricles bilaterally (*white arrows*). Expansile increased T2 signal of the subcortical white matter is consistent with cortical/subcortical tubers (*black arrows*). A hypointense tuber in the left insula is partially calcified (*white arrowhead*). **(B)** Axial fluid-attenuated inversion recovery (FLAIR) image serves to better delineate the areas of increased T2 signal with mild mass effect involving the subcortical white matter bilaterally (*arrows*). **(C)** Axial gradient recalled echo sequence demonstrates susceptibility artifact associated with some of the subependymal nodules due to internal calcifications (*black arrowheads*) and with a tuber in the left occipital lobe (*white arrowhead*). **(D)** Axial T1-weighted postcontrast image of the brain shows enhancement of many of the subependymal nodules (*arrowheads*).

■ **Differential Diagnosis**

- **Tuberous sclerosis:** The constellation of findings including cortical tubers, enhancing and often calcified subependymal nodules, and linear or wedge-shaped white matter lesions are characteristic of tuberous sclerosis (TS).
- *Subependymal gray matter heterotopia:* Also referred to as periventricular heterotopia. Migrational defect resulting in nodules of gray matter lining the ventricular surface that follow gray matter signal on all MRI sequences, do not calcify or enhance, and are not associated with cortical tubers.
- *Taylor focal cortical dysplasia:* Also known as focal cortical dysplasia type IIb. This entity exhibits a classically solitary, expansile, T2 hyperintense focus with blurring of the gray–white matter interface. A single cortical tuber is indistinguishable from a focal cortical dysplasia. However, in this case where many cortical tubers are present in association with other classic findings, TS is the favored diagnosis.

■ **Essential Facts**

- Neurocutaneous syndrome with multiorgan involvement.
- Approximately 50% are de novo and 50% follow an autosomal-dominant inheritance pattern.
- Classic clinical triad of epilepsy, mental retardation, and adenoma sebaceum.
- Most common manifestations outside of the central nervous system (CNS) include cardiac rhabdomyomas and renal angiomyolipomas.
- CNS findings:
  - Cortical/subcortical tubers: Disorganized brain tissue with dysmorphic neurons and loss of normal cortical six-layer structure. Better seen on MR imaging as expansion of the gyrus with high T2 and low T1 signal. Calcification can be seen with advancing age.
  - Subependymal nodules: Small bulges that project from the ependymal lining into the ventricles. Typically, hyperintense on T1 and hypointense on T2 and may frequently calcify and enhance.
  - White matter lesions: May present as T2 hyperintense, linear or wedge-shaped lesions that extend from the ventricles to the cortex.
  - Subependymal giant-cell astrocytoma (SEGA): Mixed signal on T1- and T2-weighted images. May occur anywhere along the ventricular lining but have a predilection for the foramina of Monro.

■ **Other Imaging Findings**

- Cortical/subcortical tubers can demonstrate mild enhancement in 3 to 5% of cases.
- SEGA are believed to arise from preexisting subependymal nodules. Therefore, interval growth of a subependymal nodule should raise concern for SEGA.
- When located at the foramina of Monro, SEGA can cause obstructive hydrocephalus.
- Occasionally, cystlike white matter lesions can be seen in the deep white matter and are considered a combination of enlarged perivascular spaces and white matter degeneration.

✓ **Pearls and** ✗ **Pitfalls**

- ✓ CT and susceptibility-weighted imaging may aid in detecting calcifications within subependymal nodules and cortical tubers.
- ✓ Imaging surveillance is useful to establish the presence of SEGA or hydrocephalus.
- ✗ Enhancement of the subependymal nodules does not indicate transformation to SEGA.
- ✗ For subependymal nodules, size > 1 cm alone, without documented growth, is not sufficient to raise suspicion for SEGA.

Case 21

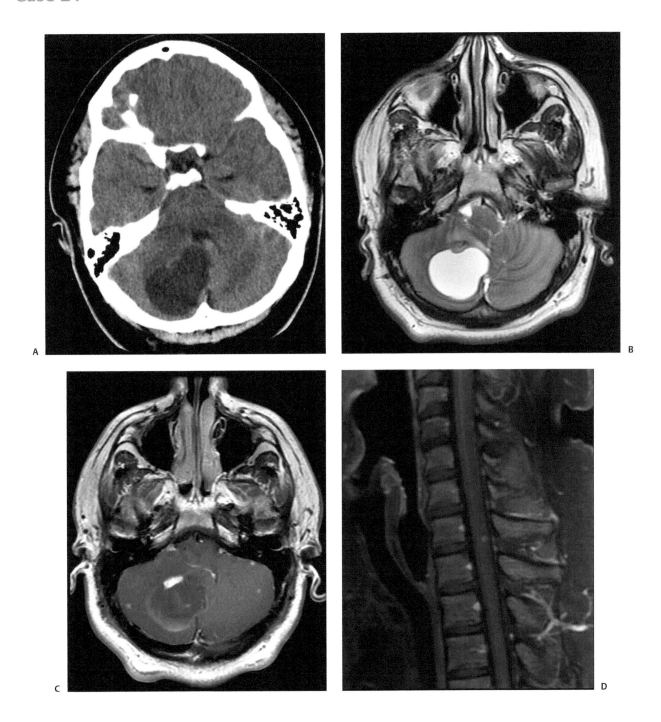

▨ Clinical Presentation

A 14-year-old boy presents with vertigo.

■ Imaging Findings

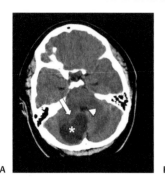 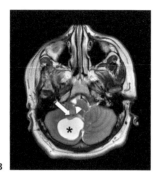 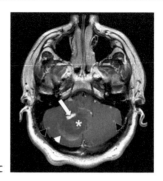 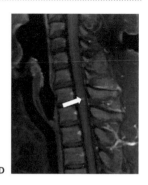

(A) Axial CT scan of the head without contrast shows a cystic lesion in the right cerebellar hemisphere (*asterisk*) with an anterior nodular component (*arrow*). The fourth ventricle is deformed by the mass effect (*arrowhead*). (B) Axial T2-weighted image (WI) shows a right cerebellar cystic lesion (*asterisk*) with an anterior nodule (*arrow*) and surrounding vasogenic edema (*arrowhead*). (C) Axial T1WI with contrast shows the cystic mass (*asterisk*) with enhancement of the anterior nodule (*arrow*) with slight peripheral enhancement of the cyst wall (*white arrowhead*). Other smaller enhancing nodules are seen in the cerebellar hemispheres (*black arrowheads*). (D) Sagittal MRI scan of the cervical spine with contrast shows a punctate area of enhancement in the cervical cord (*arrow*).

■ Differential Diagnosis

- **von Hippel–Lindau syndrome:** Autosomal-dominant familial cancer syndrome. In the central nervous system, this condition is characterized by cerebellar and posterior spinal cord hemangioblastomas (WHO I). Hemangiomas classically present as intra-axial cystic masses with a well-defined mural nodule (75%). Large cerebellar masses can displace the fourth ventricle. Mural nodule typically shows avid enhancement. Calcifications are not a common feature.
- *Cerebellar metastasis:* Most frequent malignancy of the posterior fossa in late adulthood. Extremely rare in childhood.
- *Pilocytic astrocytoma:* Most frequent posterior fossa malignancy in children. Usually seen in patients younger than 20 years old. Pylocytic astrocytomas (PA) also present as cystic posterior fossa masses with an enhancing nodule. However, unlike hemangioblastomas, PA usually have enhancement along the borders of the cyst. Twenty percent calcify. These tumors are typically located in the cerebellar hemisphere and compress the fourth ventricle. They are solitary lesions with no spinal cord involvement.

■ Essential Facts

- The presence of a cyst with a nodule that abuts the pial surface is typical; up to 40% can be solid tumors.
- Of all hemangioblastomas, 4 to 20% are associated with von Hippel–Lindau syndrome (VHL).
- Eighty percent of spinal hemangioblastomas are associated with VHL.
- The cyst wall shows no enhancement.

■ Other Imaging Findings

- On T2-weighted images, the nodule tends to be hyperintense.
- Variable amount of surrounding vasogenic edema.
- The mural nodule enhances profusely.
- The mass can show hemosiderin deposits on gradient echo/susceptibility-weighted image if bleeding occurred.
- On angiography, hemangioblastomas are visible as enhancing lesions that have a late washout.

✓ Pearls and ✗ Pitfalls

✓ Manifestations of VHL include:
  - Multiple brain hemangioblastomas (45–70%).
  - Spinal cord hemangioblastoma (15–50%).
  - Retinal hemangioblastomas (50%).
  - Renal (70%) and pancreatic (50%) simple cysts.
  - Renal cell carcinoma (30%).
  - Pheochromocytoma (12%).
  - Islet cell tumor of the pancreas (10%).
  - Endolymphatic sac tumors.
✗ Do not forget to image all of the spine.
✗ Small hemangioblastomas tend to be solid rather than cystic.

Case 22

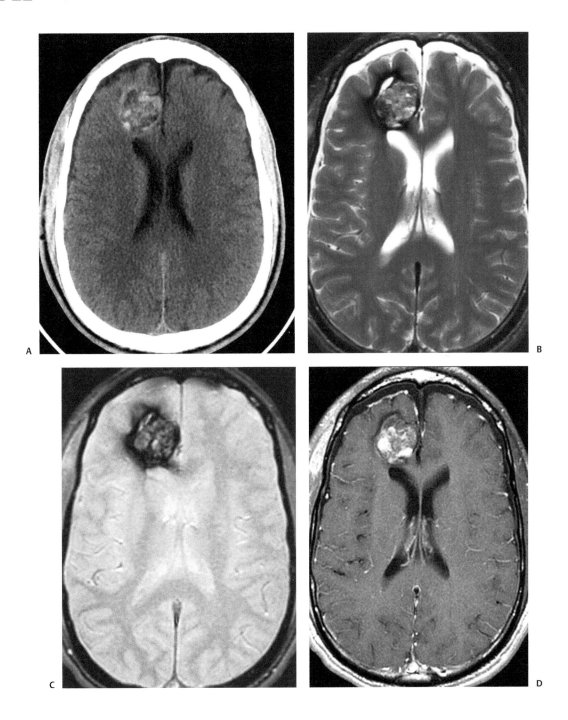

A

B

C

D

■ Clinical Presentation

A 42-year-old man presents with headaches and personality changes over 3 years.

■ Imaging Findings

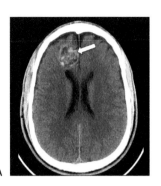 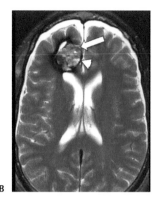 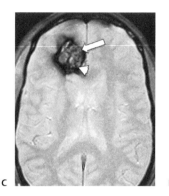 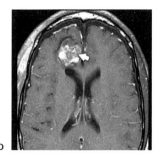

A   B   C   D

(A) Axial CT image without contrast shows a lesion with mixed densities in the right frontal lobe with minimal mass effect (*arrow*). **(B, C)** Axial T2-weighted image (WI) **(B)** and gradient echo image **(C)** show a mass on the right frontal lobe with minimal mass effect (*arrow*). The lesion shows a dark rim of hemosiderin deposits (*arrowhead*) with "popcorn"-like appearance. **(D)** Axial T1WI with contrast shows no enhancement. The areas of increased signal in the lesion (*arrow*) were present on the T1 image without contrast, related to T1 shortening from the blood products.

■ Differential Diagnosis

- **Cavernous malformation:** Vascular lesions that contain multiple immature blood vessels with no intervening neural tissue and present with blood products at different stages of evolution. These lesions are present in approximately 0.5 to 0.7% of the population. They are not seen on digital subtraction angiography. Cavernous malformations can present as either a sporadic abnormality or as part of familial cavernomatosis (25%). They tend to be associated with developmental venous anomalies.
- *Hypertensive parenchymal hematoma:* Solitary brain parenchymal hematomas account for 10 to 15% of strokes. Located in order of frequency in the basal ganglia (especially the putamen), thalamus, pons, and cerebellum.
- *Hemorrhagic metastasis:* Secondary brain tumors generally arise in the subcortical white matter and 50% are solitary lesions. They tend to hemorrhage mostly in elderly patients. Metastases from melanoma, renal cell carcinoma, choriocarcinoma, thyroid papillary carcinoma, lung carcinoma, breast carcinoma, and hepatocellular carcinoma are more likely to hemorrhage.

■ Essential Facts

- Zabramski has proposed a classification of cavernous malformations based on their imaging presentation:
  ○ Type I: Subacute hemorrhage.
  ○ Type II: Lesion with hemorrhage in different stages of evolution. Popcornlike appearance with a peripheral T2 hemosiderin rim.
  ○ Type III: Chronic hemorrhage with hemosiderin rim.
  ○ Type IV: Tiny lesions or telangiectasia seen only on gradient echo images.
- Eighty percent are supratentorial.

■ Other Imaging Findings

- CT images can be negative in one third of cases.
- Fifty percent of cavernous malformations show calcifications.
- Recent hemorrhage produces mass effect.
- When a T1 hyperintense rim is present around a hemorrhagic lesion, there is a high probability that the lesion corresponds to a cavernous malformation.

✓ Pearls and × Pitfalls

✓ Patients with familial cavernomatosis should be followed with imaging, and screening can be offered to family members.

✓ May be congenital or arise de novo after radiation, pregnancy, or brain biopsy.

✗ Recent hemorrhage in a cavernous malformation may result in an atypical appearance, with perilesional and extralesional hemorrhage outside the hemosiderin ring, increase in size with respect to prior studies, edema, or mass effect. Follow-up imaging is warranted in these cases.

Case 23

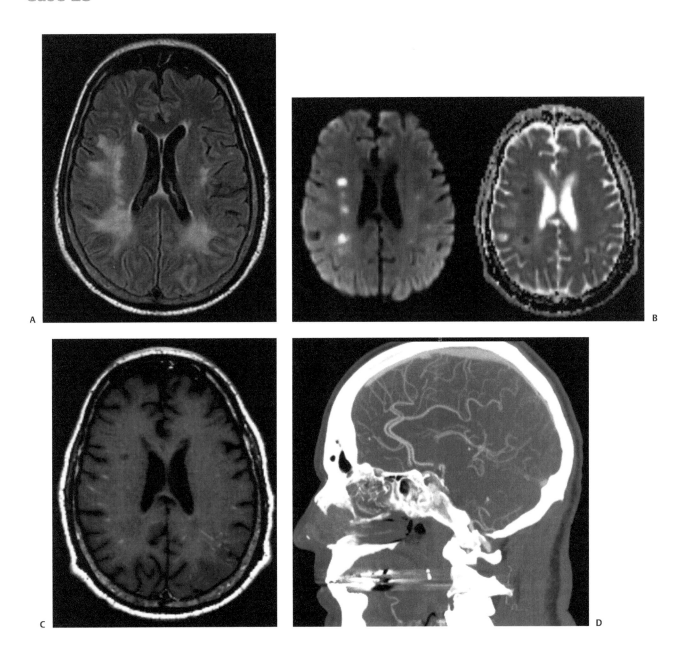

■ Clinical Presentation

A 65-year-old man presents with altered mental status.

■ Imaging Findings

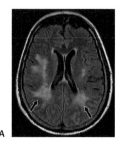
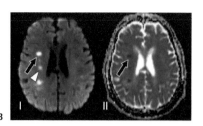
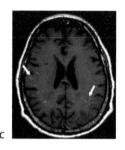
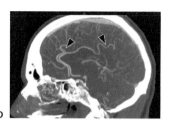

(A) Axial fluid-attenuated inversion recovery image of the brain shows ill-defined hyperintensity primarily involving the white matter and extending from the ventricular surface to the subcortical region (*black arrows*). **(B)** Axial diffusion-weighted image (DWI) (*I*) and corresponding apparent diffusion coefficient (ADC) map (*II*) show multiple punctate foci of restricted diffusion (*black arrows*) with other foci of increased DWI signal without low ADC values (*white arrowhead*), suggesting a subacute stage. **(C)** Axial T1-weighted postcontrast MR image shows multiple areas of linear enhancement in a perivascular distribution (*white arrows*). **(D)** CT angiography of the head. Sagittal maximum intensity projection image shows multiple subtle regions of stenosis involving medium- and small-caliber vessels (*black arrowheads*).

■ Differential Diagnosis

- ***Primary angiitis of the central nervous system (PACNS):*** Condition of insidious onset, seen more frequently in older men, characterized by multifocal infarcts in varying stages of evolution.
- *Reversible cerebral vasoconstriction syndrome (RCVS):* RCVS is a condition characterized by a hyperacute onset of headache with or without subarachnoid hemorrhage, with imaging showing involvement of medium to large arteries in multiple territories. Young to middle-aged females are more frequently affected. There is associated diffuse, uniform vessel wall thickening without enhancement which responds to vasodilators and is typically self-limited.
- *Lymphomatoid granulomatosis:* Lymphoproliferative disorder of the CNS seen more commonly in men between the 4th and 6th decades of life, caused by a lymphomatous infiltration of the perivascular spaces. There can be focal or linear, parenchymal, and leptomeningeal enhancement, as well as T2 hyperintense lesions that involve the white matter, deep gray nuclei, and the brainstem.

■ Essential Facts

- Inflammatory disease of the small to medium-sized arteries of the CNS.
- Peak of incidence is the 5th to 6th decades of life.
- There is generally multifocal short-segment wall thickening with associated enhancement.
- Cerebrospinal fluid studies may show increased proteins and white blood cells.
- Patients tend to clinically deteriorate, in contrast to the self-limited course of RCVS.
- Hemorrhagic complications are uncommon, which is another distinguishing factor from RCVS.

- Generally there is no response to vasodilators on conventional angiography.
- Patients are treated with high-dose steroids and cytotoxic agents.

■ Other Imaging Findings

- CT can have subtle findings, including ill-defined hypodensities secondary to ischemia.
- MRI:
  - Supra- and infratentorial involvement.
  - White matter lesions in the periventricular and subcortical regions.
  - Irregularity affecting the parenchymal and leptomeningeal vessels.
  - Infarcts in multiples stages of evolution.
- Digital subtraction angiography (DSA):
  - Focal or multifocal segmental stenosis.
  - May be negative

✓ Pearls and ✗ Pitfalls

✓ The vessel walls are thickened and demonstrate associated enhancement that can be evaluated with vessel wall MRI.

✓ Prompt treatment with steroids prevents sequela from repeated microinfarcts.

✗ Patients with PACNS may have an unremarkable angiography. A negative DSA does not exclude a diagnosis of PACNS.

✗ Infusion of vasodilators during DSA, and the corresponding response, may aid in differentiating between PACNS and RCVS.

✗ Occasionally, brain biopsy is required to establish a diagnosis.

Case 24

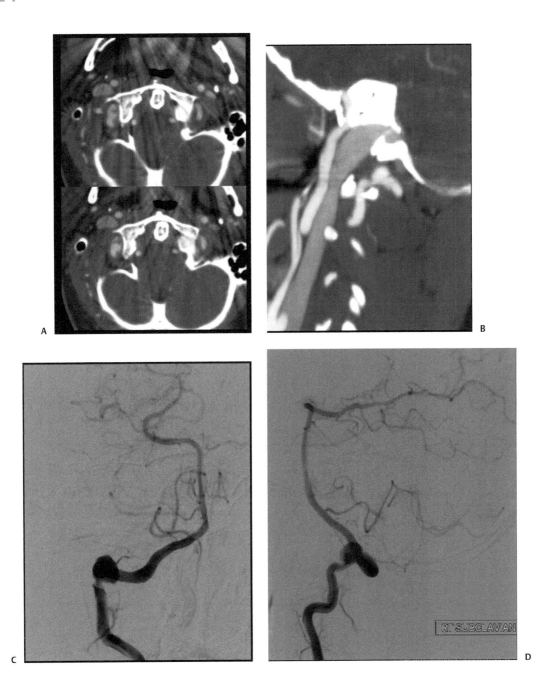

A

B

C

D

■ Clinical Presentation

A 34-year-old woman is undergoing a work-up for a recent left posterior cerebral artery infarct.

■ Imaging Findings

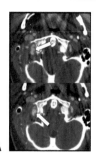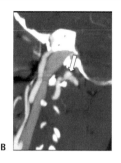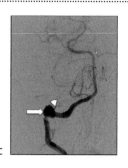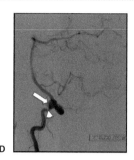

A   B   C   D

(A) Axial CT angiography (CTA) source images demonstrate an outpouching of the medial wall of the V3 segment of the right vertebral artery (*arrows*). **(B)** Sagittal reformatted CTA image demonstrates an outpouching of the V3 segment of the right vertebral artery (*arrow*), flanked by areas of segmental narrowing of the vessel. **(C)** Frontal view of a digital subtraction angiography (DSA) image of the right vertebral artery demonstrates aneurysmal dilatation of the V3 segment of the right vertebral artery (*arrow*). A muscular branch arises from the dome of the aneurysm (*arrowhead*). **(D)** Lateral view of a DSA image of the right vertebral artery demonstrates aneurysmal dilatation of the V3 segment of the right vertebral artery (*arrow*), with proximal stenosis (*arrowhead*).

■ Differential Diagnosis

- **Dissecting aneurysm:** Aneurysm in a nonbranching location with associated signs of dissection, including the presence of a false lumen, stenosis with dilatation (pearl with string sign), or, less reliably, stenosis alone.
- *Blood blister aneurysms*: These aneurysms are infrequent but are associated with increased morbidity and mortality. Blood blister aneurysms can resemble pseudoaneurysms and are acquired secondary to hemodynamic stresses and focal weakening of the vessel wall. These aneurysms are often covered only by a thin cap of fibrous tissue/adventitia. They appear as a broad-based, shallow outpouching of the vessel wall in a nonbranching location. They are frequently occult on CT angiography (CTA). On digital subtraction angiography (DSA) imaging, they may only be seen as a broad-based bulge in one projection.
- *Infectious aneurysm:* Infectious aneurysms, formerly called mycotic aneurysms, are abnormal dilatations of the blood vessels, associated with infections, most commonly bacterial. They may be multiple and variable in size, and they typically present in nonbranching locations of the arteries.

■ Essential Facts

- Dissecting intracranial aneurysms result in blood accumulation within the vessel wall through a tear in the intima and internal elastic lamina. Intramural hematoma may extend into the subadventitial plane, forming a saclike outpouching.
- If the mural hematoma ruptures the vascular layers of the intradural artery, a subarachnoid hemorrhage will occur.
- If the intramural hematoma reopens distally into the parent vessel, ischemic embolic events may happen following intramural clot formation.

- The vessel wall may dilate, leading to occlusion of perforator branches and local ischemia.
- Organization of the mural hematoma may result in a chronic dissecting process which may eventually lead to formation of a "giant partially thrombosed" aneurysm with thrombus of varying ages within the vessel. This may lead to ingrowth of the vasa vasorum and recurrent dissections, with subsequent growth of the aneurysm from the periphery.

■ Other Imaging Findings

- DSA with 3D reconstructions facilitates analysis of the angioarchitecture of the aneurysm, including the relationship to branching vessels and the presence of vessels at the dome.

✓ Pearls and ✗ Pitfalls

✓ True aneurysms are described as outpouches of all layers of a vessel associated with degenerative changes of the aneurysmal wall.

✓ False aneurysms, which can have saccular or fusiform morphologic features, are characterized by incomplete or complete disruption of the vessel wall, with formation of a lumen that can be contained by a layer of the wall or by a cavitated clot (pseudoaneurysm).

✗ The V3 and V4 segments of the vertebral arteries near the craniocervical junction and the cavernous segments of the internal carotid arteries near the skull base may be difficult to delineate in reformatted CTA images. Careful analysis of the source images is needed for a full evaluation of these segments.

✗ Bone subtraction techniques are helpful in these areas.

Case 25

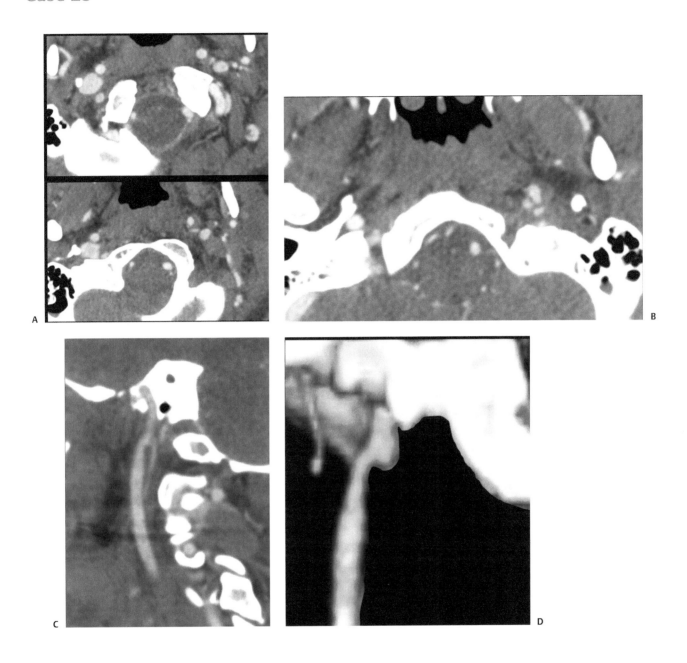

A

B

C

D

■ Clinical Presentation
....

A 24-year-old man presents with neck pain and a left eye ptosis after a motor vehicle accident.

■ Imaging Findings

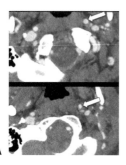 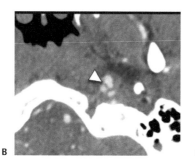 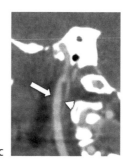 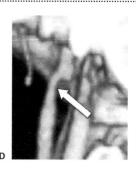

(A) CT scan with contrast shows an irregularity of the posterior and medial contour of the left internal carotid artery (ICA) (*arrows*). **(B)** CT scan with contrast slightly more cephalad demonstrates a flap (*arrowhead*) in the left ICA. **(C)** CT angiography sagittal reformatted image shows increase in diameter of the left ICA (*arrow*) with a central intraluminal flap (*arrowhead*) that defines a true lumen anteriorly and a false posterior lumen. **(D)** Volume-rendered CT scan with contrast shows irregularity of the posterior wall of the left ICA (*arrow*).

■ Differential Diagnosis

- ***Traumatic carotid dissection:*** Characterized by fusiform dilatation or stenosis of the carotid artery not associated with atheromas. Dissections are usually located distal to the carotid bifurcations and may present with an intraluminal flap. They are more common in the carotid arteries than in the vertebral circulation. 15% of patients have involvement of multiple arteries.
- *Atherosclerosis:* Atheromatous plaques occur close to the carotid bifurcations. Ulcerated plaques can cause dissections and thrombus formation. Narrowing tends to occur in short segments, at vessel origins, or at sites of turbulent flow. Atherosclerosis is usually bilateral and may be associated with dissection but not with trauma.
- *Vasospasm:* Narrowing of the vascular lumen, may be wavy in appearance, and typically related to catheter contact with the intima. This finding is typically reversible. No mural thrombus or intraluminal flap is seen.

■ Essential Facts

- Incidence is 2% in cases of blunt trauma.
- These injuries are caused by a tear in the intima of the vessel, which allows intraluminal blood to dissect along the layers of the vessel wall or, alternatively, direct hemorrhage from the vasa vasorum of the media into the arterial wall.
- Luminal narrowing or total occlusion occurs if the hematoma lies just beneath the intima.
- If the hematoma dissects just beneath the adventitia, a pseudoaneurysm forms. The presence of a thin intraluminal flap defines a true and a false lumen.
- Contrast can fill both lumina.
- Can present as Horner syndrome due to the presence of the sympathetic plexus around the internal carotid artery (ICA).
- Associated with a 60% stroke rate.

■ Other Imaging Findings

- CT is helpful to identify adjacent fracture sites.
- CT angiography detects the luminal defect. Contrast can fill the vasa vasorum surrounding the mural hematoma.
- MRI can show an intramural hematoma, which may have a crescent or concentric/target shape.
- The residual lumen can show a flow void.
- Common locations:
  ○ Cervical ICA 2 to 3 cm distal to the carotid bulb.
  ○ Vertebral artery at the level of the first and second cervical vertebrae.
  ○ Multiple-vessel disease.

✓ Pearls and ✗ Pitfalls

✓ Can be associated with:
  - Pseudoaneurysms.
  - Trauma of the cervical spine.
  ✓ Other vascular dissections.
✓ Thrombosis of a false lumen may become a source of distal emboli presenting as a transient ischemic attack or stroke.
✗ When a thrombus is present, it is difficult to define if it is associated with a dissection.
✗ An acute intramural hematoma can be hypointense on T2- and T1-weighted images and therefore is difficult to delineate from an area of flow void. The intramural hematoma may therefore be missed on MRI within the first 24 to 48 hours after an ICA dissection.

Case 26

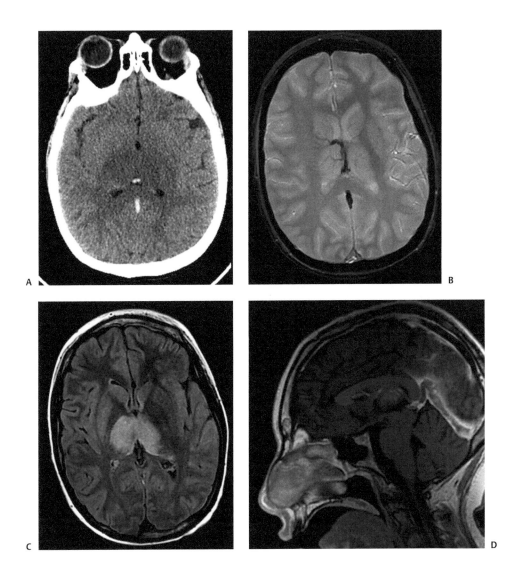

■ Clinical Presentation

A 16-year-old girl with acute lymphocytic leukemia presents with a 1-week history of headache and nausea.

■ Imaging Findings

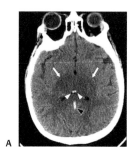 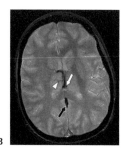 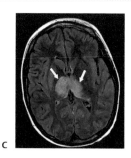 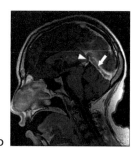

A   B   C   D

(A) Axial noncontrast CT image of the head shows diffuse hypodensity of the bilateral thalami (*white arrows*). There is hyperdensity of the internal cerebral veins (*white arrowheads*) and of the straight sinus (*black arrowhead*). **(B)** Axial T2* image demonstrates susceptibility artifact involving the thalamostriate veins (*white arrowhead*), internal cerebral veins (*white arrow*), and the straight sinus (*black arrow*). **(C)** Axial fluid-attenuated inversion recovery image shows diffuse T2 hyperintensity of the bilateral thalami (*arrows*) secondary to subacute ischemia. **(D)** Sagittal T1 postcontrast image shows a filling defect within an expanded vein of Galen (*arrowhead*) and straight sinus (*arrow*).

■ Differential Diagnosis

- **Deep cerebral venous thrombosis:** Relatively uncommon disorder in which there is occlusion of the internal cerebral veins, of the vein of Galen, and/or of the straight sinus that typically leads to bilateral thalamic edema with or without infarction.
- *Artery of Percheron territory infarct:* The artery of Percheron is a rare anatomic variant of the thalamic paramedian arteries. These vessels typically arise from the bilateral P1 segments of the posterior cerebral arteries. The artery of Percheron consists of a single artery arising from either side, forming a dominant thalamoperforating artery that supplies the circulation to the medial thalami bilaterally. When this artery becomes thrombosed, there is characteristic infarction of the bilateral paramedian thalami.
- *Top of the basilar syndrome:* Syndrome characterized by occlusion of the basilar tip with variable extension to the bilateral P1 segments with involvement of the ventral midbrain and thalami. The distribution of the infarction largely depends on the size of the occlusion and on the individual's arterial anatomy. In patients with prominent posterior communicating arteries, the PCA territory can be spared. Occasionally, the clot can affect the pontine perforators and the superior cerebellar arteries.

■ Essential Facts

- The pathophysiology of brain injury secondary to venous thrombosis begins with increased venous pressure that may ultimately lead to hemorrhage or to the development of altered arterial perfusion pressure and infarct.
- The mechanism by which the brain attempts to regulate increased venous pressure is by the use of collateral pathways.
- The classic imaging finding of thrombosis on noncontrast CT is hyperattenuation within the thrombosed vessel, a finding seen in only 25% of cases.

- On contrast-enhanced studies, a filling defect and expansion of the affected vein or sinus is a characteristic finding. This sign has been termed the "empty delta" sign.
- On an MR image, loss of a flow void within the affected vessel is a typical finding.
- The thrombus can show variable signal intensity depending on its age.
- Edema of the thalami is the characteristic pattern for deep venous occlusion. Extension into the caudate nuclei and deep white matter can also occur.

■ Other Imaging Findings

- The most commonly used imaging modalities for the evaluation of the venous system include time-of-flight MR venography, contrast-enhanced MR venography, and CT venography.
- When deoxyhemoglobin and methemoglobin are present, susceptibility artifact on gradient echo sequences within the thrombus can aid in diagnosis.
- Unilateral thalamic edema may occur in deep venous occlusion but it is highly uncommon.
- Thalamic edema can be a reversible process, with patients resolving without associated sequelae.

✓ Pearls and ✗ Pitfalls

- ✓ Parenchymal abnormalities in cerebral venous thrombosis include focal edema, both cytotoxic or vasogenic, and bleeding, which may occur in combination with either.
- ✓ Parenchymal enhancement may occur in the setting of venous thrombosis.
- ✗ Hyperdensity on CT within the venous system may occur in patients with dehydration or elevated hematocrit level.
- ✗ The appearance of postgadolinium MR studies can be confounding. Enhancement secondary to intrinsic vascularization within an organized thrombus, as well as enhancement in collateral channels, can simulate a patent sinus.

Case 27

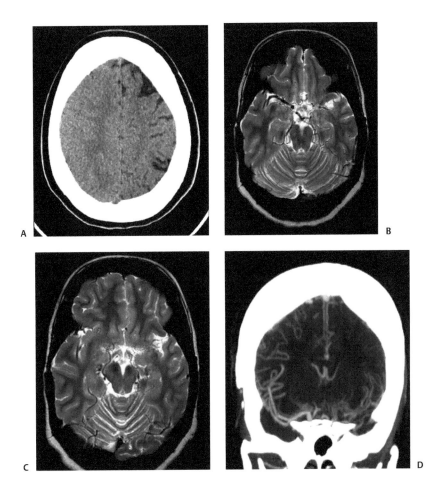

■ Clinical Presentation

A 30-year-old woman with history of sickle cell anemia presents with headaches.

■ Imaging Findings

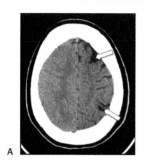 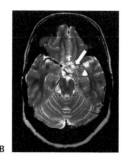 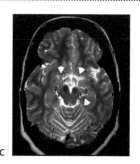 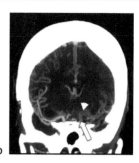

(A) Axial CT image demonstrates multiple areas of cortical atrophy in the left cerebral hemisphere resulting in compensatory enlargement of the peripheral sulci (*arrows*). **(B)** Axial T2-weighted image (WI) shows a diminutive left internal carotid artery (ICA) (*arrow*). The left middle cerebral artery is smaller than the right (*arrowhead*). **(C)** Axial T2WI shows numerous prominent leptomeningeal collateral vessels around the basal cisterns (*arrowheads*). **(D)** Coronal reformatted CT image shows a diminutive left ICA (*arrow*), surrounded by multiple small leptomeningeal collaterals that appear as diffuse enhancement in the subarachnoid space (*arrowhead*).

■ Differential Diagnosis

- ***Moyamoya disease:*** Occlusive changes in the distal internal carotid arteries (ICAs) or proximal anterior or middle cerebral arteries. Hypertrophy of leptomeningeal collaterals results in a "puff of smoke" appearance on conventional angiography.
- *Chronic left ICA dissection:* ICA dissection is a tear or rupture of the intima, allowing blood to gain access to the subintima and media. There is an intimal flap or double lumen. Aneurysmal dilatation can be seen in 30% of cases. Flame-shaped ICA occlusion occurs in the acute phase. Most commonly originates in the ICA 2 to 3 cm distal to the carotid bulb and variably involves the distal ICA.
- *Cerebral hemiatrophy (Dyke–Davidoff–Masson syndrome):* Unilateral cerebral atrophy occurring early enough in cerebral development that it leads to changes in the skull. The ipsilateral paranasal sinuses and mastoid air cells are hyperpneumatized. Ipsilateral calvarial thickening occurs. MR may be helpful for determining the etiology of the hemiatrophy, including: vascular/infectious insult, encephalomalacia/gliosis.

■ Essential Facts

- Moyamoya angiopathy is characterized by a progressive stenosis of the terminal portion of the ICAs and the development of a network of abnormal collateral vessels.
- The collateral network results in "puff of smoke" appearance on angiography.
- Affects children in the first decade of life or adults in the third or fourth decades of life.

- Mainly leads to brain ischemic events in children, and to ischemic and hemorrhagic events in adults.
- Conditions that may be associated with the development of Moyamoya disease include: sickle cell anemia, Down syndrome, Fanconi's anemia, brain radiation therapy, familial occurrence, neurofibromatosis type I.

■ Other Imaging Findings

- MR angiography can delineate the occlusive changes and collateral networks.
- CT, MR, and single-photon emission CT perfusion studies provide information regarding the cerebrovascular reserve, which may aid in management decisions.
- Findings on cerebral angiography include:
  ○ Stenosis or occlusion at the terminal portion of the ICA or at the proximal portion of the anterior or middle cerebral arteries.
  ○ Abnormal vascular networks in the vicinity of the occlusive or stenotic areas.

✓ Pearls and ✗ Pitfalls

✓ The term "moyamoya disease" should be reserved for cases in which the characteristic angiographic pattern is idiopathic.
✓ "Moyamoya syndrome" is used when the underlying condition is known.
✗ In a T2-weighted image, attention to the flow voids can help identify the leptomeningeal collaterals as tiny vessels around the circle of Willis.

Case 28

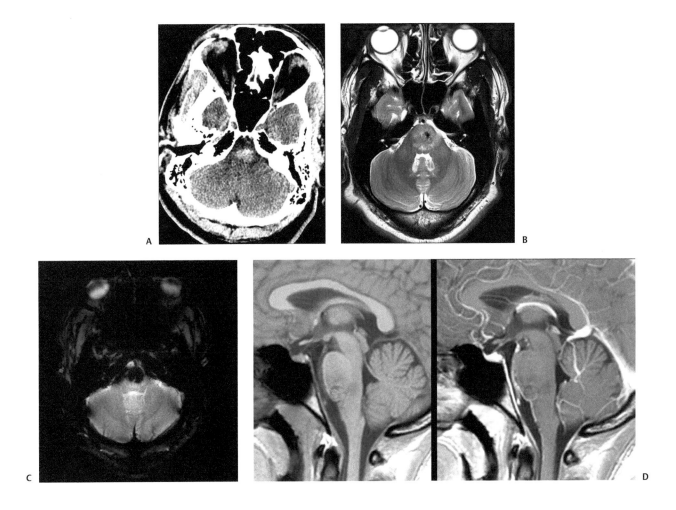

■ Clinical Presentation

A 48-year-old patient with hypertension presents with decreased level of consciousness and multiple bilateral cranial nerve palsies.

■ Imaging Findings

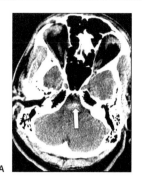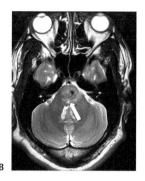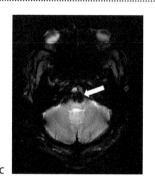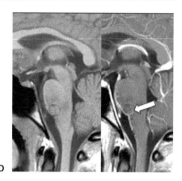

(A) Noncontrast CT image of the head shows an area of increased density seen centrally in the pons (*arrow*). **(B)** Axial T2-weighted image (WI) shows an ill-defined area of hyperintensity in the pons (*arrow*) with a central punctate area of low signal related to hemosiderin deposits. **(C)** Axial gradient echo WI shows an area of susceptibility artifact in the pons (*arrow*). **(D)** Sagittal T1 without (*left*) and with (*right*) contrast shows a slight amount of peripheral enhancement in the pontine lesion (*arrow*).

■ Differential Diagnosis

- **Hemorrhagic pontine stroke:** Brainstem strokes are typically located in the inferior aspect of the pons, at the pontomedullary junction or in the central aspect of the tectum. Hemorrhage will be accompanied by increased surrounding edema and expansion of the pons.
- *Pontine cavernous malformation:* Cavernous malformations show hemosiderin deposits in a popcornlike configuration. These lesions can be either solitary or multiple. With acute hemorrhage, expansion of the lesion can be seen. Generally, surrounding edema is not identified. Cavernous malformations are associated with adjacent developmental venous anomalies (DVAs).
- *Hemorrhagic pontine mass:* Pontine masses are typically diffuse astrocytomas. They generally present as diffuse enlargement of the pons and can show heterogeneous enhancement. These masses are better delineated on fluid-attenuated inversion recovery (FLAIR) sequences and rarely hemorrhage.

■ Essential Facts

- Hemorrhagic pontine lesions may originate from hypertensive angiopathy, as in this case. Other causes include cavernous malformations, arteriovenous malformations, primary glial neoplasms, metastases, or Duret hemorrhages in trauma.
- The basilar perforating arteries are median and paramedian branches that provide the majority of the circulation to the pons.

■ Other Imaging Findings

- CT images can demonstrate increased density.
- MR with contrast is the imaging modality of choice for evaluating hemorrhagic pontine strokes.
- In the acute stages of hemorrhage, it may be impossible to know if an underlying neoplasm is present; follow-up imaging is necessary.

✓ Pearls and ✗ Pitfalls

✓ Pontine hemorrhages can extend to the fourth ventricle and cause hydrocephalus.
✓ The hemorrhage typically spares the medulla and the mesencephalon.
✓ Pontine strokes are not associated with DVAs.

Case 29

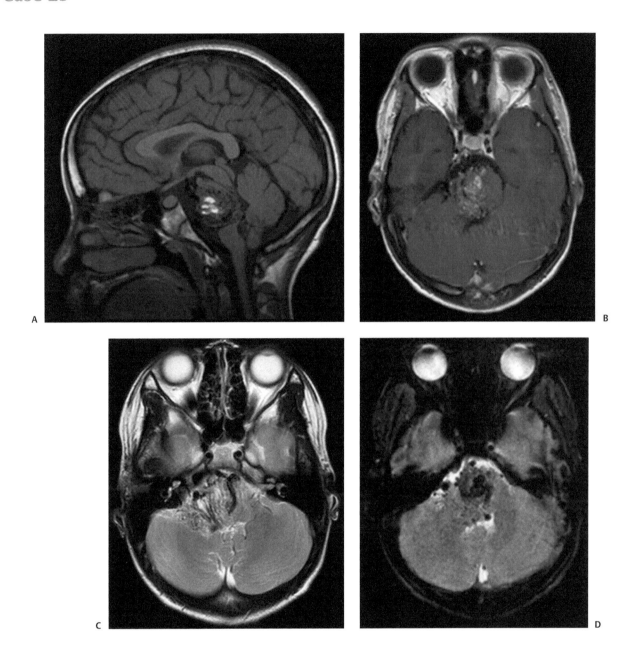

A

B

C

D

■ Clinical Presentation

A 21-year-old woman presents with headaches.

■ Imaging Findings

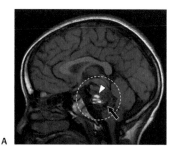
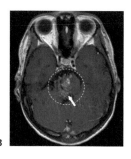
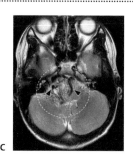
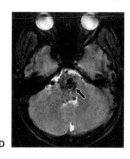

(A) Sagittal T1 image shows a heterogeneous vascular nidus in the pons (*circle*) with internal areas of intrinsic high T1 signal intensity (*white arrowhead*) that may represent blood products and/or calcifications. There are abnormal vascular flow voids within the tangle of vessels and in the surrounding basal cisterns (*black arrow*). **(B)** Axial T1 postcontrast image shows a tightly packed vascular nidus within the brain tissue centered in the right side of the pons and slightly extending into the right middle cerebellar peduncle (*circle*) with vascular opacification (*white arrow*). **(C)** Axial T2 shows numerous flow voids within the vascular nidus indicating rapid flow (*circle*). Large draining veins are seen extending from the pons to the pre-pontine cistern (*arrowheads*). **(D)** Axial susceptibility-weighted imaging shows areas of susceptibility artifact within the lesion itself indicating calcifications and/or remote blood products (*arrow*).

■ Differential Diagnosis

- ***Arteriovenous malformation (AVM):*** Tangle of abnormal vessels within the brain parenchyma characterized by direct artery to vein shunting with prominent draining veins and without an intervening capillary network.
- *Cavernous malformation*: Vascular malformation characterized by dilated vessels without intervening brain tissue. Does not show vascular flow voids or prominent draining veins. Typically presents as a popcorn-like, multilobulated heterogeneous lesion with blood products in multiple stages of evolution, a dark T2 hemosiderin rim, internal fluid–fluid levels, and blooming on susceptibility-weighted imaging.
- *Hemorrhagic neoplasm (i.e., glioblastoma)*: The heterogeneous nature and marked angiogenesis of high-grade neoplasms can mimic AVMs. Unlike glioblastoma, no discernable mass lesion is associated with the abnormal vessels in AVMs. Furthermore, the presence of a prominent draining vein is not characteristic of high-grade hemorrhagic neoplasms.

■ Essential Facts

- Congenital malformations of vascular development.
- Majority are supratentorial (85%) and solitary lesions.
- Can vary greatly in size from tiny lesions to large malformations that affect up to entire cerebral hemispheres.
- AVMs most frequently are tightly packed and show no intervening brain tissue (glomerular type) or, less commonly, can be loosely arranged within the parenchyma (diffuse or proliferative type).
- Interspersed brain tissue is generally gliotic.
- Often heterogeneous density on CT and signal intensity on MRI due to internal dystrophic calcifications, blood products, and thrombus.
- Superficial lesions: pial artery suppliers and cortical vein drainage.
- Deep lesions: perforator or choroidal suppliers and deep venous drainage.

■ Other Imaging Findings

- Approximately half of AVMs show internal aneurysmal dilatations.
- High-velocity turbulent flow from dilated feeding vessels may induce proximal aneurysms that can resolve spontaneously after treatment of the AVM.
- Mass effect from the nidus itself and/or from associated hemorrhage and edema can lead to a wide range of complications including hydrocephalus and herniation.
- Digital subtraction angiography (DSA) aids in better depicting the organization of the vessel mass by clearly delineating the feeding vessels, draining veins, and associated aneurysms.
- Bleeding can occur from aneurysm rupture or venous thrombosis that can lead to congestion and hemorrhage.

✓ Pearls and ✗ Pitfalls

- ✓ Heterogeneous imaging features due to thrombus, calcifications, and blood products.
- ✓ High risk of bleeding.
- ✓ Spetzler–Martin grading system:
  - Helps predict the likelihood of a satisfactory outcome if surgical resection is attempted.
  - Grades are assigned depending on the size of the nidus, eloquence of the adjacent brain parenchyma, and deep versus superficial venous drainage.
  - Eloquent areas include the sensorimotor, language and visual cortex, thalami, hypothalamus, internal capsules, brainstem, cerebellar peduncles, and deep cerebellar nuclei.
- ✗ The heterogeneous nature of the nidus can mimic hemorrhagic neoplasms. The presence of neighboring dilated vessels and the absence of a discernable mass helps to differentiate the two.
- ✗ A complete peripheral hemosiderin rim and multiple internal fluid–fluid levels indicate a cavernous malformation.

Case 30

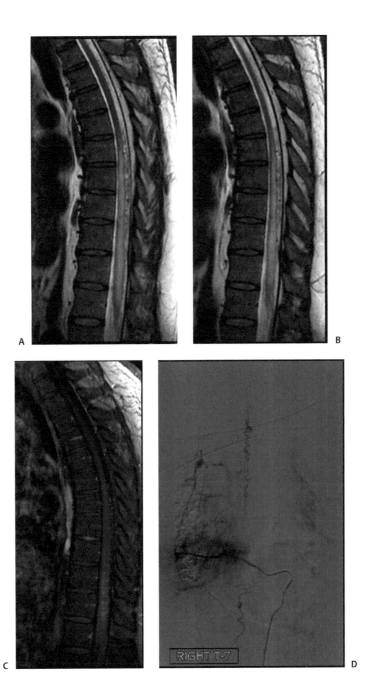

▪ Clinical Presentation

A 56-year-old man presents with back pain and thoracic radiculopathy.

■ Imaging Findings

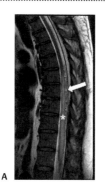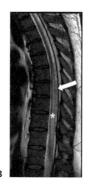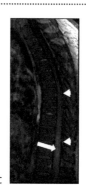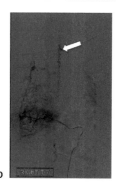

A B C D

(A, B) Sagittal T2-weighted images (WIs) demonstrate a longitudinally extensive area of increased cord signal spanning six levels (*asterisk*). Enlarged vessels in the subarachnoid space in the vicinity are demonstrated (*arrow*). **(C)** Sagittal postcontrast T1WI shows patchy enhancement within the cord lesion (*arrow*). Enhancement within the prominent vessels in the subarachnoid space is also noted (*arrowheads*). **(D)** Digital subtraction angiography frontal view with injection of the right T7 segmental artery shows opacification of a dural arteriovenous fistula in the spinal canal (*arrow*).

■ Differential Diagnosis

- **Spinal arteriovenous fistula (AVF):**
  - Spinal vascular malformations are abnormal arteriovenous (AV) communications in the spinal cord or dura mater.
  - They may have extramedullary/extradural components and parenchymal cord components.
- *Cord infarct:*
  - Cord infarction secondary to vessel occlusion (radicular artery).
  - Diffusion-weighted image: Hyperintense signal with apparent diffusion coefficient correlation.
  - T2-weighted image: Hyperintense central gray matter or entire cross-sectional area.
  - Not associated with abnormal flow voids in the subarachnoid space.
- *Neuromyelitis optica:*
  - Idiopathic inflammatory demyelinating disorder of the central nervous system characterized by severe attacks of optic neuritis and myelitis.
  - Cord lesions with longitudinal extension ≥ 3 vertebral segments.
  - T2 hyperintensity within the cord with patchy contrast enhancement.
  - T2 abnormality tends to involve the entire cross-section of the cord, unlike more focal involvement of multiple sclerosis.
  - Not associated with abnormal flow voids in the subarachnoid space.

■ Essential Facts

- Spinal AV lesions are abnormal connections between arteries (radicular, anterior spinal, posterior spinal) and veins in the epidural space, intradural space, or cord/conus medullaris.

- Multiple classifications have been used. Currently the lesions are described based on location of the lesion (extradural or intradural; ventral, dorsal, or intramedullary), and on the presence of single or multiple feeding branches.
- In most spinal AV lesions, direct AVFs occur in the extra-axial spaces; however, intramedullary arteriovenous malformations (AVMs) (analogous to intracranial AVMs) and extradural-intradural AVMs (juvenile or metameric AVMs) have shunts within the spinal cord parenchyma.

■ Other Imaging Findings

- Conventional MRI shows cord hyperintensity on T2-weighted images, gadolinium enhancement within the cord, and multiple vascular flow voids along the surface of the cord.
- MR angiography with contrast can be used to better characterize the AVF-AVM and help localize the feeders prior to angiography.
- Digital subtraction angiography characterizes the arterial feeders and venous drainage.

✓ Pearls and ✗ Pitfalls

✓ Three pathophysiologic mechanisms underlying spinal AV lesions can cause neurologic injury: hemorrhage, mass effect, and vascular steal.

✓ Venous hypertension tends to be associated with either intradural spinal AVFs or conus medullaris–type spinal AVMs.

✗ Flow voids from normal vessels in the epidural space should not be confused with spinal AVMs.

Case 31

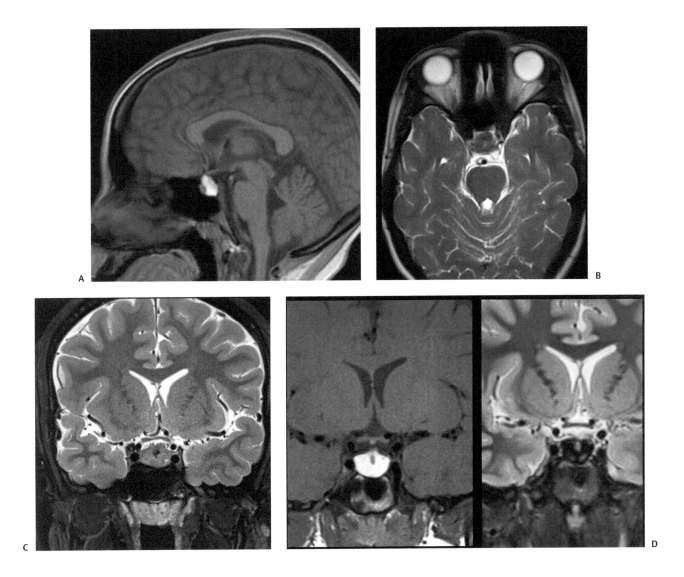

■ Clinical Presentation
....

A 16-year-old girl presents with acute visual disturbances and strabismus.

■ Imaging Findings

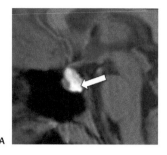 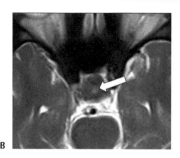 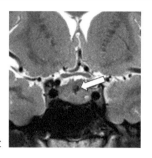 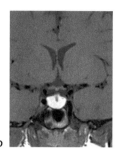

(A, D) Sagittal **(A)** and coronal **(D)** T1-weighted images show an enlarged pituitary gland (*arrow*) that is hyperintense and contacts the optic chiasm.
(B, C) Axial **(B)** and coronal **(C)** T2 fast spin echo demonstrate an enlarged pituitary gland with a punctate central hypointensity (*arrow*).

■ Differential Diagnosis

- **Pituitary apoplexy:**
  - Abrupt hemorrhage or infarct of the pituitary gland, typically within an adenoma.
  - 2 to 12% of adenomas undergo apoplexy.
  - More common in men in the 5th to 6th decades of life.
  - Variable morphology.
- *Rathke cleft cyst:*
  - Endoderm-lined cyst.
  - No enhancement.
  - Usually located in the sella. However, approximately 50% can extend to the suprasellar region.
  - Claw sign with the normal pituitary gland.
  - Content may be hyperintense on T1-weighted image (50%).
  - Slight female predominance.
- *Parasellar aneurysm:*
  - Giant aneurysms in the intracavernous portion of the carotid artery or arising from the anterior communicating artery may invade the sella.
  - Variable signal intensity from flowing blood or blood clots.
  - Communication with the parent vessel may be established with MR angiography.

■ Essential Facts

- Believed to be caused by the propensity of pituitary tumor cells to glucose deprivation along with the fragility of tumoral blood vessels.
- Sudden increase in sellar contents compresses surrounding structures and portal vessels, resulting in acute, severe headache, visual disturbances, and impairment in pituitary function.

- Clinical presentation includes:
  - Headache (80%).
  - Visual disturbances.
  - Visual field defects.
  - Ocular paresis.
  - Visual images acuity.
  - Meningeal irritation, if subarachnoid spread.

■ Other Imaging Findings

- CT can detect hemorrhage.
- MR is the imaging modality of choice.
- Gradient echo imaging can detect susceptibility effect of blood.
- T1 hyperintensity begins in the center of the mass.

✓ Pearls and ✗ Pitfalls

✓ The adenoma may be destroyed by the hemorrhage or it may regrow.
✓ Pituitary apoplexy can be precipitated by head trauma, hypotension, surgical procedures, dynamic pituitary testing, and insulin-induced hypoglycemia.
✓ Initial management of patients with pituitary tumor apoplexy includes supportive therapy (intravenous fluids and corticosteroids).
✓ Urgent surgical decompression in unstable patients.
✗ Hemorrhage into a Rathke cyst may be indistinguishable from pituitary tumor apoplexy, both clinically and by imaging.

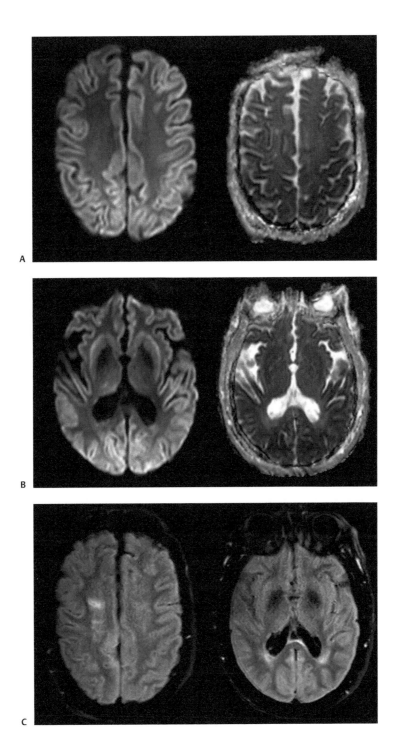

Case 32

■ Clinical Presentation

A 65-year-old man is found down.

■ Imaging Findings

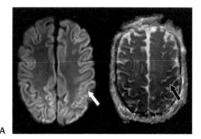 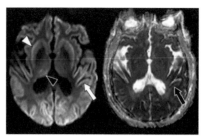 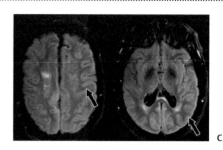

(A) Axial diffusion-weighted imaging (DWI) (*left*) and apparent diffusion coefficient (ADC) map (*right*) through the brain demonstrate diffusely increased DWI signal (*white arrow*) with corresponding low ADC values (*black arrow*) consistent with restricted diffusion involving the cortex of the frontal and parietal lobes. **(B)** Axial DWI (*left*) and ADC map (*right*) show generalized cortical restricted diffusion (*white* and *black arrows*), as well as involving the basal ganglia (*white arrowhead*) and right thalamus (*black arrowhead*). **(C)** Axial FLAIR images through the brain demonstrate increased gray–white matter differentiation due to cortical edema (*black arrows*).

■ Differential Diagnosis

- ***Hypoxic-ischemic injury (HII):*** Decreased blood flow and/or blood oxygenation resulting in infarcts involving vulnerable sites including watershed regions, as well as deep and superficial gray matter structures with associated restricted diffusion and diffuse edema with effacement of the subarachnoid spaces.
- *Creutzfeldt–Jakob disease:* Prion-mediated spongiform encephalopathy that affects the basal ganglia, thalami, cortex, and white matter with increased T2 signal and associated restricted diffusion. Signal abnormality of the dorsomedial thalamic nuclei results in the classic pulvinar sign or "hockey stick" sign. Clinical history typically reveals a progressive course rather than an acute event.
- *Hypoglycemic encephalopathy:* Brain injury resulting from prolonged or severe hypoglycemia with preferred involvement of the parieto-occipital and insular cortex, as well as the deep gray nuclei, internal capsule, and hippocampi.

■ Essential Facts

- Caused by a wide range of insults that ultimately lead to a decrease in blood flow and blood oxygen saturation.
- In adults, HII is most commonly due to cardiac arrest or cerebrovascular disease.
- Imaging findings depend on the age of the patient, the severity of the insult, the time between onset to image acquisition, and the modality obtained.
- In general, regions of brain with greater energy demands are the first to suffer injury from energy depletion. This first wave of insult results in death from tissue necrosis.
- Tissue with a lesser degree of energy deficit will show delayed injury secondary to programmed cell death (apoptosis) and will appear involved on imaging at a later time.
- Most commonly affected brain tissue includes watershed zones in mild to moderate insults and gray matter structures in more severe injury.

■ Other Imaging Findings

- CT:
  - Diffuse cerebral edema leads to decreased ventricular size and effacement of the subarachnoid spaces.
  - Loss of gray–white matter differentiation due to diffuse reduction in gray matter attenuation.
- MR:
  - Diffusion-weighted imaging (DWI) shows increased signal in the affected cortex and deep gray matter structures that typically lasts for approximately 7 days.
  - The perirolandic and occipital cortices are involved most frequently.
  - Initially, T1- and T2-weighted imaging may be normal. After cortical swelling ensues, edema may become evident on T2-weighted images as increased signal intensity.

✓ Pearls and ✗ Pitfalls

- ✓ Patients generally present after cardiac or cerebrovascular event, possibly requiring cardiopulmonary resuscitation.
- ✓ Initial CT imaging may be normal or show diffuse cerebral edema with decrease in size of cerebrospinal fluid–containing spaces.
- ✓ MRI exhibits restricted diffusion on DWI primarily involving the cortex and deep gray matter structures with eventual increase in T2 signal due to edema.
- ✓ Special predilection for the perirolandic and occipital cortices.
- ✗ Normal-appearing brain imaging in the hyperacute setting does not exclude HII.
- ✗ Follow-up exams may be warranted 24 to 72 hours after the insult to assess extent of damage.
- ✗ Symmetric, diffuse findings may make detection of abnormality more difficult to establish.

Case 33

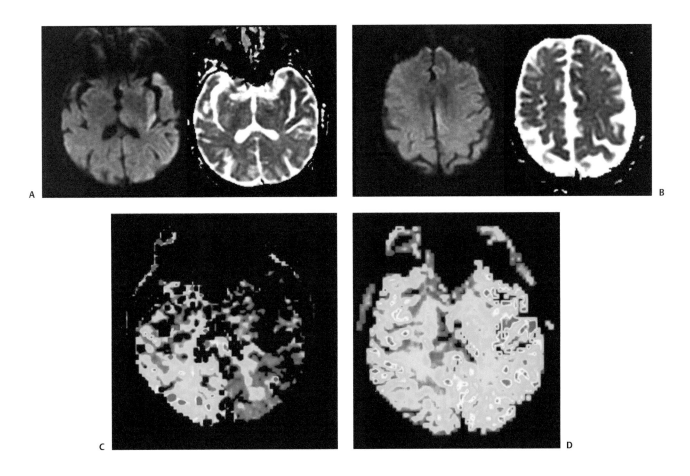

■ Clinical Presentation

A 68-year-old woman with a history of cirrhosis presents with aphasia, left facial droop, and left-sided weakness.

■ Imaging Findings

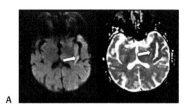 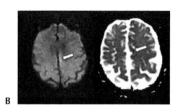 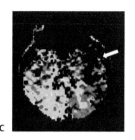 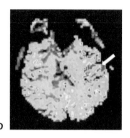

A   B   C   D

(A) Diffusion-weighted image (DWI) demonstrates restricted diffusion in the left insular cortex and inferior frontal gyrus, with corresponding signal dropout in the apparent diffusion coefficient (ADC) map (*arrows*). **(B)** DWI demonstrates restricted diffusion in the left cingulate gyrus, with corresponding signal dropout in the ADC map (*arrows*). **(C)** MR perfusion, mean transit time map, shows delayed cerebral blood flow in the left cerebral hemisphere (*arrow*). **(D)** MR perfusion, negative enhancement integral map, shows increased cerebral blood volume in the left cerebral hemisphere (*arrow*).

■ Differential Diagnosis

- ***Postictal diffusion-weighted image (DWI) and perfusion changes:***
  - MRI changes after generalized tonic-clonic seizure or status epilepticus include transient increase of signal intensity and swelling at the cortical gray matter, subcortical white matter, corpus callosum, basal ganglia, cerebellum, or hippocampus on postictal T2-weighted sequences and DWIs.
  - Contrast enhancement may be present.
  - These findings reflect transient cytotoxic and vasogenic edema induced by seizure.
  - The reversibility and typical location of lesions can help exclude the epileptogenic structural lesions.
- *Left middle cerebral artery infarct:*
  - Restricted diffusion and T2 signal increase in a typical vascular distribution in a patient with corresponding acute neurologic deficit.
  - Most changes are not reversible.
- *Limbic encephalitis:*
  - Limbic encephalitis is the most common clinical paraneoplastic syndrome.
  - T2-weighted image: Hyperintensity in mesial temporal lobes (hippocampus, amygdala), insula, cingulate gyrus, subfrontal cortex, inferior frontal white matter.
  - Diffusion restriction is uncommon.

■ Essential Facts

- Postictal paresis (Todd's paresis) describes a transient motor malfunction following partial seizures with or without secondary generalization.
  - Usually unilateral, affecting the extremities.
  - It usually subsides completely within 48 hours.
  - May also affect speech, gaze, or vision.
  - It may occur in up to 13% of seizure cases.

■ Other Imaging Findings

- In patients with postictal paralysis, MR perfusion may show reversible global hemispheric hypoperfusion.
- Hyperperfusion pattern (increased cerebral blood flow and cerebral blood volume, decreased mean transit time) has been observed in status epilepticus.
- Irreversible changes that evolve into atrophy and gliosis have also been reported.

✓ Pearls and ✗ Pitfalls

- ✓ Acute onset hemiparesis should always raise the suspicion of stroke, although it is not an infrequent symptom in postictal states.
- ✗ Acute seizures or status epilepticus may mimic other pathology, such as tumor progression or cerebritis. Clinical information and follow-up imaging help differentiate them from other etiologies.
- ✗ Seizure-related changes usually resolve within days to weeks.

Case 34

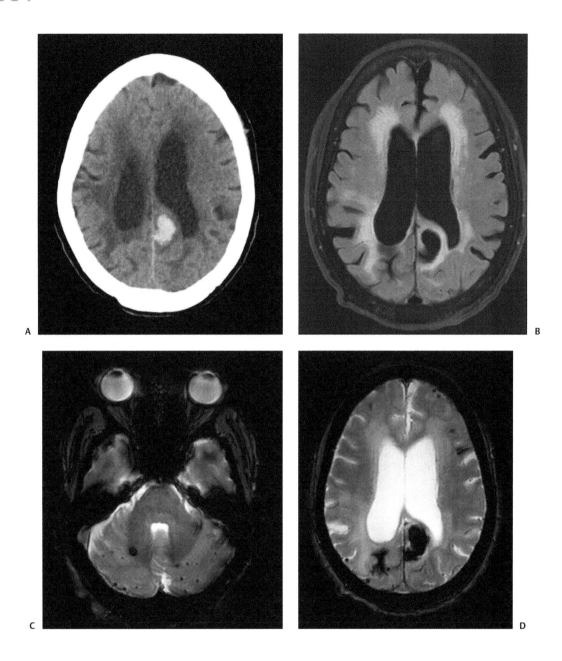

A

B

C

D

■ Clinical Presentation

A 76-year-old presents with leg weakness and mental status changes.

■ Imaging Findings

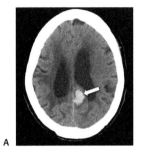 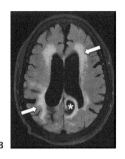 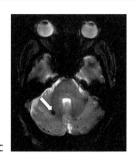 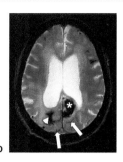

A   B   C   D

(A) Axial CT of the brain demonstrates an acute parenchymal hemorrhage in the left parietal lobe (*arrow*). **(B)** Axial FLAIR demonstrates confluent areas of high T2 signal in the periventricular white matter (*arrows*). The left parietal hematoma demonstrates low signal (*asterisk*). **(C)** Axial gradient echo (GRE) in the posterior fossa demonstrates multiple foci of magnetic susceptibility in both cerebellar hemispheres (*arrow*). **(D)** Axial GRE at the level of the lateral ventricles. In addition to the left parietal hemorrhage (*asterisk*), there are hemosiderin deposits in the right parietal deep white matter (*arrowhead*), bilateral cortical hemosiderin deposits, and superficial siderosis (*arrows*).

■ Differential Diagnosis

• **Cerebral amyloid angiopathy:**
  ○ Generally presents as multiple or solitary hemorrhages in a predominantly cortical and subcortical distribution that can be associated with focal or disseminated superficial siderosis.
  ○ Age ≥ 55 years.
  ○ Absence of other causes of hemorrhage.
• *Hypertensive hemorrhage:*
  ○ Hypertension is the most common cause of intracerebral hemorrhage (ICH). Located in order of frequency in the basal ganglia (especially the putamen), thalamus, pons, and cerebellum.
  ○ Patients may have hemosiderin deposits in the basal ganglia, thalamus, centrum semiovale, and cerebellum. These foci overlap with areas of small-vessel disease attributed to chronic hypertension.
• *Venous sinus thrombosis:* May result in hemorrhagic venous infarct. Hemorrhages are usually subcortical, adjacent to the occluded sinus. Risk factors include: dehydration, pregnancy, and use of oral contraceptives.

■ Essential Facts

• Cerebral amyloid angiopathy (CAA) is characterized by cerebrovascular amyloid deposition and is classified into several types according to the amyloid protein involved.
• Seven amyloid proteins have been reported in CAA. Among these, sporadic CAA of the Aβ type is most commonly found in older individuals and patients with Alzheimer disease.
• CAA-associated vasculopathies lead to development of hemorrhagic lesions (lobar intracerebral macrohemorrhage, cortical microhemorrhage, and cortical superficial siderosis/focal convexity subarachnoid hemorrhage), ischemic lesions (cortical infarction and ischemic changes of the white matter), and encephalopathies that include subacute leukoencephalopathy caused by CAA-associated inflammation/angiitis.

■ Other Imaging Findings

• MRI sequences detecting magnetic susceptibility, such as gradient echo T2* imaging and susceptibility-weighted imaging, are useful for detecting cortical microhemorrhages and cortical superficial siderosis.
• Amyloid imaging with amyloid-binding positron emission tomography ligands, such as Pittsburgh compound B, can detect CAA, although they cannot discriminate vascular from parenchymal amyloid deposits.

✓ Pearls and ✗ Pitfalls

✓ CAA-related inflammation is a disease subtype characterized by rapidly progressive cognitive decline, seizures, headaches, T2-weighted hyperintense MRI lesions, and neuropathologic evidence of CAA-associated vascular inflammation. Many patients with the disease respond to immunosuppressive therapy.

✗ Cerebral microbleeds are most commonly found in patients with severe hypertension and CAA. However, they can be present in patients with cerebral autosomal-dominant arteriopathy, subcortical infarcts, and leukoencephalopathy (CADASIL), moyamoya disease, fat embolism, cerebral malaria, and infective endocarditis.

Case 35

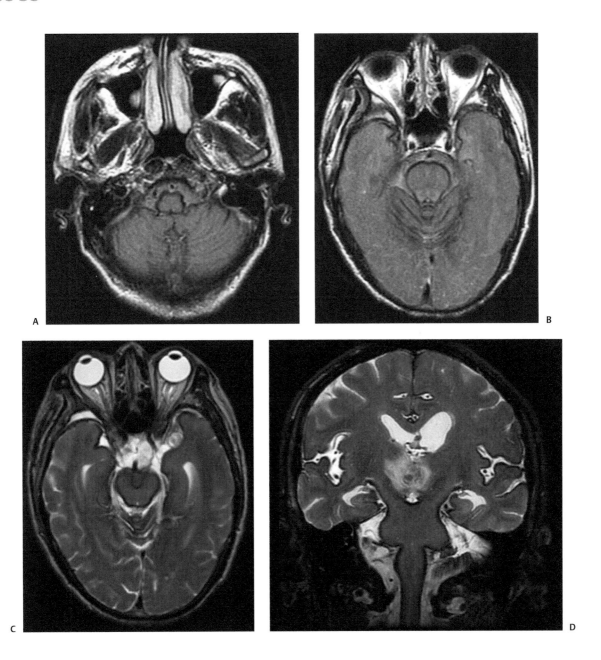

A 70-year-old woman presents with hearing loss.

■ Imaging Findings

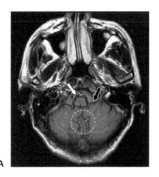 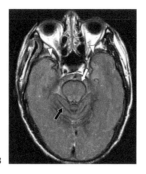 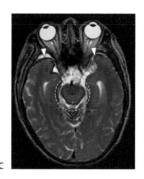 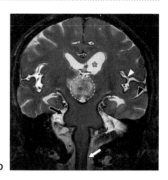

(A) Axial T2* image through the posterior fossa demonstrates markedly low signal representing susceptibility artifact surrounding the medulla (*white arrow*), along the anterior surface of the inferior cerebellar hemispheres (*black arrow*) and within the fourth ventricle (*circle*) in a linear fashion. **(B)** Axial T2* image at the level of the superior pons shows linear susceptibility artifact outlining the pons (*white arrow*), cerebellar folia (*black arrow*), and anterior temporal poles (*white arrowheads*). **(C)** Axial T2-weighted image of the brain demonstrates very low, linear signal intensity outlining the anterior temporal poles (*white arrowheads*) and midbrain (*circle*). **(D)** Coronal T2 image shows linear low signal along the surface of the insular cortices (*white arrowhead*), temporal lobes (*black arrowhead*), cerebral peduncles, brainstem (*black arrow*), and superior cervical cord (*white arrow*). Centered in the third ventricle is a heterogeneous mass with surrounding increased T2 signal (*circle*) resulting in mild dilatation of the lateral ventricles (*asterisk*).

■ Differential Diagnosis

- **Superficial siderosis (SS):** Deposition of hemosiderin along the leptomeninges due to a variety of sources of recurrent or silent subarachnoid hemorrhage, resulting in low signal on T2 and T2* images. In this particular case, the neoplasm in the third ventricle is the likely source of bleeding.
- *Neurocutaneous melanosis:* Rare neurocutaneous syndrome characterized by accumulation of melanin-containing cells along the leptomeninges, appearing as linear or nodular increased T1 signal and decreased T2 signal intensity seen primarily at the anterior temporal poles. The intrinsic T1 shortening and common associated enhancement differentiate this entity from SS.
- *Meningioangiomatosis:* Rare neurocutaneous syndrome presenting with proliferation of pial hamartomas that are generally moderately hypointense on T2. Unlike SS, meningioangiomatosis shows serpentine enhancement along the surface of the gyri and sulci, as well as gliosis and/or edema of the underlying parenchyma.

■ Essential Facts

- Hemosiderin deposits that accumulate in the subpial layers of the brain, with a special predilection for the brainstem, cerebellum, and cranial nerves. Supratentorial involvement is less common.
- Sensorineural hearing loss and ataxia are the most frequent presenting symptoms.
- Many patients have no recollection of prior events of subarachnoid hemorrhage.
- Iron deposition results in free radical damage leading to neuronal injury.

- Common causes include trauma, vascular malformations, neoplasms, and amyloid angiopathy. However, in many cases no clear etiology is identified.
- Hemosiderin exhibits low signal intensity on T1- and T2-weighted sequences.
- Gradient echo and susceptibility-weighted images show low signal and associated blooming outlining the involved structures.

■ Other Imaging Findings

- Imaging the entire neuroaxis is recommended to determine the source of bleeding.
- Susceptibility-weighted imaging shows greater sensitivity to signal drop from hemosiderin.
- Occasionally, volume loss and gliosis can be seen at the sites of deposition.

✓ Pearls and ✗ Pitfalls

- ✓ Linear low signal intensity on T2 and T2* images.
- ✓ Predilection for the posterior fossa.
- ✓ In up to 50% of cases, no clear source of hemorrhage is detected.
- ✓ Correction of the causative condition can aid in preventing deafness and progressive ataxia.
- ✗ Lack of enhancement in SS can help to differentiate this entity from neurocutaneous syndromes such as meningioangiomatosis and neurocutaneous melanosis.

Case 36

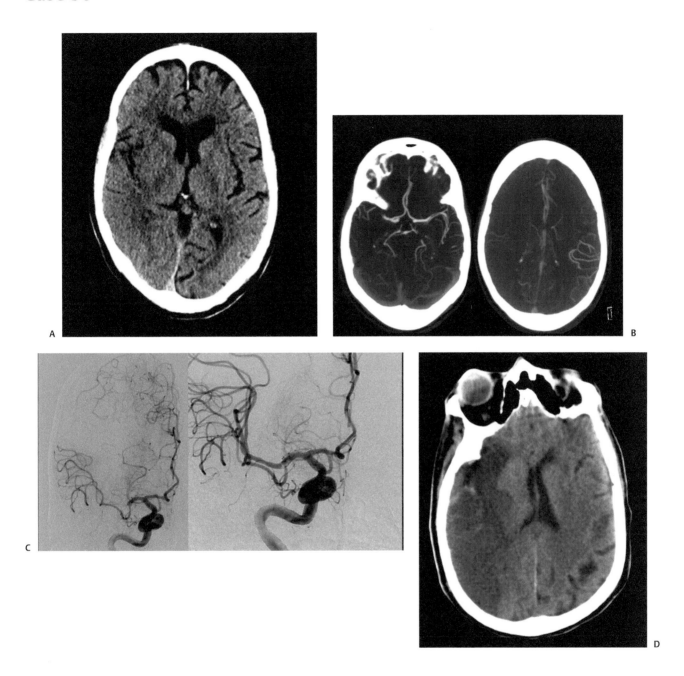

■ Clinical Presentation

A 76-year-old presents with left-sided weakness.

■ Imaging Findings

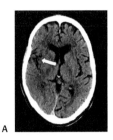 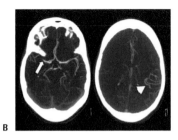 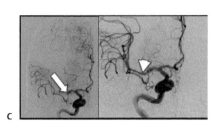 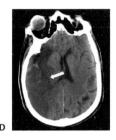

(A) Axial CT demonstrates low attenuation in the right insula, with absent gray–white matter distinction (*arrow*), consistent with early ischemia. **(B)** Axial CT angiography maximum intensity projection reconstructions show occlusion of the M1 segment of the right middle cerebral artery (MCA) (*arrow*) after the takeoff of the temporal branch. There is poor opacification of distal MCA branches as compared to the left MCA (*arrowhead*). **(C)** Right internal carotid artery digital subtraction angiography anteroposterior views before and after intra-arterial recanalization. There is occlusion of the right M1 segment (*arrow*) with poor distal collateral vessels. Postintervention view shows recanalization of the MCA (*arrowhead*). **(D)** Axial CT 2 days later shows an extensive infarct in the right MCA territory (*arrow*) in spite of the previously achieved MCA recanalization.

■ Differential Diagnosis

- *Middle cerebral artery (MCA) occlusion with poor leptomeningeal collaterals:*
  - Cerebral collaterals can partially maintain blood flow to ischemic tissue when primary conduits are blocked.
  - Patients with good and intermediate collaterals who achieve recanalization with intra-arterial therapy do well when compared with those who do not achieve recanalization.
  - Patients with poor collaterals do not do well even if recanalization is achieved with intra-arterial therapy.
- *Reversible cerebral vasoconstriction syndrome:*
  - Characterized by thunderclap headache and reversible vasoconstriction of cerebral arteries, which can either be spontaneous or related to an exogenous trigger.
  - Alterations in cerebral vascular tone.
  - Patients may develop ischemic stroke or intracranial hemorrhage.
  - Digital subtraction angiography shows cerebral vasoconstriction and may demonstrate reversibility of vasoconstriction following intra-arterial vasodilator therapy.
  - MRI vessel wall imaging may demonstrate arterial wall thickening without wall enhancement.
- *Chronic atherosclerotic occlusion of the MCA:*
  - Chronic intracranial occlusions usually demonstrate areas of encephalomalacia from prior infarction. The distal end of the vessel tapers before it occludes.

■ Essential Facts

- After occlusion of a cerebral artery, anastomoses connecting the distal segments of the MCA with distal branches of the anterior and posterior cerebral arteries (known as leptomeningeal or pial collaterals) allow

for partially maintained blood flow in the ischemic penumbra and delay or prevent cell death.
- Collateral status at baseline is an independent determinant of clinical outcome among patients with acute ischemic stroke.

■ Other Imaging Findings

- While invasive, conventional angiography is the reference standard for evaluation of collateral circulation.
- Single-phase CT angiography (CTA) and multiphasic CTA are commonly used modalities for evaluation of collateral circulation.
- Fluid-attenuated inversion recovery images may show distal hyperintense vessels corresponding to leptomeningeal collaterals.
- Vessel-encoded arterial spin labeling can be used for collateral evaluation but may be affected by contamination from the partial labeling of the nearby vessels or antegrade flow.

✓ Pearls and ✕ Pitfalls

✓ Revascularization encompasses all treatment-related improvements in blood flow, including recanalization of the proximal arterial occlusion and reperfusion of the downstream territory. Recanalization is required for antegrade tissue reperfusion, but recanalization may not necessarily lead to reperfusion in regions where distal emboli or established infarctions are present.

✕ Routine CTA is a single snapshot of contrast-filled blood vessels. Early timing of image acquisition with respect to that of bolus injection could potentially result in underestimation of true collateral status.

Case 37

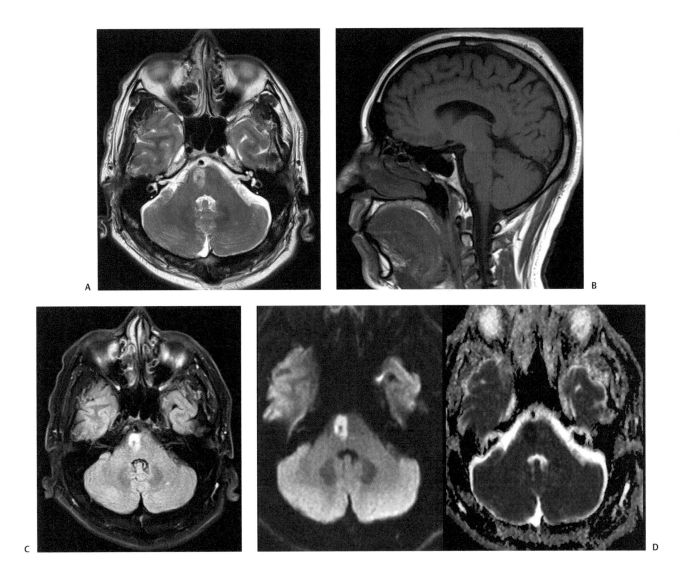

■ Clinical Presentation

A 52-year-old presents with two days of focal sixth right cranial nerve palsy and a "clumsy hand."

■ Imaging Findings

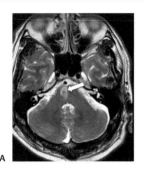 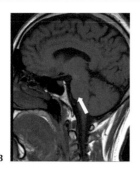 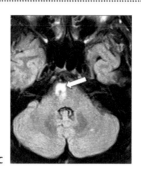 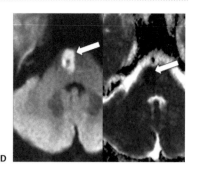

(A) T2-weighted image (WI) shows an area of increased signal on the right pons (*arrow*) with no significant mass effect. (B) Sagittal T1WI shows an ill-defined area of hypointensity in the inferior aspect of the left pons (*arrow*). (C) Axial fluid-attenuated inversion recovery WI shows an area of increased signal in the right pons (*arrow*). (D) Diffusion-weighted image (*left*) and apparent diffusion coefficient map (*right*) show restricted diffusion in the right pontine lesion (*arrows*).

■ Differential Diagnosis

- ***Pontine basilar perforator stroke:***
  - ○ Stroke in the territory of the basilar artery perforators.
  - ○ Unilateral lesions typically located in the inferior aspect of the pons or in the pontomedullary junction.
  - ○ Rarely bilateral.
- *Acute demyelinating plaque:*
  - ○ Multiple sclerosis is an autoimmune inflammatory neurologic disease characterized by demyelination and axonal injury.
  - ○ Demyelinating lesions can mimic stroke both clinically and in the imaging studies.
  - ○ Acute demyelinating lesions more frequently show T2 shine-through rather than true restricted diffusion.
- *Chronic lymphocytic inflammation with pontine perivascular enhancement responsive to steroids (CLIPPERS):*
  - ○ Affects the brainstem, mostly the pons.
  - ○ Punctate bilateral enhancement.
  - ○ Faint increase in T2 signal.
  - ○ No mass effect.
  - ○ No restricted diffusion.

■ Essential Facts

- Strokes involving the vertebrobasilar system are focal and asymmetric when smaller branches and perforators are involved. If a major branch occlusion occurs, infarcts tend to be bilateral and involve the cerebellum, brainstem, thalami, and occipital lobes.
- The basilar perforating arteries are median and paramedian branches that provide the majority of the circulation to the pons.

■ Other Imaging Findings

- CT is limited in the evaluation of the pons, due to beam hardening artifact.
- Early strokes have normal CT findings in the first 12 hours.
- MRI is the imaging modality of choice for evaluating basilar perforator strokes.
- Angiograms can be normal.

✓ Pearls and ✗ Pitfalls

- ✓ Always perform an MRI scan if suspecting a posterior fossa syndrome. Misinterpretation of lesions using CT is frequent due to artifacts.
- ✗ Acute small vessel infarcts in the brainstem and cerebellum may be less conspicuous in the MRI scan obtained in the first 24 hours compared to infarcts in the anterior circulation.
- ✗ Obtaining a second diffusion-weighted imaging sequence with larger B value and using diffusion tensor imaging sequences increases the sensitivity for the detection of these lesions. Alternatively, a follow-up MRI scan tends to show these small infarcts in the subacute stage.

Case 38

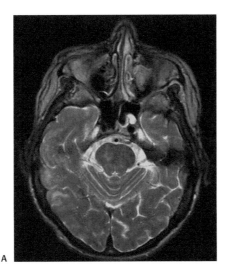

A

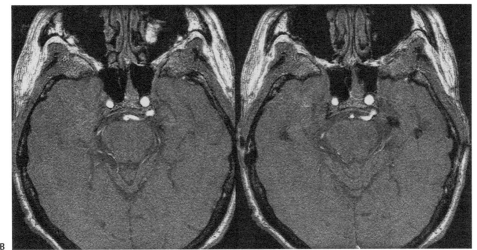

B

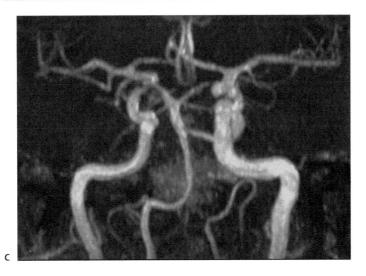

C

■ Clinical Presentation

History withheld.

■ Imaging Findings

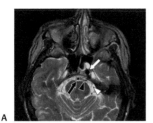 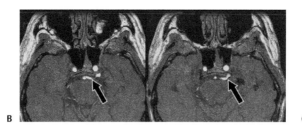 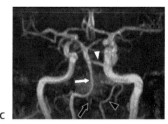

(A) Axial T2-weighted image shows a variant vessel (*black arrowhead*) that communicates the cavernous segment of the left internal carotid artery (ICA) (*white arrow*) with the midbasilar artery (*black arrow*) at the level of the pons, medial to the left trigeminal nerve (*white arrowhead*). (B) Time-of-flight MR angiography of the brain again demonstrates the small carotid-basilar anastomotic vessel (*black arrows*) between the proximal left cavernous ICA and the basilar system. (C) Three-dimensional reconstruction shows the variant carotid-basilar anastomosis (*white arrowhead*). The basilar artery proximal to the anastomosis is of normal caliber (*white arrow*). In addition, the left vertebral artery terminates predominantly in the left posterior inferior cerebellar artery (*black arrowhead*) with a hypoplastic distal V4 segment (*black arrow*).

■ Differential Diagnosis

- **Persistent trigeminal artery (PTA):** A variant carotid-vertebrobasilar anastomosis where a variant vessel communicates the internal carotid artery (ICA) with the midbasilar artery.
- *Persistent hypoglossal artery:* The second most common carotid-vertebrobasilar anastomosis. The variant artery arises from the ICA, generally at the level of C1–C3, and communicates to the basilar artery after coursing through the hypoglossal canal.
- *Fetal origin of the posterior cerebral artery (PCA):* Although not classified as a variant carotid-vertebrobasilar anastomosis but rather a variant of the posterior communicating artery, the fetal origin of the PCA can easily simulate a PTA. In fetal origin of the PCA, a prominent posterior communicating artery is the main blood supply for the occipital lobes. The P1 segment is classically hypoplastic or can be absent (uncommon), and the communication is between the anterior circulation and the PCA rather than the basilar artery as we see in this case.

■ Essential Facts

- The most common of the carotid-vertebrobasilar anastomoses.
- Occurs due to failure of regression of communications between the anterior and posterior circulation during embryonic life. These anastomoses are named according to their neighboring structures.
- The PTA, named because it courses parallel to the trigeminal nerves, can be subclassified as either medial or lateral. The medial variant courses medially to the trigeminal nerve and the lateral variant courses posteriorly and lateral to the nerve.

- The medial PTA can course through the sella and can even compress the pituitary gland.
- Typically, the basilar artery proximal to the anastomosis is hypoplastic, although its caliber can be normal as is the case in this example.

■ Other Imaging Findings

- A PTA has shown association with other vascular malformations such as aneurysms.
- The detection and description of a medial PTA is important when planning for transsphenoidal surgery because it can present an operative hazard.
- The PTA can either supply the entire vertebrobasilar circulation distal to its anastomosis (Saltzman type 1) or it can coexist with a fetal origin of the PCA with a hypoplastic ipsilateral P1 segment (Saltzman type 2).

✓ Pearls and ✗ Pitfalls

✓ Variant artery that communicates the ICA, typically the clinoid segment, with the midbasilar artery.

✓ The anastomosis is at the level of the trigeminal nerves, giving the variant artery its name.

✓ The PTA can course either medial or lateral to the nerve.

✓ The basilar artery proximal to the anastomosis can be hypoplastic.

✗ Anastomoses between the carotid and vertebrobasilar system can occur throughout the cervical segment.

✗ It is important to look out for other vascular malformations because they can be associated with PTA.

✗ When the course of the PTA is transsellar, this can pose a risk for transsphenoidal surgery and should be accurately identified and described in the report.

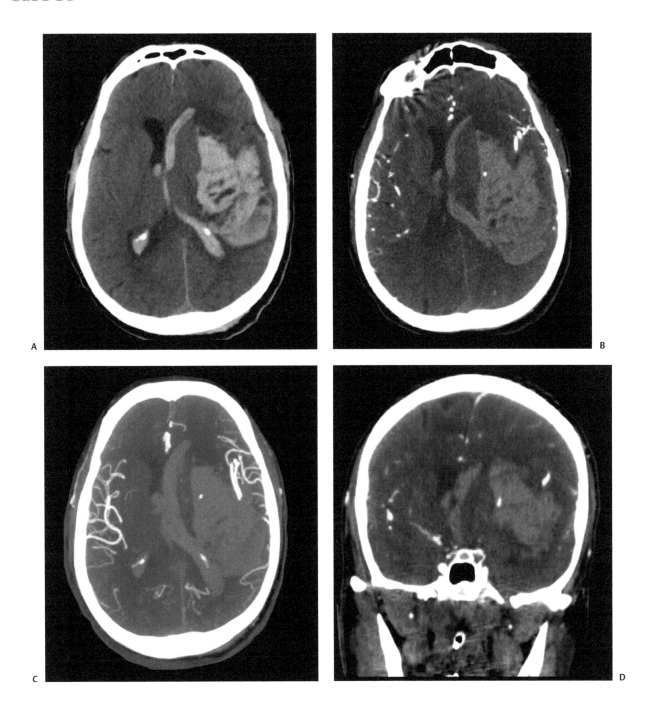

Case 39

■ Clinical Presentation

A 50-year-old man is found down.

■ Imaging Findings

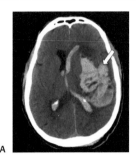
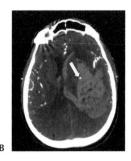
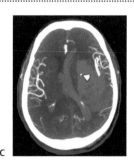
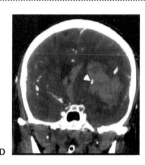

(A) Axial CT demonstrates a large parenchymal hematoma in the left cerebral hemisphere (*arrow*). Intraventricular hemorrhage is also noted. **(B)** Axial CT angiography (CTA) source image shows an oval-shaped area of enhancement within the hematoma, with attenuation similar to the contrast in the vessels (*arrow*). **(C)** Axial CTA maximum intensity projection (MIP) image shows an enhancing structure with attenuation similar to the vascular structures, but not connected to any vessel (*arrowhead*). **(D)** Coronal CTA MIP image shows an enhancing structure with attenuation similar to the vascular structures but not connected to any vessel (*arrowhead*).

■ Differential Diagnosis

- ***Intracerebral hemorrhage (ICH) with spot sign:***
  - ○ Spot sign is defined as:
    - ▪ A focus of contrast pooling within the intraparenchymal hemorrhage.
    - ▪ Attenuation ≥ 120 Hounsfield units.
    - ▪ Discontinuous from normal or abnormal vasculature adjacent to the hemorrhage.
    - ▪ Any size and morphology.
- *Arteriovenous malformation (AVM):*
  - ○ AVMs are congenital vascular malformations characterized by a nidus forming the transition between the feeding artery and draining vein.
  - ○ If ruptured they present with parenchymal hemorrhage, which may extend to the subarachnoid space, ventricles, or subdural space.
  - ○ CT angiography (CTA) demonstrates vascular enhancement in feeding arteries, nidus, and draining veins.
- *Hemorrhagic tumor:*
  - ○ Various types of brain tumors may cause hemorrhage.
  - ○ Increased tumor vascularization with dilated, thin-walled vessels and tumor necrosis are the most important mechanisms of hemorrhage.
  - ○ CTA does not typically show vascular enhancement within the tumor.

■ Essential Facts

- Nontraumatic ICH accounts for 10 to 15% of cases of acute stroke in the United States and has a worse prognosis than ischemic stroke.

- The spot sign, defined as the presence of active contrast extravasation into the hematoma at the time of multidetector CTA, is an indicator of active hemorrhage and has been associated with an increased risk of hematoma expansion and mortality in patients with ICH.
- Hematoma size has been shown to be one of the most important predictors of 30-day mortality. Hematoma expansion is highly predictive of neurologic deterioration.

■ Other Imaging Findings

- Additional features in the evaluation of ICH include:
  - ○ ICH location (lobar, deep gray matter, or infratentorial).
  - ○ Presence of associated intraventricular hemorrhage.
  - ○ Presence of calcifications within or adjacent to the ICH.

✓ Pearls and ✗ Pitfalls

- ✓ Important etiologic factors in the elderly population in whom ICH is more common are hypertension, amyloid angiopathy, and anticoagulation.
- ✗ The frequency of spot signs in the delayed CTA acquisitions is significantly higher than in the first-pass CTA. Acquiring delayed images through the ICH approximately 2 to 3 minutes after contrast injection, either routinely or if a spot sign is not identified in the first-pass CTA, is likely to increase the sensitivity of the exam.

Case 40

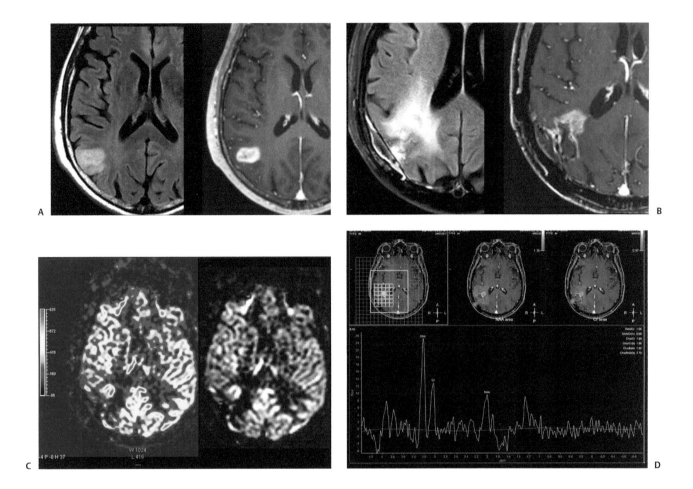

■ Clinical Presentation

A 67-year-old man presents with a diagnosis of glioblastoma. He is treated with surgery, temozolomide (TMZ), and radiation (XRT).

■ Imaging Findings

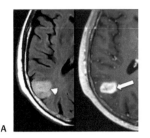
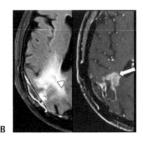
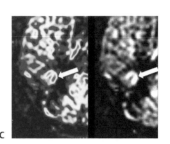
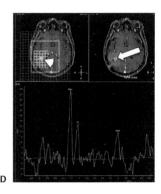

A   B   C   D

(A) Axial T2 fluid-attenuated inversion recovery (FLAIR) and T1 with contrast show a T2 hyperintense lesion in the cortical/subcortical region of the right parietal lobe (*arrowhead*) that thickens the gyrus. The T2 signal extends to the pial surface, unlike with vasogenic edema. The lesion shows diffuse enhancement after administration of contrast with the presence of a center of lower enhancement (*arrow*). **(B)** Nine months after resection and treatment with chemoradiotherapy, increased T2 FLAIR signal is noted around the surgical cavity with a nodular area of lower signal (*arrowhead*). The T1 postcontrast sequence shows a new area of nodular enhancement at the medial and anterior aspect of the resection cavity (*arrow*). **(C)** Color and grayscale arterial spin-labeled perfusion maps show that the nodular area of enhancement has increased perfusion (*arrows*). **(D)** Multivoxel MR spectroscopy (MRS) interrogates the area of nodular enhancement (*arrowhead*). The N-acetylaspartate (NAA) color map shows depletion of NAA compared to the adjacent brain (*arrow*) and the MRS demonstrates an increased choline peak, inversion of the choline:creatine ratio (approximately 2:1), and a decreased NAA peak.

■ Differential Diagnosis

- **Glioblastoma tumor recurrence:**
  - New area of growth of tumor at the surgical site.
  - Increase of 25% or more in the enhancing component (response assessment in neuro-oncology criteria [RANO]) after 12 weeks following completion of chemoradiation.
  - Tumors can recur as nonenhancing T2/fluid-attenuated inversion recovery (FLAIR) hyperintensities.
  - Mass effect is noted in the surrounding structures.
  - Tumor shows higher apparent diffusion coefficient values than treated radiation changes.
  - May have subependymal spread of disease.
- *Tumor pseudoprogression:*
  - A process of new areas of enhancement that are not tumor progression.
  - Occurs in the first 6 months of treatment.
  - More frequent in O-6-methylguanine-DNA methyltransferase (MGMT) hypermethylation (deactivated tumors).
  - More commonly seen in patients treated with a combination of chemotherapy and radiation rather than with radiation alone.
  - May represent a less severe or self-limiting form of radiation necrosis.
- *Delayed radiation necrosis:*
  - New focus of enhancement.
  - Typically seen between 9 and 12 months after chemoradiotherapy.
  - Hypoperfused on relative cerebral blood volume maps with low choline and N-acetylaspartate (NAA) peaks on MR spectroscopy (MRS).

■ Essential Facts

- Differentiating tumor progression from pseudoprogression or radiation necrosis is not always possible through imaging, but the utilization of advanced imaging techniques can provide useful information.

■ Other Imaging Findings

- MRS:
  - In tumors with high cell proliferation there is a shift in the concentrations of choline versus NAA (decrease of NAA with increase in choline—inversion of the normal Hunter's angle).
  - In a rapid-growing tumor with necrosis, a free lipid peak may be identified.
  - Lactic acid is a marker of ischemia.

✓ Pearls and ✗ Pitfalls

- ✓ T2/FLAIR hyperintensities typically represent a mixture of vasogenic edema and tumoral infiltration; conventional imaging is limited in making this differentiation.
- ✗ Perfusion (cerebral blood volume [CBV]) is less effective in differentiating tumor progression from pseudoprogression in MGMT hypermethylated tumors.
- ✗ Treatment with bevacizumab can normalize or decrease the CBV in patients with tumoral recurrence.

Case 41

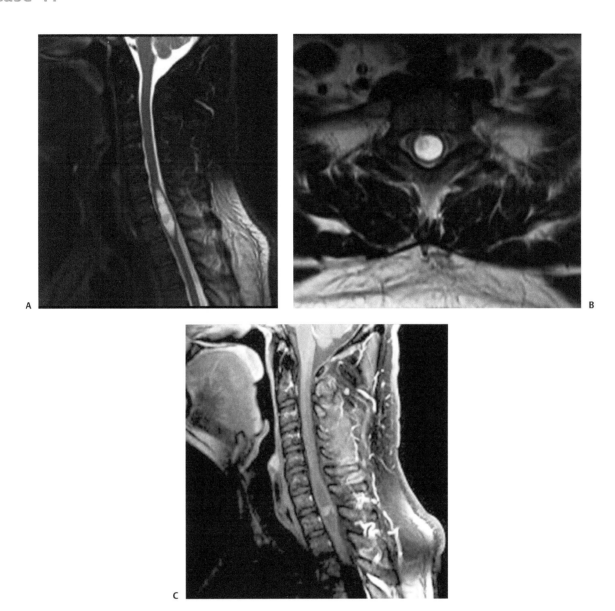

A 40-year-old man presents with bilateral upper extremity weakness.

■ Imaging Findings

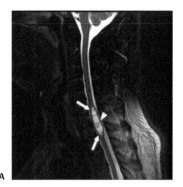 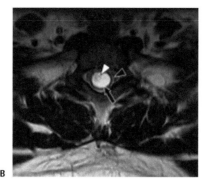 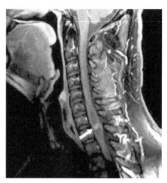

(A) Sagittal T2 image of the cervical and upper thoracic spine demonstrates an isointense mass within the central ependymal canal at T1 (*arrowhead*) with associated syrinx extending from C6 to T1 (*arrows*). **(B)** Axial T2 image demonstrates dilatation of the central ependymal canal (*black arrow*) with a small isointense nodule (*white arrowhead*) located eccentrically within the canal. There is effacement of the subarachnoid space surrounding the cord (*black arrowhead*). **(C)** Sagittal T1 postcontrast image shows the intramedullary mass with relatively homogeneous enhancement (*arrow*).

■ Differential Diagnosis

- **Ependymoma:** Ependymomas represent the most common intramedullary tumor in adults. On imaging, these masses are well circumscribed, are located centrally within the cord, generally enhance, and can commonly be associated with syringohydromyelia and hemorrhage.
- *Astrocytoma:* Astrocytomas are the second most common intramedullary tumor in adults and are the most common cord mass in children. Unlike ependymomas, astrocytomas are peripherally located within the cord, rarely hemorrhage, are infiltrating masses, and are generally ill-defined.
- *Cavernous malformation:* Cavernous malformations of the spine can repeatedly bleed and therefore show associated blood products. However, unlike ependymomas, cavernous malformations show a complete hemosiderin ring instead of the characteristic "hemosiderin cap" seen in ependymomas. Furthermore, whereas ependymomas generally enhance, cavernous malformations do not.

■ Essential Facts

- Ependymomas represent approximately 60% of intramedullary tumors in adults.
- These tumors generally present in early adults and have been reported to show a slight male predominance.
- The most common location is the cervical cord, with or without extension into the thoracic region. The second most common location is the thoracic spine and, lastly, the conus medullaris or distal cord.
- On CT, ependymomas tend to be isodense to slightly hyperdense and generally show intense contrast enhancement.
- On MRI, these tumors show intermediate to low signal intensity on T1 and intermediate to high signal intensity on T2-weighted images.
- Although not truly encapsulated, ependymomas are typically well-defined.

- Approximately one third of patients show a "hemosiderin cap sign" due to accumulation of remote blood products at the poles of the tumors secondary to the tumor's high vascularity.
- The majority of these tumors originate at the central portion of the cord.

■ Other Imaging Findings

- Cyst formation and associated syringohydromyelia are additional features of variable prevalence.
- A variant of ependymoma, termed myxopapillary ependymoma, generally originates from ependymal remnants near the filum terminale.
- Plain radiography can show scoliosis or canal widening as secondary features that may alert to this diagnosis.
- Myelography can reveal obstruction to flow due to expansion of the cord and effacement of the subarachnoid space.

✓ Pearls and ✗ Pitfalls

✓ Well-defined, oval-shaped, enhancing intramedullary mass.
✓ Most commonly seen in the cervical cord.
✓ Highly vascular leading to hemorrhage and the development of a "hemosiderin cap" presenting as very low signal intensity at the poles of the tumor on T2-weighted imaging.
✗ Not all hemorrhagic intramedullary masses are ependymomas. Cavernous malformations can also exhibit hemosiderin, yet in cavernous malformations the hemosiderin generally forms a complete ring.
✗ Astrocytomas are the more common intramedullary tumor in children. Unlike ependymomas, astrocytomas are ill-defined and do not tend to bleed.

Case 42

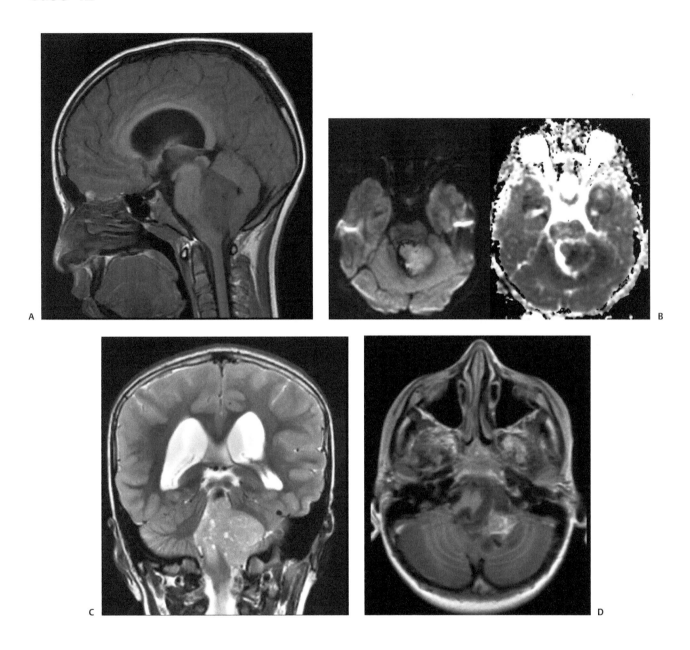

An 11-year-old boy presents with vomiting and headache.

■ Imaging Findings

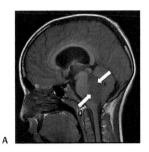 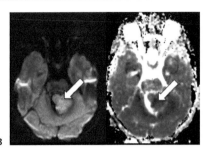 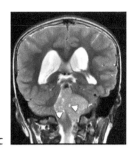 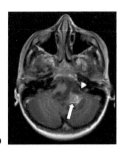

(A) Sagittal T1-weighted image (WI) demonstrates a heterogeneous low signal mass (*arrows*) expanding the fourth ventricle and causing hydrocephalus. **(B)** Axial diffusion-weighted imaging with corresponding apparent diffusion coefficient map show areas of restricted diffusion in the superior aspect of the mass (*arrows*). **(C)** Coronal T2WI shows multiple small cystic components within the mass (*arrowheads*), which extends toward the left cerebellopontine angle. **(D)** Axial postcontrast T1WI shows heterogeneous enhancement of the mass (*arrow*) as well as extension to the left cerebellopontine angle (*arrowhead*).

■ Differential Diagnosis

- ***Medulloblastoma (MB):***
  - MB, the most frequent malignant brain tumor of childhood, is an invasive embryonal tumor of the cerebellum with an inherent tendency to metastasize via the subarachnoidal space.
  - It accounts for approximately 20 to 25% of all pediatric brain tumors and 40% of all posterior fossa tumors.
  - Because of the fast growth, clinical symptoms mostly develop rapidly and are typically related to intracranial hypertension and cerebellar ataxia.
- *Ependymoma:*
  - Fourth most common posterior fossa tumors in children.
  - Peak incidence in young children (3–5 years), with slight predominance in males.
  - Imaging typically shows a mass filling the fourth ventricle. The tumor tends to be iso- to hypointense on T1 and hyperintense on T2, with heterogeneous enhancement and variable calcifications and hemorrhage.
- *Pilocytic astrocytoma:*
  - Cerebellar astrocytomas are the most frequent posterior fossa tumors in children (30–35% of cases).
  - Peak incidence between the ages of 5 and 13 years, equally frequent in boys and girls.
  - Cerebellar astrocytomas are mostly benign, low-grade, and slow-growing.
  - Pilocytic astrocytomas arise from the vermis cerebelli or the cerebellar hemispheres.
  - MRI: Approximately 50% of the tumors are cystic with a mural nodule; 40 to 45% of the tumors are composed of a rim of solid tumor with a cystic-necrotic center; and 10% are solid, non-necrotic tumors.
  - The solid components tend to enhance.

■ Essential Facts

- There are four histologic variants of MB: desmoplastic/nodular, with extensive nodularity, large-cell, and anaplastic.
- Four genetically defined groups of MB:
  - Wnt-activated
  - SHH-activated and TP53-mutant
  - SHH-activated and TP53-wildtype
  - Non-Wnt/Non-SHH-activated:
    - Group 3
    - Group 4
- Associated with specific clinical course and prognosis.
- If no markers are available, it is defined as a MB NOS (medulloblastoma not otherwise specified).

■ Other Imaging Findings

- CT: Hyperdense or isodense.
- Calcifications in up to 20% of cases; cysts/necrosis in approximately 50%.
- Intratumoral hemorrhage is rare.
- The tumor on MRI is round, slightly lobulated, and T1-iso-/hypointense; On T2, the mass is often hypo- to isointense compared with the gray matter.
- Variable contrast enhancement.

✓ Pearls and ✗ Pitfalls

- ✓ MBs arise from the roof of the fourth ventricle, in contrast to ependymomas, which arise from the floor of the fourth ventricle.
- ✓ Extension through the foramina of Magendie and Luschka is typical for ependymomas but has also been reported in MBs.
- ✗ Direct foraminal extension in ependymomas must be differentiated from the normal enhancement of the choroid plexus in the foramen of Luschka and from cerebrospinal fluid seeding of a primary MB.

Case 43

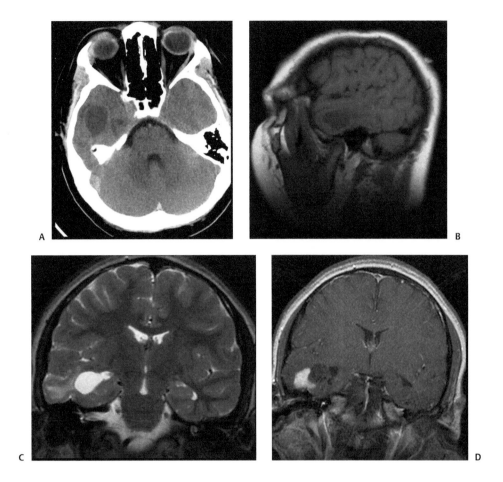

A 13-year-old boy presents with seizures.

■ Imaging Findings

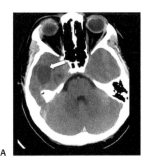 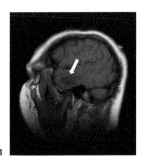 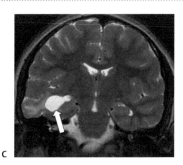 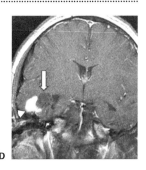

(A) Axial CT scan of the head without contrast shows a cystic lesion in the right temporal lobe (*arrow*). **(B)** Sagittal T1-weighted image (WI) shows a cystic mass in the temporal lobe (*arrow*). **(C)** Coronal T2WI shows the cystic mass in the right temporal lobe (*arrow*). **(D)** Coronal T1WI with contrast shows the cystic lesion in the right temporal lobe (*arrow*) with a lateral nodular component that enhances (*arrowhead*).

■ Differential Diagnosis

- *Ganglioglioma:*
  - Mixed cortically based neuronal and glial tumor.
  - Cystic mass (50%).
  - Most commonly located in the temporal lobe (70%), followed by the parietal lobe.
  - Solid enhancing mural nodule (40–50%).
  - Most commonly occur in children and young adults.
  - Calcification in 40%.
  - If located in the periphery, can indent the inner skull.
- *Dysembryoplastic neuroepithelial tumor (DNET or DNT):*
  - The cystic component of DNET has a multicystic, "bubbly" appearance.
  - It presents in the same age population.
  - A rim of high signal is seen in the fluid-attenuated inversion recovery (FLAIR) image, rarely present in ganglioglioma.
  - DNET are frequent in the temporal and frontal lobes, rarely in the parietal lobe.
  - Calcifies in < 20%.
  - Does not show vasogenic edema.
- *Pleomorphic xanthoastrocytoma:*
  - Superficial astrocytic tumor.
  - 1% of astrocytomas.
  - Peripheral location.
  - Mural nodule in contact with meninges.
  - Most frequently seen in the temporal lobe.
  - Enhancement is a characteristic.
  - Dural enhancement "dural tail" (70%).
  - Rarely calcifies.

■ Essential Facts

- Multiple locations have been described in the neural axis for ganglioma; most are supratentorial.

■ Other Imaging Findings

- CT:
  - Can detect calcification (rare).
  - Evaluate for inner table scalloping.
  - Can be undetected in CT.
- MRI:
  - Nonspecific findings.
  - Cystic component follows cerebrospinal fluid.
  - Does not show a rim on FLAIR (DNET does).
- Spectroscopy: Increased choline:creatine ratio; does not correlate with histology.

✓ Pearls and ✗ Pitfalls

- ✓ Gangliogliomas tend to be larger and more cystic in children.
- ✗ Dysembryoplastic infantile gangliogliomas are a variant of ganglioglioma seen in predominantly male patients younger than 18 months of age. They also present as a cystic mass with a mural nodule. The prognosis is very good.

Case 44

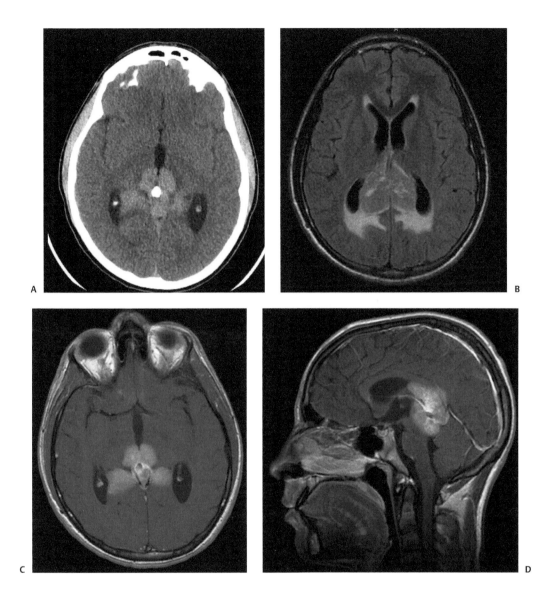

A

B

C

D

■ Clinical Presentation

A 16-year-old boy presents with double vision.

■ Imaging Findings

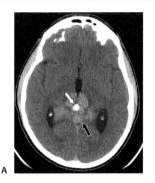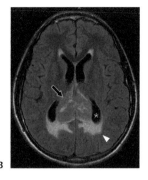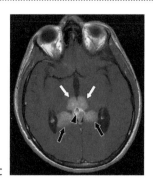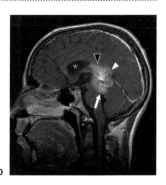

(A) Axial CT image demonstrates a relatively well-defined, hyperdense mass (*black arrow*) with a coarse central calcification (*white arrow*) centered in the pineal region. **(B)** Axial T2 fluid-attenuated inversion recovery image shows a heterogeneous, slightly hypointense mass (*black arrow*) above the pineal gland causing dilatation of the ventricles (*asterisk*) with transependymal flow of cerebrospinal fluid (*white arrowhead*). **(C)** Axial T1 postcontrast image shows a multilobulated enhancing mass centered in the pineal gland with extension into the bilateral thalami (*white arrows*) and parahippocampal gyri (*black arrows*). A central hypointensity corresponds to the coarse calcification better appreciated on CT (*black arrowhead*). **(D)** Sagittal T1 postcontrast image demonstrates an enhancing multilobulated mass involving the pineal gland and invading the tectal plate causing compression on the cerebral aqueduct (*white arrow*) and obstruction hydrocephalus (*asterisk*). The mass extends superiorly to the lateral ventricles (*black arrowhead*) and compresses the splenium of the corpus callosum posteriorly (*white arrowhead*).

■ Differential Diagnosis

- **Pineal germinoma:** Malignant tumors that occur more frequently in males in the second and third decades of life. These tumors present as hyperdense masses that engulf a centrally located, calcified pineal gland. On MRI scans, germinomas have variable T1 and T2 signal with enhancement. On CT images, they show a central dense calcification.
- *Pineoblastoma:* Pineoblastomas are World Health Organization (WHO) grade IV pineal parenchymal tumors that generally occur in the first two decades of life. The majority of masses measure > 3 cm at the time of presentation and are generally associated with obstructive hydrocephalus. These masses are hyperdense due to high cellularity and demonstrate heterogeneous enhancement. Unlike pineal germ cell tumors that engulf the pineal calcification, pineoblastomas disperse fragmented calcification to the periphery of the mass.
- *Pineocytoma:* The pineocytoma is a WHO grade I primary pineal parenchymal tumor seen in young adults. These tumors are characterized by a well-defined mass generally measuring < 3 cm in size and occasionally presenting with internal cystic components. Like the pineoblastoma, pineocytomas also show peripheral dispersal of pineal calcifications toward the periphery.

■ Essential Facts

- Germ cell tumors comprise > 50% of pineal region tumors.
- Can be subdivided into germinomas and nongerminomatous germ cell tumors.

- Found throughout the body typically in midline locations.
- In the central nervous system, the most common locations include the pineal and the suprasellar regions.
- Tumors may demonstrate growth into neighboring structures as well as seeding by cerebrospinal fluid (CSF).
- Imaging of the entire neuroaxis is recommended.

■ Other Imaging Findings

- Hyperdensity on CT images is due to lymphocyte hypercellularity within the tumor.
- High cellularity generally results in restricted diffusion on MRI scans.
- Germinomas are typically solid masses but may demonstrate internal cystic components.

✓ Pearls and ✗ Pitfalls

- ✓ Germinomas can be subdivided into pure germinoma and germinoma with syncytiotrophoblastic cells. With the latter, CSF levels of human chorionic gonadotropin may be elevated.
- ✓ Most of pineal tumors present with obstructive hydrocephalus.
- ✓ Germinomas generally have a favorable prognosis and are highly sensitive to radiation therapy.
- ✗ Unlike pineal region germinomas that occur 10 times more commonly in males, suprasellar region germinomas do not have a gender predilection.
- ✗ Most of pineal region masses enhance due to lack of a blood–brain barrier.

Case 45

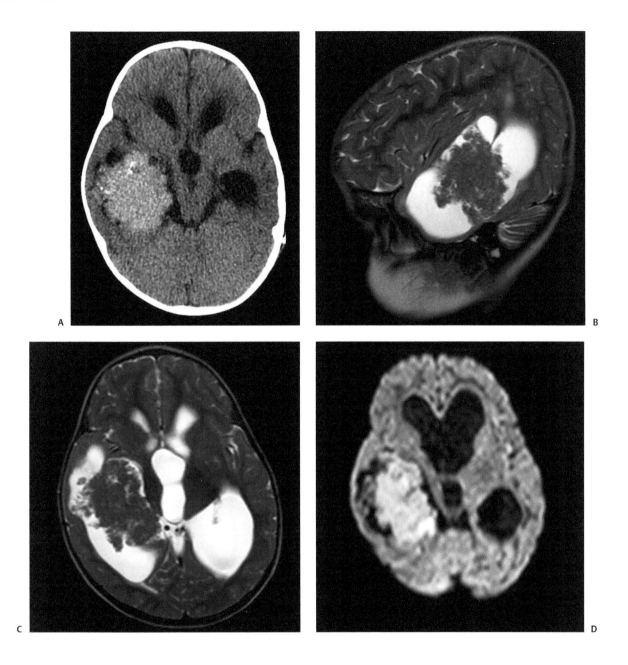

■ Clinical Presentation

A 12-year-old boy presents with headache.

■ Imaging Findings

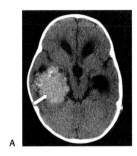
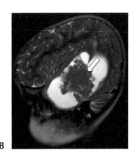
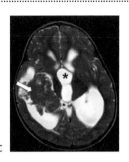
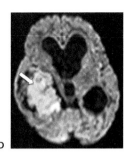

A   B   C   D

(A) Axial CT image demonstrates a large, lobulated hyperattenuating mass (*arrow*) in the right atrium, with punctate calcifications. Hydrocephalus is also noted. **(B)** Sagittal T2-weighted image (WI) shows a well-circumscribed lobulated cauliflower-like mass in the right atrium (*arrow*), which is enlarged. **(C)** Axial T2WI shows a well-circumscribed lobulated cauliflower-like mass in the right atrium (*arrow*), arising in the choroid plexus, not the ventricular wall. Notice the enlargement of the third (*asterisk*) and lateral ventricles. **(D)** Axial diffusion-weighted image shows restricted diffusion in the right atrial mass (*arrow*).

■ Differential Diagnosis

• ***Choroid plexus papilloma (CPP):***
  ○ Peak incidence: young children.
  ○ Typically located in the trigone in children and in the fourth ventricle in adults.
  ○ Associated with hydrocephalus.
  ○ Highly lobulated.
  ○ Avidly enhancing.
  ○ Choroid plexus carcinoma (CPC) can appear identical although usually there is evidence of heterogeneity (necrosis/hemorrhage) and brain invasion.
• *Intraventricular meningioma:*
  ○ Arises from the arachnoid cap cells within the choroid plexus, usually seen within the atria of the lateral ventricles.
  ○ Age group of 30 to 60 years, with female predilection.
  ○ Generally benign: World Health Organization grade I tumors.
  ○ Pediatric meningiomas have higher tendency for sarcomatous transformation.
  ○ Imaging similar to dural meningiomas: hyperdense on CT, calcifications in 50% of cases, isointense to hypointense on T1-weighted image (WI), hyperintense on T2WI, with avid postcontrast enhancement.
• *Subependymoma:*
  ○ Rare benign WHO grade I tumors arising from the ependymal-glial precursor cells.
  ○ Most tumors are located in the fourth ventricle (50–60%) followed by the ventricular margins or septum pellucidum of the lateral ventricle (30–40%).
  ○ Imaging: well-circumscribed lobulated appearance on both CT and MRI scans.
  ○ Associated hydrocephalus in 80%.
  ○ Calcification in 30%.
  ○ No parenchymal invasion and poor-to-absent contrast enhancement.

■ Essential Facts

• Choroid plexus tumors are divided on histology as typical CPP (WHO grade I), atypical CPP (WHO grade II), and CPC (WHO grade III).
• CPCs are found exclusively in children.
• Derived from the neuroepithelial cells of the choroid plexus and present as well-circumscribed lobulated cauliflower-like masses.
• There is marked overproduction of cerebrospinal fluid (CSF) by all these tumors resulting in hydrocephalus and signs of increased intracranial pressure.

■ Other Imaging Findings

• CT: Iso- to hyperdense with "frond-like" appearance and calcification in around 24% of cases.
• MRI: Isointense to hypointense intraventricular masses on T1WI, variable T2 signal. They are very well circumscribed and tend to engulf the normal choroid plexus.
• Avid enhancement, prominent intralesional flow voids, enlarged choroidal arteries.
• MR spectroscopy has shown elevated myoinositol in cases of CPP and elevated choline peak in CPC.

✓ Pearls and ✗ Pitfalls

✓ In the analysis of intraventricular tumors, it is useful to distinguish those arising in the ventricular wall (central neurocytoma, ependymoma, subependymoma, subependymal giant cell astrocytoma [SEGA], glioma, metastasis, primitive neuroectodermal tumor, solitary fibrous tumor, rosette-forming glioneural tumor) versus those arising in the choroid plexus (CPP/CPC, meningioma).
✓ The frequency of lateral ventricular tumors varies by location. Central neurocytoma, SEGA, metastasis, and subependymoma favor the frontal horns, whereas CPP, CPC, metastasis, and meningioma generally arise in the trigone.
✗ Parenchymal invasion and CSF seeding are highly suspicious of CPC.

Case 46

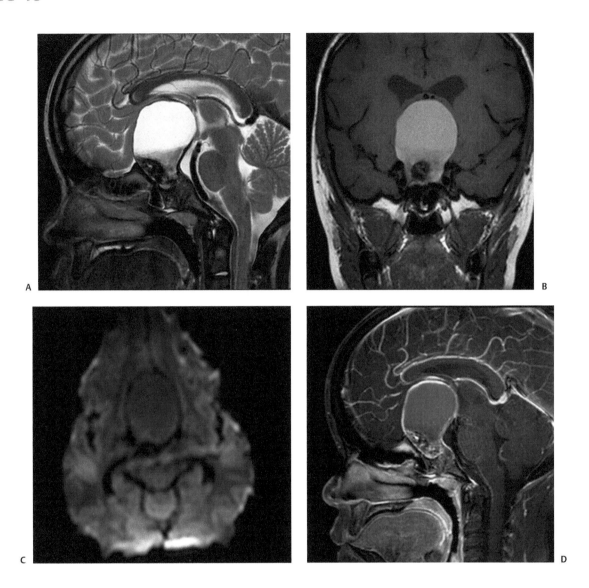

A

B

C

D

■ Clinical Presentation

Child presents with headaches.

■ Imaging Findings

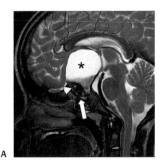 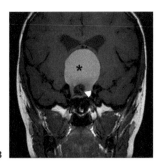 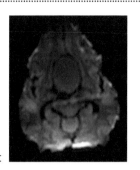 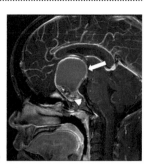

(A) Sagittal T2-weighted image (WI) shows a large cystic mass (*asterisk*) that has an inferior solid component (*arrowhead*). The sella is small and the pituitary gland is separate from the mass (*arrow*). **(B)** Sagittal T1WI without contrast. The cyst's content shows high T1 signal (*asterisk*). The solid component has calcifications (*arrowhead*). **(C)** Diffusion-weighted image shows no restricted diffusion. **(D)** On sagittal T1WI with contrast, the mass shows a rim of peripheral enhancement (*arrow*). The solid component demonstrates heterogenous enhancement (*arrowhead*).

■ Differential Diagnosis

- *Craniopharyngioma (adamantinomatous):*
  - Sella/suprasellar mass derived from Rathke's pouch.
  - Typically cystic with nodular component.
  - Reticulated enhancement.
  - 90% calcify.
  - Two types:
    - Adamantinomatous: Hyperintense cyst on T1-weighted image with a heterogeneous solid component.
    - Papillary: Rarely cystic, no calcification.
- *Cystic pituitary adenoma:*
  - Adenoma is the most common mass in the sella/parasellar region.
  - Rare in early childhood.
  - Signal parallels white matter and enhances homogenously with gadolinium.
  - Can have necrosis, cystic degeneration, or hemorrhage.
  - If soft in consistency, these masses can exhibit the "snowman" appearance as they extend superiorly through the diaphragma sellae.
- *Rathke's cleft cyst:*
  - Benign epithelium-lined cyst thought to be a remnant of Rathke's pouch.
  - Cyst may have increased T1 signal.
  - Thin rim or no enhancement.
  - No calcification.
  - Arises at the pars intermedia.
  - May show a small, nonenhancing, peripherally located intracystic nodule representing debris.

■ Essential Facts

- Adamantinomatous craniopharyngiomas are more common in the pediatric population.
- They contain stratified squamous epithelium from Rathke's pouch.
- The distribution by age is bimodal with the peak incidence in children at 5 to 14 years and in adults at 65 to 74 years of age.

■ Other Imaging Findings

- Suprasellar (75%), supra- and infrasellar (20%), and infrasellar (5%) regions.
- Part-solid, part-cystic calcified mass lesion.
- Reticular enhancement in the solid portion.
- Superior extension compressing the third ventricle.

✓ Pearls and ✗ Pitfalls

- ✓ Malignant transformation is rare.
- ✓ Lateral extent beyond the lateral wall of the internal carotid artery may be seen in adenomas and craniopharyngiomas but not in Rathke's cleft cyst.
- ✗ Arrested pneumatization of the sphenoid sinus appears as a nonexpansile lesion with internal soft or fatty tissue, curvilinear calcifications, and sclerotic well-defined margins. This may be mistaken for a mass lesion or an extension of a pituitary lesion.

Case 47

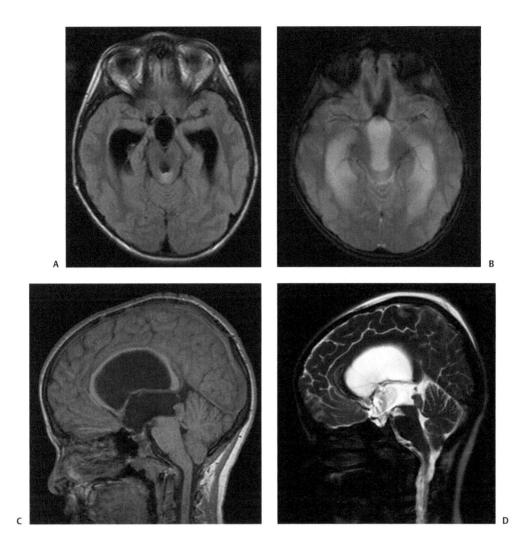

Clinical Presentation

A 5-year-old boy presents with headaches and vomiting.

■ Imaging Findings

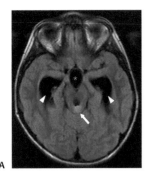
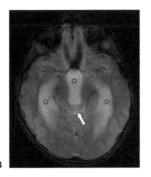
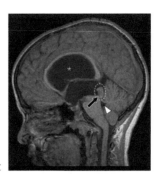
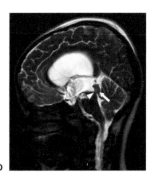

A   B   C   D

(A) Axial fluid-attenuated inversion recovery image shows an ill-defined T2 hyperintense mass in the tectal plate (*arrow*). The temporal horns of the lateral ventricles (*arrowheads*) and the third ventricle (*asterisk*) are dilated secondary to obstructive hydrocephalus from compression on the cerebral aqueduct. **(B)** Axial gradient echo sequence shows no susceptibility artifact within the mass in the tectal plate (*arrow*). Again seen is the dilatation of the supratentorial ventricles (*asterisks*). **(C)** Sagittal T1-weighted image (WI) of the brain demonstrates a T1 hypointense, ill-defined mass expanding the tectal plate (*oval*) and causing compression on the cerebral aqueduct (*black arrow*). The supratentorial ventricles are dilated (*asterisk*), whereas the fourth ventricle is normal in size (*white arrowhead*). **(D)** Sagittal T2WI shows increased signal intensity within the expansile lesion in the tectal plate (*arrow*). Also, there is better depiction of the site of obstruction to flow in the cerebral aqueduct from the mass (*arrowhead*).

■ Differential Diagnosis

- **Tectal glioma:** Ill-defined expansile mass within the tectal plate, usually corresponding to a low-grade astrocytoma, with low T1 signal, high T2 signal, absent enhancement, and secondary obstruction of the cerebral aqueduct.
- *Aqueductal stenosis:* This entity can be either acquired or congenital. Aqueductal stenosis also causes obstructive hydrocephalus at the level of the cerebral aqueduct; however, unlike tectal gliomas, the tectum has normal thickness and no discernable expansion or mass is identified.
- *Pineal tumor:* In general this group includes pineal parenchymal tumors and germ cell tumors. Pineal tumors can also cause compression on the cerebral aqueduct; however, the mass in this case expands the tectal plate. The pineal gland, seen more cephalad, is normal in size and signal intensity.

■ Essential Facts

- Tectal gliomas are generally low-grade astrocytomas, typically grade I or II. The most common pathology for resected tectal gliomas is pilocytic astrocytoma.
- Tectal gliomas commonly expand the tectal plate and cause obstructive hydrocephalus.
- These tumors occur more frequently in children, who generally present with signs of hydrocephalus, including headache and vomiting.
- On MRI scans, tectal gliomas are usually iso- to hypointense on T1, hyperintense on T2, and show little to no enhancement on postcontrast imaging.
- Occasionally, tectal gliomas may extend posteriorly beyond the limits of the tectum in an exophytic fashion.

■ Other Imaging Findings

- In general, these tumors have a better prognosis than diffuse pontine gliomas, now referred to as diffuse midline gliomas.
- These tumors rarely progress or require surgical resection, chemotherapy, or radiation therapy.
- Generally, these children require only cerebrospinal fluid diversion either by shunting or endoscopic third ventriculostomy and close follow-up with imaging.
- Occasionally, tectal gliomas enlarge. No imaging feature has been directly correlated to the likelihood of progression.

✓ Pearls and ✗ Pitfalls

✓ Although these tumors are midline and represent gliomas, tectal gliomas do not fall under the new World Health Organization (WHO) 2016 classification of *diffuse midline glioma, H3 K27M–mutant*. Whereas tectal gliomas are generally pilocytic astrocytomas and have a favorable prognosis, diffuse midline gliomas (previously referred to as diffuse intrinsic pontine glioma, or DIPG) are typically WHO grade IV tumors with 2-year survival rates of < 2%.

✗ Because of the close proximity between the quadrigeminal plate and the pineal gland, it can be difficult to determine the origin in the case of large masses in this region.

✗ Special scrutiny must be paid to the signal intensity of the tectum in cases of apparent acquired aqueductal stenosis. Often, tectal gliomas are subtle and ill-defined. Furthermore, characteristic lack of contrast enhancement can make them more difficult to detect.

Case 48

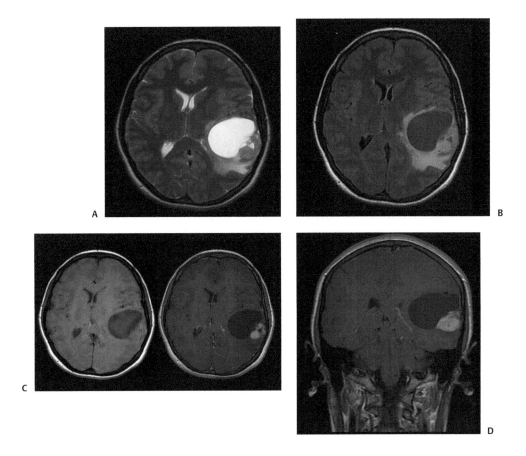

■ Clinical Presentation

A 12-year-old boy presents with new-onset seizure.

■ Imaging Findings

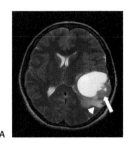 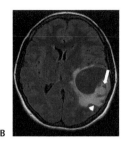 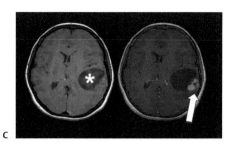 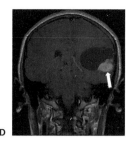

(A) Axial T2-weighted image (WI) demonstrates a cystic tumor with a solid mural nodule (*arrow*) in the left temporal lobe. Notice the surrounding vasogenic edema (*arrowhead*). **(B)** Axial fluid-attenuated inversion recovery image demonstrates a cystic tumor with a solid mural nodule (*arrow*) in the left temporal lobe. Notice the vasogenic edema (*arrowhead*). **(C)** Axial pre- and postcontrast T1WI demonstrate a cyst (*asterisk*) with an enhancing mural nodule (*arrow*), which abuts the pial surface. **(D)** Coronal T1WI after contrast demonstrates a left temporal cyst with an enhancing mural nodule (*arrow*), which abuts the pial surface.

■ Differential Diagnosis

- **Pleomorphic xanthoastrocytoma (PXA):**
  - Peripheral supratentorial tumors that appear during childhood.
  - Cysts, inner table scalloping, marked vasogenic edema, and meningeal enhancement are common features.
  - Relatively low apparent diffusion coefficient (ADC) values and ADC ratios may be present.
  - PXAs represent grade II tumors histologically.
- *Embryonal tumor with multilayered rosettes (C19MC-altered or not otherwise specified [NOS]); previously, primitive neuroectodermal tumor (PNET):*
  - Embryonal tumor composed of undifferentiated neuroepithelial cells.
  - Complex hemispheric mass in infants and young children.
  - Hemispheric PNETs tend to be larger than suprasellar or pineal PNETs.
  - Heterogeneous density/signal intensity, enhancement.
  - Minimal or absent peritumoral edema.
  - Calcifications are common (50–70%).
  - Restricted diffusion is common.
- *Ganglioglioma:*
  - Well-differentiated, slowly growing neuroepithelial tumor composed of neoplastic ganglion cells and neoplastic glial cells.
  - Partially cystic, enhancing cortically based mass in child/young adult with temporal lobe epilepsy.
  - Commonly superficial hemispheres, temporal lobe (> 75%).
  - Calcification is common (up to 50%).
  - Superficial lesions may expand cortex, remodel bone.

■ Essential Facts

- PXAs are rare neoplasms comprising < 1% of all astrocytic tumors.
- Most patients have longstanding epilepsy, often partial complex seizures (temporal lobe).

- They are more frequently encountered in childhood and young adulthood.
- 99% are supratentorial and tend to be superficial in the cerebral hemispheres.
- 40 to 50% involve the temporal lobes.

■ Other Imaging Findings

- CT:
  - Cystic, mixed, or solid mass.
  - Calcification or hemorrhage is not frequent.
  - Can create scalloping of the inner table.
- MRI:
  - Diffusion-weighted image: May show ADC hypointensity in solid portions.
  - Enhancement of adjacent meninges, dural "tail" common (~ 70%).
  - Enhancing nodule often abuts the pial surface.

✓ Pearls and ✗ Pitfalls

- ✓ The 2016 World Health Organization (WHO) Classification of Tumors of the Central Nervous System added anaplastic PXA, WHO grade III, as a distinct entity, to replace the previous descriptive title of PXA with anaplastic features. Patients with such tumors have shorter survival times when compared to those with WHO grade II PXAs.
- ✗ Common tumors that present as a cyst with a mural nodule include hemangioblastoma, pilocytic astrocytoma, ganglioglioma, and PXA.
- ✗ Uncommon tumors that can have similar features include tanycytic ependymoma, intraparenchymal schwannoma, desmoplastic infantile ganglioglioma, and cystic metastasis.

Case 49

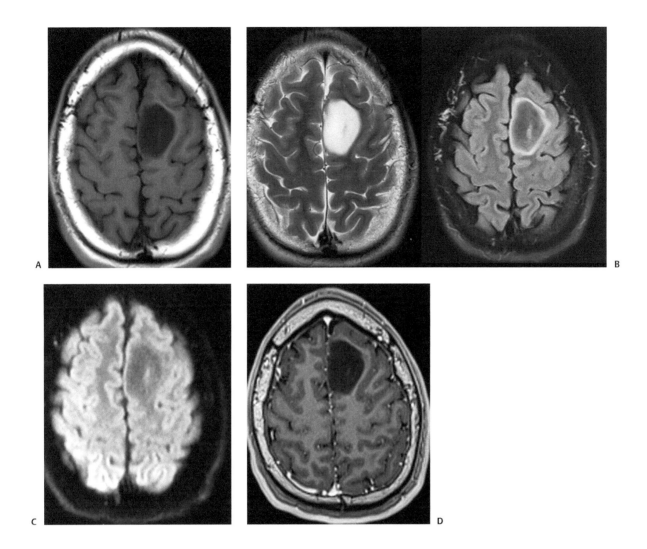

A

B

C

D

■ Clinical Presentation

A 22-year-old woman presents with headaches.

■ Imaging Findings

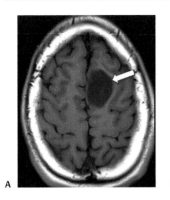
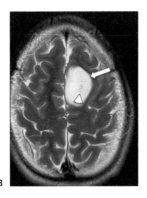
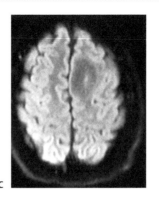
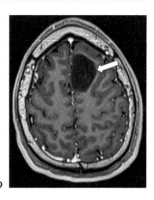

A   B   C   D

(A) Axial T1-weighted image (WI) shows a well-defined hypointense intra-axial lesion in the left superior frontal gyrus (*arrow*). A small area of hyperintensity is noted in the center of the lesion. **(B)** Axial T2WI shows the left frontal lesion (*arrow*) with central hypointensity (*arrowhead*). No surrounding edema is noted. **(C)** Axial diffusion-weighted image shows that the lesion has no restricted diffusion. **(D)** Axial T1WI with contrast; the left frontal lesion shows no enhancement (*arrow*).

■ Differential Diagnosis

• **Oligodendroglioma:**
  ○ Well-marginated mass in the cortex or subcortical white matter.
  ○ Coarse calcifications (20–90%).
  ○ Occasional cystic degeneration or hemorrhage.
  ○ Subtle enhancement seen in 20%.
  ○ Supratentorial location (90%).
  ○ Vasogenic edema is uncommon.
• *Arachnoid cyst:*
  ○ Extra-axial focal fluid collection with arachnoid lining.
  ○ Most common location is in the middle cranial fossa, followed by the posterior fossa.
  ○ No enhancement.
  ○ No calcifications.
  ○ No vessels are noted crossing it.
  ○ No restricted diffusion.
• *Ganglioglioma:*
  ○ Neuroepithelial origin mass with both ganglionic and glial components.
  ○ Cortical-based lesion most commonly seen in the temporal lobe.
  ○ Cystic component with a solitary nodule.
  ○ 50% calcify.

■ Essential Facts

• Genetically defined oligodendrogliomas by the most recent World Health Organization (WHO) classification of brain tumors (2016) are glial tumors that are isocitrate dehydrogenase (IDH)-mutant and present the 1p/19q codeletion.
• Most common location is in the frontal lobe (70%), the parietal lobe (17%), and the temporal lobe (6%).
• Oligodendrogliomas can be classified as WHO grade II or grade III.

■ Other Imaging Findings

• Bright signal on T2-weighted image is frequent.
• Susceptibility sensitive sequences can demonstrate calcification.
• Calcification is generally curvilinear or gyriform in morphology.
• In a recent series, oligodendrogliomas tend to have less distinct borders than their astrocytic counterparts.

✓ Pearls and ✗ Pitfalls

✓ Knowing the genetic characteristics of tumors allows one to understand the pathogenesis and behavior of these tumors and to tailor therapies.
✓ Grade III (anaplastic) oligodendrogliomas can present with hemorrhage or a lactate peak on MR spectroscopy.
✗ The term *oligoastrocytoma* should be avoided.
✗ If the genetic footprint is not known, and the lesion shows histologic characteristics of oligodendroglioma, the term *oligodendroglioma NOS* (not otherwise specified) should be used.

Case 50

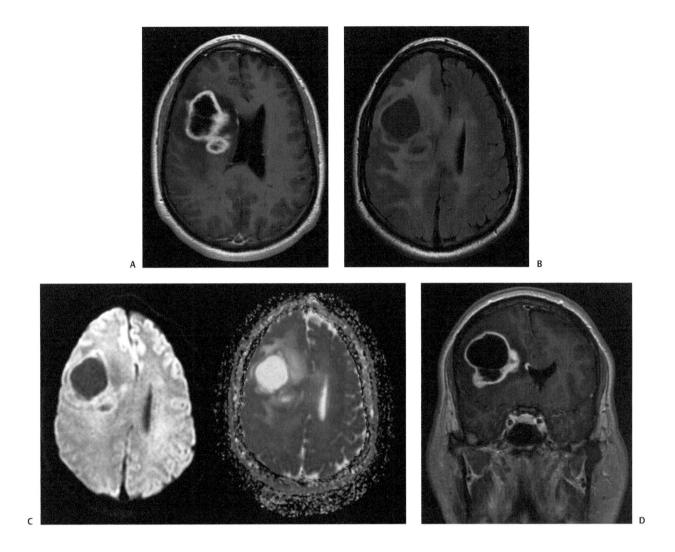

■ Clinical Presentation

A 53-year-old man presents with forgetfulness and confusion.

■ **Imaging Findings**

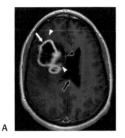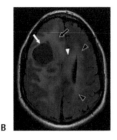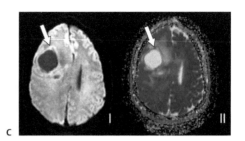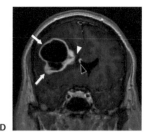

(A) Axial T1 postcontrast image demonstrates a centrally necrotic, multiloculated mass with thick peripheral enhancement (*white arrow*) and small satellite nodules (*white arrowheads*) centered in the right frontal lobe. There is secondary mass effect with midline shift to the left (*black arrow*) and partial effacement of the right lateral ventricle. Linear enhancement is seen along the ependymal surface of the body of the right lateral ventricle (*black arrowhead*). **(B)** Axial T2 fluid-attenuated inversion recovery image shows the heterogeneous mass in the right frontal lobe with low internal signal intensity (*white arrow*) and extensive surrounding T2 hyperintensity (*black arrow*) extending across the corpus callosum (*white arrowhead*) to the contralateral hemisphere (*black arrowheads*). **(C)** Axial diffusion-weighted image (*I*) and corresponding apparent diffusion coefficient map (*II*) shows mild restricted diffusion along the margins of the mass (*white arrows*) without internal areas of diffusion restriction. **(D)** Coronal T1 postcontrast image demonstrated the irregularly enhancing margins of the mass (*white arrows*) with thin linear projections emanating from the outer edges (*white arrowhead*). There is enhancement of the ependymal lining of the right lateral ventricle (*black arrowhead*) and significant midline shift to the left.

■ **Differential Diagnosis**

- **Glioblastoma:** Glioblastoma is classified by the World Health Organization (WHO) as a grade IV tumor and is the most common primary brain malignancy in adults. Imaging classically demonstrates a peripherally enhancing, centrally necrotic hemispheric mass. Subependymal enhancement is a classical feature, and linear projections emanating from the tumor generally suggest perivascular space invasion.
- *Solitary brain metastasis:* Brain metastases typically arise at the gray–white matter interface and are better circumscribed than glioblastomas. Surrounding vasogenic edema can often be disproportionate to the size of the lesion. Unlike glioblastoma, signal abnormality does not cross commissures or the corpus callosum. It is uncommon for a solitary brain metastasis to grow to this size without developing other additional sites of brain metastasis.
- *Abscess:* Similar to glioblastoma, brain abscess can demonstrate peripheral, ringlike enhancement and central necrosis. Extensive surrounding edema that does not cross commissures can also be present and may be difficult to differentiate from metastasis. In the case of pyogenic abscess, the central portion of the mass demonstrates restricted diffusion, whereas in glioblastoma and metastasis, the central necrotic component does not.

■ **Essential Facts**

- The WHO 2016 classification of brain tumors has recently included both histopathologic and molecular markers in the terminology for glioblastoma.
- Currently, glioblastoma has three separate subtypes: glioblastoma isocitrate dehydrogenase (IDH)-wildtype, glioblastoma IDH-mutant, and glioblastoma NOS (not otherwise specified) when an IDH status has not been established.

- Glioblastoma IDH-wildtype accounts for approximately 90% of cases. These tumors generally present de novo in patients older than 55 years of age.
- Glioblastoma IDH-mutant are less common and may develop from lower grade gliomas that have dedifferentiated. This variant is generally seen in younger patients.

■ **Other Imaging Findings**

- On CT and MRI scans, glioblastomas are generally seen within the cerebral hemispheres and have a heterogeneous appearance.
- Necrosis, hemorrhage, and enhancement are highly variable.
- Tumors may extend across commissures, including the corpus callosum, to the contralateral hemisphere.
- MR perfusion techniques demonstrate elevation of cerebral blood flow, cerebral blood volume, and K^{trans}.
- MR spectroscopy shows elevation of choline and depression of the *N*-acetylaspartate (NAA) peak with inversion of choline to creatine and choline:NAA ratios.

✓ **Pearls and** ✗ **Pitfalls**

- ✓ Multifocal glioblastoma refers to multiple areas of contrast enhancement that are connected by increased T2/fluid-attenuated inversion recovery (FLAIR) signal.
- ✓ Multicentric glioblastoma are tumors with different foci of enhancement that have no apparent connection by T2/FLAIR hyperintensity and are separated by normal intervening brain.
- ✗ The accompanying T2 hyperintensity surrounding glioblastomas often represents infiltrative tumor rather than edema. Unlike vasogenic edema that spares the cortex, this abnormal T2 signal may extend to the pial surface.

Case 51

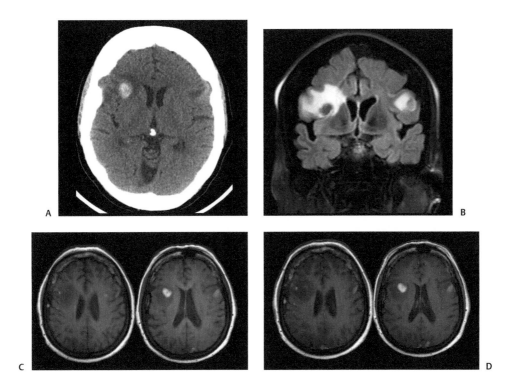

■ Clinical Presentation

An 86-year-old with a history of headache, with previously removed melanoma of the mouth, presents with bumps developing on the scalp.

■ Imaging Findings

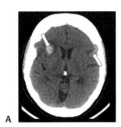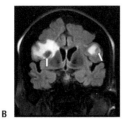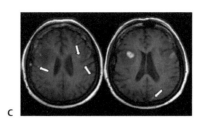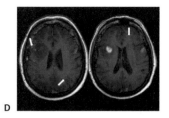

(A) Axial CT demonstrates hyperattenuating lesions in both frontal lobes (*arrows*), with surrounding vasogenic edema. **(B)** Coronal fluid-attenuated inversion recovery image shows low signal within the lesions and better delineates the extent of vasogenic edema (*arrows*). **(C)** Axial T1-weighted image (WI) without contrast. There are multiple additional parenchymal lesions with intrinsic high T1 signal (*arrows*). **(D)** Axial T1WI with contrast. Multiple enhancing foci in both cerebral hemispheres become evident after contrast administration (*arrows*).

■ Differential Diagnosis

- **Melanoma metastasis:** Multiple lesions with intrinsic T1 hyperintensity can be secondary to subacute hemorrhage; however, with the history of prior melanoma, melanotic metastatic deposits are the main concern.
- *Hemorrhagic metastasis:*
  ○ Most frequent primary tumors to present with hemorrhagic metastases include melanoma, renal cell carcinoma, choriocarcinoma, thyroid carcinoma (highest rate of hemorrhage for papillary carcinoma of thyroid), and lung carcinoma.
  ○ However, of all the primary tumors to present with hemorrhagic metastases, lung and breast cancers are the most common etiologies due to their higher overall prevalence.
- *Septic emboli:*
  ○ Infarcts in multiple arterial distributions from embolic source, often cardiac origin.
  ○ Frequently hemorrhagic.
  ○ May result in micro abscesses.

■ Essential Facts

- Melanoma is the third most common cause of brain metastases, after lung and breast cancer.
- Melanoma brain metastases occur late in the disease course and have a poor prognosis.
- On MRI, melanin decreases T1 relaxation time, causing T1 hyperintensity. Melanin may also shorten the T2* relaxation time. Melanotic lesions have a reduced T2 signal, making them less conspicuous, with an appearance similar to blood products.

■ Other Imaging Findings

- On unenhanced CT examination, melanoma metastases tend to be hyperdense (from melanin and/or hemorrhage) in relation to normal brain parenchyma.
- Melanoma metastases can be amelanotic, in which case they do not demonstrate intrinsic T1 hyperintensity.

✓ Pearls and ✕ Pitfalls

✓ Lesions with intrinsic high T1 signal on MRI scans include:
- Hemorrhage.
- Protein-containing lesions: colloid cyst, craniopharyngioma, Rathke's cleft cyst, and atypical epidermoid.
- Fat-containing lesions: lipoma, dermoid, and lipomatous meningioma.
- Calcification or ossification: endocrine-metabolic disorder, calcified neoplasm, infection.
- Other mineral deposits: acquired hepatocerebral degeneration and Wilson disease.
- Melanin-containing lesions: metastasis from melanoma and leptomeningeal melanosis.
- Miscellaneous: ectopic neurohypophysis, chronic stages of multiple sclerosis, and neurofibromatosis type I.

Case 52

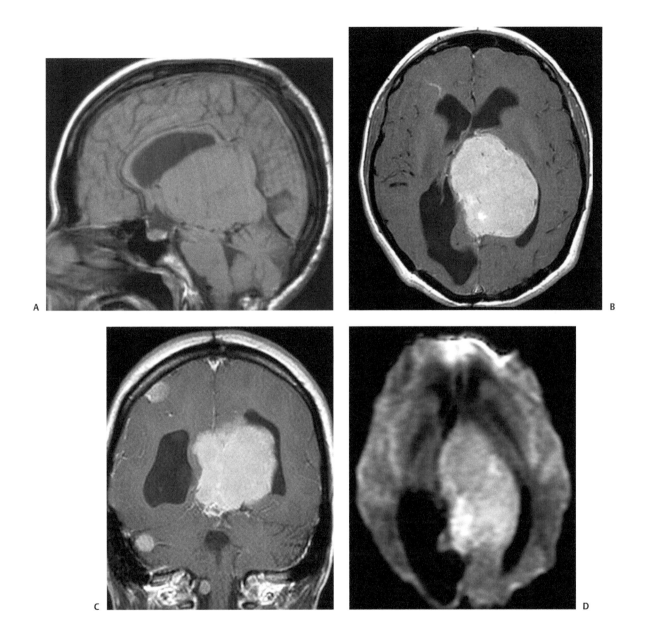

A 28-year-old with history of headaches; imaging revealed normal cerebellopontine angles and internal auditory canals.

■ Imaging Findings

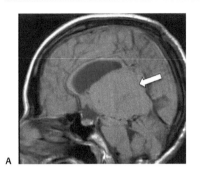 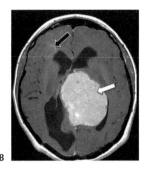 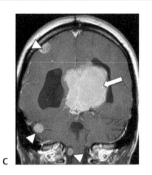 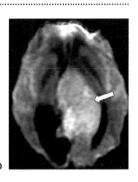

(A) Sagittal T1-weighted image (WI) shows a large central mass isointense to the brain parenchyma (*arrow*). The mass compresses the third ventricle and tectum, and causes dilatation of the lateral ventricles. **(B)** Axial T1WI with contrast shows avid enhancement of the left parafalcine mass (*white arrow*). An incidental small developmental venous anomaly is noted in the right frontal lobe (*black arrow*). **(C)** Coronal T1WI with contrast shows the left parafalcine mass (*arrow*) and multiple smaller extra-axial masses (*arrowheads*) with similar imaging characteristics. The lateral ventricles are dilated. **(D)** Diffusion-weighted image shows increased signal in the mass (*arrow*), a feature indicative of hypercellularity.

■ Differential Diagnosis

- **Meningiomatosis (multiple meningiomas):**
  - Multiple dural-based meningiomas.
  - Meningiomatosis does not course with schwannomas.
  - Associated with mutation of chromosome 22 (50%).
  - *SMARCB1* mutation is common.
  - Slight female predominance.
- *Neurofibromatosis type 2 (NF2):*
  - Congenital syndrome that results in multiple intracranial schwannomas, meningiomas, and ependymomas: "MISME."
  - Can also present in the spine.
  - Mutation in chromosome 22.
  - Mean age of presentation is 25 years old.
- *Dural metastasis:*
  - Tumor infiltration can involve the dura and/or leptomeninges.
  - Dural disease generally involves the skull.
  - They can present with hemorrhage which is not seen in meningiomas.
  - Can present as smooth enhancement or nodular areas.
  - Primary tumor cannot be identified in 2 to 4% of cases.
  - Tumor cells disseminate in the cerebrospinal fluid (CSF).
  - MRI and lumbar puncture must be performed.
  - If increased cellularity, high signal on diffusion-weighted image (DWI).

■ Essential Facts

- Multiple meningiomas can be seen as an isolated entity or as part of the NF2 syndrome.
- Meningiomas account for 15% of intracranial primary tumors.

- Multiple meningiomas are seen in only 1 to 5% of the cases.
- They have similar imaging characteristics as isolated meningiomas.
- Most are benign, World Health Organization grade I lesions.
- Rarely bleed.

■ Other Imaging Findings

- CT: Meningiomas tend to have adjacent hyperostosis. Calcification is seen in 25%.
- MRI: May show a "spoke wheel" or "sunburst" pattern on T2-weighted image due to their dural-based vascular pedicle.
- MRI with contrast: Most enhance homogeneously. May show a dural tail.
- DWI: If the tumor is hypercellular, it demonstrates increased signal.

✓ Pearls and ✗ Pitfalls

✓ Meningiomas can be seen in patients exposed to whole-brain radiation or in children with a history of radiation exposure in utero.
✓ Growth of the masses is associated with steroid hormone receptors.
✓ Meningiomas are the most common intracranial primary tumors.
✗ Absence of a CSF cleft may indicate brain invasion.
✗ A dural tail does not always indicate tumor spread.
✗ Dural sinus involvement should always be evaluated.

Case 53

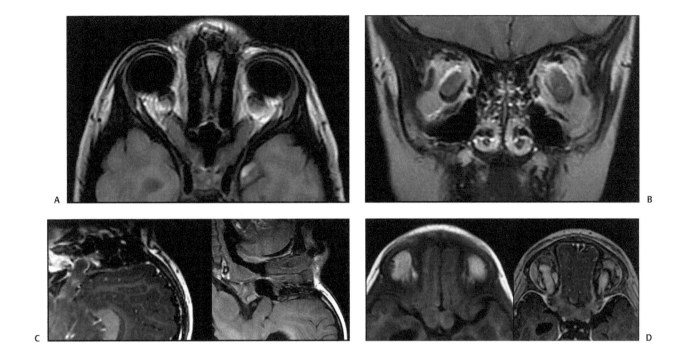

■ Clinical Presentation

A 3-year-old girl presents with vision loss.

■ Imaging Findings

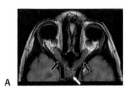 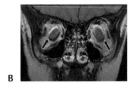 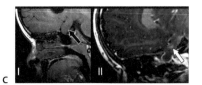 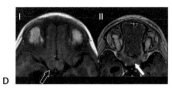

(A) Axial fluid-attenuated inversion recovery (FLAIR) image through the orbits shows enlargement, undulation, and increased T2 signal involving the intra-orbital, intracanalicular, and prechiasmatic optic nerves bilaterally (*black arrows*) and extending posteriorly to the optic chiasm (*white arrow*). (B) Coronal FLAIR image through the orbit demonstrates the bilateral enlargement of the intraorbital segments of the orbital nerves (*black arrows*). (C) Sagittal T1 (*I*) and sagittal T1 with contrast (*II*) show thickening of the optic nerves extending posteriorly to the optic chiasm with intermediate signal intensity on pre-contrast imaging (*black arrow*) and patchy, irregular enhancement following contrast administration (*white arrow*). (D) Axial T1 noncontrast image through the orbits (*I*) and axial T1 postcontrast image (*II*) demonstrate the globular appearance of the optic chiasm with isointense signal on T1 (*black arrow*) and patchy enhancement following contrast injection (*white arrow*).

■ Differential Diagnosis

- **Optic nerve glioma (ONG):** ONG represents the most common intraconal tumor of childhood and can involve any portion of the optic pathway. On imaging, these masses typically present as diffuse enlargement of the optic nerve with variable signal intensity and enhancement. When bilateral, these tumors are generally associated with neurofibromatosis type 1 (NF1).
- *Optic nerve meningioma:* Benign tumors that arise from the optic nerve sheath are generally unilateral and typically enhance, revealing the "tram-track sign" which corresponds to intense enhancement of the enlarged sheath, in contrast to the nonenhancing nerve. Unlike ONG, these tumors are generally seen in the adult population rather than in children.
- *Optic neuritis:* Inflammation of the optic nerves due to infectious and noninfectious causes, seen most frequently in young adults. Bilateral optic neuritis can be seen in patients with multiple sclerosis. On imaging, this condition can present with swelling and enhancement of the optic nerve, but the size and appearance of the nerves does not tend to be masslike as seen in this case.

■ Essential Facts

- Also referred to as optic pathway/hypothalamic gliomas because they are not exclusive to the optic nerves and can occur anywhere along the optic pathway.
- Histologically, ONGs are World Health Organization grade I pilocytic astrocytomas.
- ONGs are associated with NF1 in > 50% of patients.
- Usually, these tumors present during the 1st and 2nd decade of life.
- A slight female predominance has been reported of ~ 60%.
- On imaging, the optic nerve shows fusiform enlargement with iso- to hypodensity on CT images.
- Undulation and tortuosity of the enlarged nerve is a common finding.

- Uncommon features include eccentric growth of the mass, hyperdensity, and calcifications.
- On MRI, ONGs are iso- to hypointense on T1 and mildly hyperintense on T2 images.
- Enhancement is variable in intensity and pattern.

■ Other Imaging Findings

- ONGs related to NF are significantly different than ONGs not related to NF. Some of the differences include:
  ○ Tendency is for the tumor to grow in patients without NF, whereas stability is more common in patients with NF.
  ○ Optic chiasm involvement in patients with NF presents with enlargement; however, the general anatomy of the structure is preserved. On the other hand, in patients without NF, the optic chiasm involvement is more masslike, with cystic degeneration and extension to structures outside the optic pathway.
  ○ Patients without NF are generally more symptomatic at the time of diagnosis of ONG.

✓ Pearls and ✗ Pitfalls

- ✓ Bilateral ONGs are essentially pathognomonic for NF1.
- ✓ Fusiform enlargement of the optic nerves is seen with intermediate density and signal intensity on T1 and mildly increased signal intensity on T2.
- ✓ Enhancement is variable and is seen in approximately 50% of cases.
- ✗ It is important to distinguish enlargement and enhancement of the nerve itself, as is the case in ONG, compared to enhancement of the optic nerve sheath seen in meningiomas.
- ✗ The appearance of ONG related and not related to NF can vary greatly.

Case 54

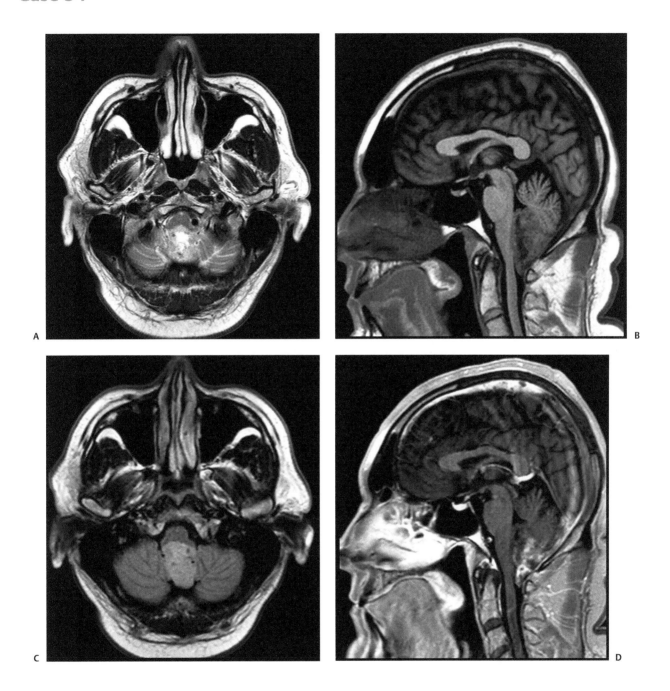

A

B

C

D

■ Clinical Presentation

A 62-year-old presents with drowsiness.

■ Imaging Findings

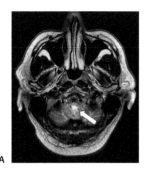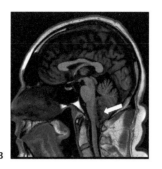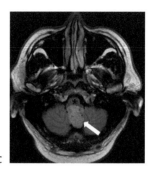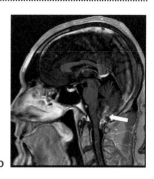

(A) Axial T2-weighted image (WI) shows a mass with heterogeneous signal filling the inferior fourth ventricle (*arrow*), deforming the dorsal surface of the medulla oblongata (*asterisk*). **(B)** Sagittal T1WI without contrast demonstrates a mass with heterogeneous low signal in the inferior fourth ventricle (*arrow*). **(C)** Axial fluid-attenuated inversion recovery image shows a mass filling the inferior fourth ventricle (*arrow*), deforming the dorsal surface of the medulla oblongata (*asterisk*). **(D)** Sagittal T1WI with contrast demonstrates a heterogeneous enhancing mass in the inferior fourth ventricle (*arrow*).

■ Differential Diagnosis

- ***Subependymoma:***
  - Typically well-circumscribed solid lobular mass within the fourth (60%) and lateral ventricles in middle-aged or elderly patients (typically 5th–6th decades).
  - Tend to be small: 1 to 2 cm.
  - When large, may have cysts, hemorrhage, or calcifications.
- *Ependymoma:*
  - Slow-growing tumor of ependymal cells.
  - Location:
    - Two thirds in posterior fossa (most in fourth ventricle).
    - One third supratentorial, the majority outside ventricles, in periventricular white matter.
  - Avidly enhance.
  - Peak incidence in young children (3–5 years), with slight predominance in males.
  - Ependymomas may progressively fill up the fourth ventricle and extend through the foramina of Magendie and Luschka into the perimedullary cisterns and upper cervical spinal canal.
- *Epidermoid cyst:*
  - Also known as ectodermal inclusion cyst.
  - Location:
    - Intradural (90%), primarily in basal cisterns (cerebellopontine angle 40–50%).
    - Fourth ventricle (17%).
    - Parasellar/middle cranial fossa (10–15%).
  - Lobulated, irregular, cauliflower-like mass with "fronds."
  - MRI: T1-weighted image (WI) slightly hyperintense to cerebrospinal fluid, T2WI isointense to slightly hyperintense, fluid-attenuated inversion recovery image usually does not completely suppress minimal marginal to absent enhancement.

■ Essential Facts

- The majority of these benign (World Health Organization grade I) tumors occur within the fourth (60%) and lateral ventricles in middle-aged or elderly patients.
- Subependymomas are typically < 2 cm and asymptomatic.
- Recurrence after surgical resection is rare.

■ Other Imaging Findings

- CT:
  - Isoattenuated to slightly hypoattenuated compared with the brain parenchyma. Internal cystic areas are frequent.
  - Calcifications and hemorrhage are not common.
- MRI:
  - Homogeneous solid masses, hypointense on T1WI and hyperintense on T2WI, without edema observed in the adjacent brain parenchyma.
  - Mild or no enhancement.

✓ Pearls and ✗ Pitfalls

✓ Common masses in the fourth ventricle include ependymoma, subependymoma, choroid plexus papilloma/carcinoma, epidermoid cyst, neurocysticercosis, and rosette-forming glioneuronal tumor.

✗ Subependymomas are most commonly seen in the fourth ventricle but can arise anywhere there is ependymal lining. Distribution by location: fourth ventricle, 50 to 60%. Lateral ventricles (usually frontal horns), 30 to 40%. Third ventricle and central canal of the spinal cord: rare.

Case 55

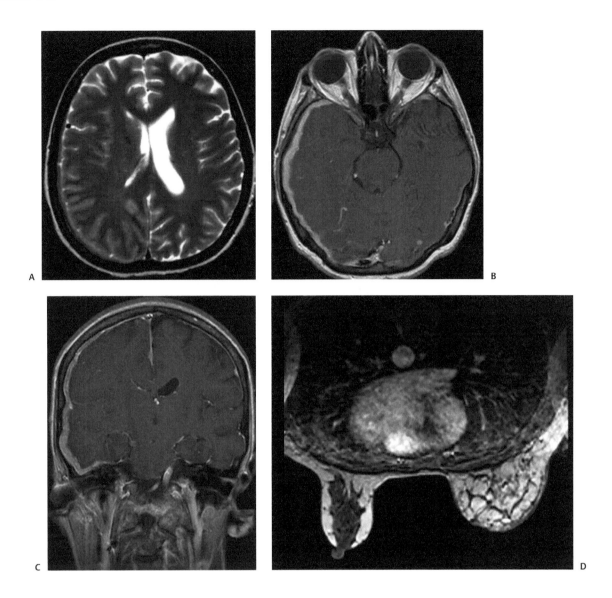

■ Clinical Presentation

A 59-year-old woman presents with headache and breast asymmetry.

■ Imaging Findings

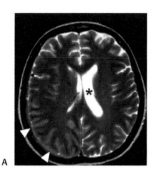 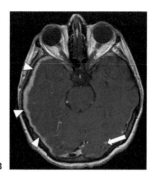 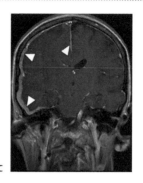 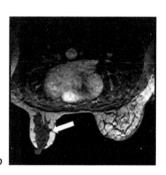

(A) Axial T2-weighted image (WI) shows asymmetry of the lateral ventricles (*asterisk*). The sulci on the right are slightly effaced due to a lesion replacing the cerebrospinal fluid in the convexity (*arrowheads*). **(B, C)** Axial **(B)** and coronal **(C)** T1WI of the brain with contrast show abnormal thick enhancement along the meninges on the right side (*arrowheads*). A nodular enhancing lesion is seen in the left occipital lobe (*arrow*). **(D)** Axial MRI scan of the breast shows asymmetry of the breast tissue with a mass on the smaller right breast (*arrow*).

■ Differential Diagnosis

- ***Meningeal carcinomatosis:***
  - Dural or leptomeningeal infiltration of malignant cells.
  - Avid enhancement.
  - Dural disease tends to spread to the calvarium.
  - Leptomeningeal disease causes seeding of the arachnoid layer and pial surface.
  - Adjacent sulcal effacement.
- *Bacterial meningitis:*
  - Infectious inflammatory process of the meninges.
  - Thick nodular enhancement.
  - Can be associated with cerebritis and abscess formation.
  - Hydrocephalus.
- *En-plaque meningioma:*
  - Specific macroscopic appearance of meningiomas characterized by diffuse and extensive dural involvement.
  - Usually with extracranial extension into the calvarium, orbit, and soft tissues.

■ Essential Facts

- Meningeal seeding is typically hematogenous.
- In children, the primary lesions to result in meningeal carcinomatosis are medulloblastoma and lymphoma. In adults, metastases from breast carcinoma, lymphoma, and prostate carcinoma.

■ Other Imaging Findings

- CT is not a good imaging tool for the detection of meningeal carcinomatosis.
- MR with contrast is the imaging modality of choice.
- Postcontrast fluid-attenuated inversion recovery sequences are helpful to identify leptomeningeal disease.

✓ Pearls and ✗ Pitfalls

- ✓ Meningeal carcinomatosis may involve the spine. "Sugar coating" and nodular enhancement of the nerve roots are typical imaging findings.
- ✗ Lumbar puncture (LP) can be negative in > 50% of the cases on the first attempt. Sensitivity increases to 90% with three repetitive LPs.

Case 56

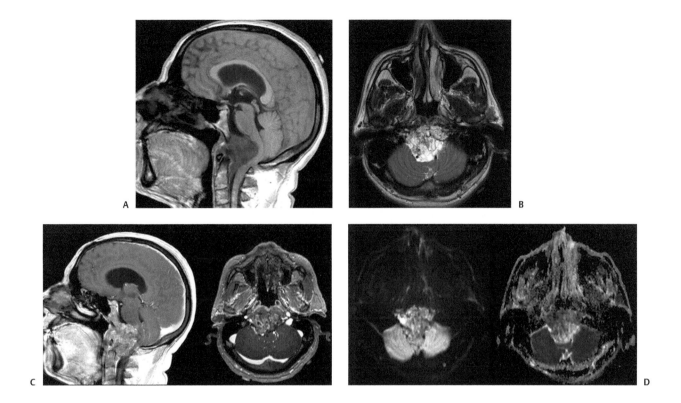

■ Clinical Presentation

A 60-year-old man presents with headaches.

■ Imaging Findings

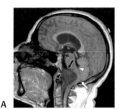 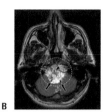 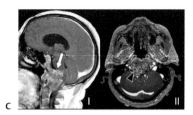 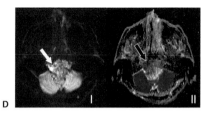

(A) Sagittal T1-weighted image (WI) shows a relatively well-defined hypointense mass (*black arrow*) arising from the inferior tip of the clivus (*black arrowhead*) and extending to the ventral basal cisterns causing posterior displacement of the medulla and inferior cerebellum (*white arrow*), leading to obstructive hydrocephalus due to compression on the outflow of the fourth ventricle (*white arrowhead*). **(B)** Axial T2WI demonstrates markedly high T2 signal intensity within the mass (*circle*) with thin hypointense septations (*black arrowhead*). The mass displaces the medulla and cerebellum posteriorly as well as the bilateral vertebral arteries, which are also partially encased (*black arrows*). **(C)** Sagittal (*I*) and axial (*II*) T1 postcontrast images demonstrate heterogeneous enhancement within the mass (*white arrow*), giving the mass a "honeycomb" pattern secondary to multiple internal areas of absent enhancement (*black arrowhead*). **(D)** Diffusion-weighted image (DWI) (*I*) and corresponding apparent diffusion coefficient (ADC) map (*II*) show heterogeneous areas of increased DWI signal with low ADC values consistent with regions of restricted diffusion (*white* and *black arrows*).

■ Differential Diagnosis

- **Clival chordoma:** Malignant tumor that arises from notochordal remnants typically along the midline. Chordomas are characteristically bright on T2 and classically show a "honeycomb" pattern of enhancement due to internal nonenhancing septations.
- *Chondrosarcoma:* Chondrosarcomas of the skull base typically arise off of the midline, originating from the petrooccipital fissure. Furthermore, chondrosarcomas are not typically as bright on T2-weighted imaging because of their internal gelatinous matrix, and approximately 50% show internal calcifications.
- *Skull base metastasis:* Metastases at the skull base generally show intermediate signal on T1- and T2-weighted images and tend to show more bone destruction. They are typically seen in the setting of patients with known primary cancers and tend to occur along with osseous metastases elsewhere.

■ Essential Facts

- Rare, malignant tumor.
- Arise from small remnants of the notochord that remain trapped in bone along the midline.
- Usually occur in the adult population, typically around the 4th decade of life.
- Locally invasive and do not tend to metastasize.
- The most frequent site is the sacrum in 50% of cases, followed by the clivus in 35% and then the remainder of the spine.
- Within the clivus, chordomas that arise from the superior, middle, or inferior portion.
- CT image shows a slightly hyperdense, well-circumscribed mass arising from the midline with bone destruction.
- On MRI scans, chordomas show intermediate to low signal intensity of T1 and characteristically high signal on T2, reflecting its high fluid content with thin hypointense septations.

- Enhancement has been described as resembling a "honeycomb" because of the internal areas of low signal on postcontrast imaging.

■ Other Imaging Findings

- Sagittal MRI is especially helpful in determining anterior extension to the nasopharynx and posterior extension to the brainstem.
- Occasionally, chordomas that arise from the central portion of the clivus can extend posteriorly as a portion of tissue that resembles a "thumb" and ventrally indents the pons.
- Small foci of intrinsically high T1 signal within the mass may reflect hemorrhage or mucus.
- Fat-suppression MRI can be helpful in detecting small chordomas by decreasing the signal of adjacent fatty bone marrow.
- Displacement and partial encasement of arteries is a common feature of chordomas.
- Chordomas generally have lower apparent diffusion coefficient values than chondrosarcomas, especially poorly differentiated chordomas.

✓ Pearls and ✗ Pitfalls

- ✓ Midline mass with bony destruction of the clivus.
- ✓ Characteristically high T2 signal.
- ✓ Extension into the nasopharynx and posterior fossa.
- ✓ Heterogeneous enhancement with internal foci of low signal exhibiting a "honeycomb" pattern.
- ✗ Occasionally, intracranial chordomas can arise off of the midline from the petrous apex.
- ✗ Small fragments of sequestered bone trapped within destroyed bone in chordomas can be difficult to distinguish from the chondroid matrix of chondrosarcomas.
- ✗ Infrequently, chordomas can show little to no enhancement because of large areas of necrosis or mucinous material.

Case 57

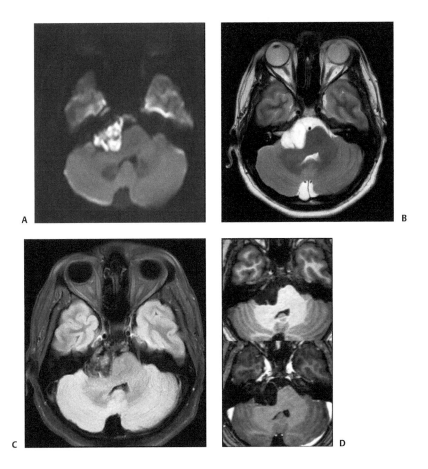

■ Clinical Presentation

A 30-year-old man presents with diagnosis of a mass.

■ Imaging Findings

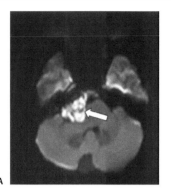
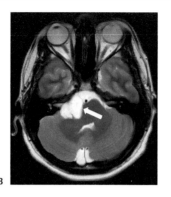
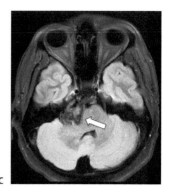
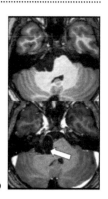

(A) Axial diffusion-weighted image demonstrates a mass in the right cerebellopontine angle (CPA) with high signal intensity (*arrow*). **(B)** Axial T2-weighted image (WI) demonstrates a mass in the right CPA with signal intensity similar to cerebrospinal fluid (CSF) (*arrow*). **(C)** Axial fluid-attenuated inversion recovery image demonstrates a mass in the right CPA with heterogeneous signal intensity, which does not match the signal of CSF (*arrow*). **(D)** Axial T1WI pre- and postcontrast demonstrate a mass in the right CPA with low signal intensity, similar to CSF, without enhancement (*arrow*).

■ Differential Diagnosis

- **Epidermoid cyst:** Epidermoid cysts are composed of epithelial cells that form a keratohyalin matrix arising from desquamation. The location is usually off midline in basal subarachnoid cisterns and ventricles. They engulf vessel and nerves.
- *Arachnoid cyst:* These are cerebrospinal fluid (CSF)-filled cysts that follow the signal in all sequences. There is no signal on diffusion-weighted image (DWI) and no enhancement. The middle cranial fossa is the most common location (50%) followed by the cerebellopontine angle (CPA) (10%). Arachnoid cysts displace cortical vessels away from the calvarium.
- *Dermoid cyst:*
  - Dermoid cysts are also ectodermal inclusion cysts that, in addition to squamous epithelium, have skin appendages that form cholesterol. They have a heterogeneous signal and are hyperintense on T1 secondary to fatty content. They tend to have a midline location.
  - Dermoid cysts grow faster than epidermoid cysts, and can rupture, causing chemical meningitis. If unruptured they do not enhance. Enhancement is seen if ruptured. Supratentorial is a more common location. Dermoid cysts do not show high signal on DWI.

■ Essential Facts

- Epidermoid cysts are congenital lesions arising from inclusion of ectodermal epithelial tissue during neural tube closure in the first weeks of embryogenesis.
- 50% of intracranial epidermoid cysts are located in the CPA. Another frequent location is the fourth ventricle.
- They grow from the slow desquamation of the stratified keratinized epithelium that lines the cyst.

■ Other Imaging Findings

- CT: Epidermoid cysts appear hypoattenuating with possible marginal calcifications.
- MRI: Low signal on T1-weighted image (WI), high signal on T2WI, slightly brighter than CSF on both T1WI and T2WI.
- On fluid-attenuated inversion recovery sequence, epidermoid cysts show mixed iso- to hypersignal intensities, but with poor demarcation.

✓ Pearls and ✗ Pitfalls

- ✓ The presence of keratin in the epidermoid cysts give the characteristic appearance on diffusion images. Because keratin shows high signal on T2WI and cannot be diffused, it appears bright on DWI and shows a positive apparent diffusion coefficient map.
- ✗ Unusual patterns of epidermoid cysts:
  - "White epidermoids" have a rich protein content and appear with homogeneous high signal intensity on T1WI and low signal intensity on T2WI.
  - Intracystic hemorrhage within an epidermoid cyst causes heterogeneous signal intensities due to blood products.
- ✗ Malignant transformation into squamous cell carcinoma should be considered in case of frank contrast enhancement.

Case 58

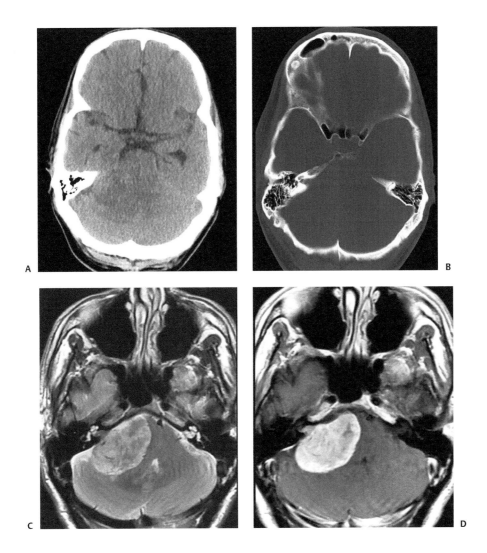

■ Clinical Presentation

A 38-year-old man presents with progressive right hearing loss.

■ Imaging Findings

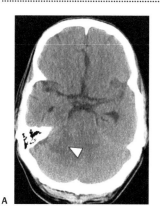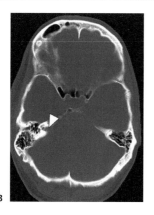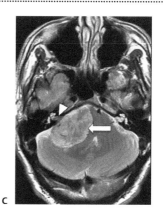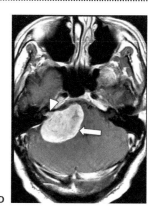

(A) CT image without contrast shows an ill-defined hypodense lesion (*arrowhead*) in the right cerebellopontine angle (CPA). There is effacement of the fourth ventricle. **(B)** CT image without contrast in bone window shows dilatation of the right internal auditory canal (IAC) (*arrowhead*). **(C)** Axial T2-weighted image (WI) shows a well-defined hyperintense mass in the right CPA with central flow voids (*arrow*). The lesion extends into the right IAC (*arrowhead*). **(D)** Axial T1WI with contrast shows homogeneous enhancement in the right CPA mass (*arrow*). The extension into the expanded right IAC canal is also evident (*arrowhead*).

■ Differential Diagnosis

- **Vestibular schwannoma:**
  - Well-defined mass that originates in the internal auditory canal (IAC) and extends to the cerebellopontine angle (CPA).
  - 70 to 80% of CPA lesions.
  - "Ice cream cone" configuration.
  - Increased T2 signal with diffuse enhancement.
  - No dural tail.
  - Depending on the size, these lesions may expand the IAC.
  - Microhemorrhage seen on the T2* image.
- *Meningioma:*
  - Second most common CPA mass.
  - Avidly enhancing CPA mass that arises from the dura of the dorsal petrous apex.
  - Rarely extends to the IAC.
  - Dural tail.
  - Calcifications are frequent.
  - Does not hemorrhage.
  - Underlying periosteal reaction/sclerosis.
- *Epidermoid inclusion cyst:*
  - 5% of CPA masses.
  - Follows the signal of cerebrospinal fluid (CSF) on T1-weighted image (WI) and T2WI.
  - Does not enhance.
  - "Dirty" (heterogeneous) fluid-attenuated inversion recovery (FLAIR) signal.
  - Vessels and nerves cross through it.
  - Increased DWI with low apparent diffusion coefficient values consistent with restricted diffusion due to keratin content.

■ Essential Facts

- Schwannomas are benign tumors derived from Schwann cells.
- If located in the CPA, these typically affect the vestibular nerve but can affect the acoustic and facial nerves as well. They arise near the porus acusticus and extend to the IAC and the CPA.
- If small, they are confined to the canalicular segment of the affected nerve.

■ Other Imaging Findings

- May be undetectable on CT image without contrast. As they grow, they remodel and expand the IAC.
- T2WI: Most show increased signal with central flow voids. Mural cysts can be present.
- A low percentage can trap CSF and create an arachnoid cyst.
- T1 with contrast: Avid enhancement.
- Gradient echo image can show the areas of hemorrhage as susceptibility artifact in 1 to 2% of cases.

✓ Pearls and ✗ Pitfalls

- ✓ Schwannomas do not tend to calcify.
- ✓ Always examine the contralateral IAC: if another schwannoma is seen, consider neurofibromatosis type 2.
- ✓ Patients with vestibular schwannomas can show increased cochlear signal on 3D FLAIR image due to increased concentration of proteins in the perilymphatic space.
- ✗ If a labyrinthine segment tail is noted, favor a facial schwannoma.
- ✗ Malignant transformation is rare.

Case 59

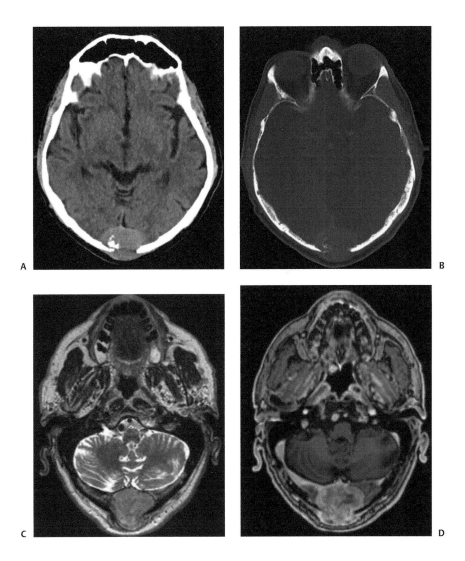

■ Clinical Presentation

A 64-year-old man presents with a painless skull mass.

■ Imaging Findings

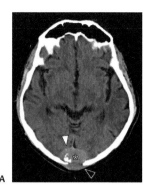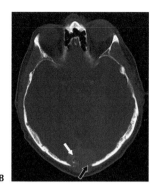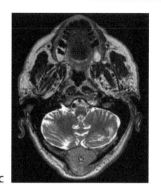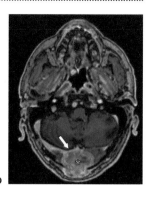

(A) Axial noncontrast CT image, brain window, shows a slightly hyperdense calvarial mass (*asterisk*) at the midline in the occipital region with extension to the epidural space (*white arrowhead*) as well as to the subcutaneous soft tissues of the scalp (*black arrowhead*). **(B)** Axial noncontrast CT image, bone window, better shows the associated bony destruction. The edges of the calvarium adjacent to the mass are irregular and nonsclerotic (*black arrow*), and there are small calcifications between the mass itself (*white arrow*), likely reflecting normal bone fragments caught within the mass rather than a frank osseous matrix. **(C)** Axial T2-weighted MR image obtained a couple of weeks later shows interval growth of the calvarial mass (*asterisk*), which demonstrates isointense signal and has well-defined contours. **(D)** Axial T1 postcontrast MR image shows heterogeneous enhancement within the mass (*asterisk*), which is located adjacent to the torcular insertion and slightly displaces the transverse sinuses (*white arrow*).

■ Differential Diagnosis

- **Plasmacytoma:** Plasmacytomas are the solitary form of multiple myeloma, which accounts for the most common malignant primary neoplasm of bone in adults, and they have a special predisposition for the axial skeleton. These masses are lytic and can cause expansion or frank cortical destruction.
- *Metastasis:* After age 50, bone metastases are the most commonly encountered malignant bone tumor. Lesions are typically asymptomatic and can be osteoblastic, osteolytic, or of mixed behavior on imaging. Furthermore, metastatic lesions can be either solitary or multiple.
- *Primary sarcoma of the skull:* Primary sarcomas of the calvarium are generally uncommon and include, among others, osteosarcoma, angiosarcoma, and chondrosarcoma. Sarcomas are aggressive-appearing masses with soft tissue components that involve both intra- and extracranial compartments, exhibit periosteal reaction, and form osseous or chondroid matrices, according to the corresponding subtype.

■ Essential Facts

- In general, calvarial lesions can be subdivided into benign or malignant.
- The location, number of lesions, patterns of destruction, contours, and associated findings (e.g., soft tissue components, periosteal reaction, matrix) serve to narrow down the differential diagnosis.
- Plasmacytomas can arise in any bone but are particularly common in the spine and other flat bones with high red-marrow content, including the skull, ribs, sternum, and clavicles.

- In general, these tumors are more common in males and have a peak incidence between the 4th and 6th decades of life.
- Lesions are generally solitary, osteolytic, and have no adjacent sclerosis.
- The adjacent cortex can demonstrate either expansion or destruction.
- Bone marrow biopsy or aspirate is required to establish the diagnosis.
- On MR imaging, plasmacytomas are generally hypo- to isointense on T1-weighted images, iso- to hyperintense on T2-weighted images, and show variable patterns of enhancement.

■ Other Imaging Findings

- The appearance on MRI scans has sometimes been referred to as a "mini brain" because of thin curvilinear hypointensities in the mass that simulate cerebral sulci.
- Imaging is fundamental in establishing tumor burden and response to treatment.

✓ Pearls and ✗ Pitfalls

✓ Plasmacytoma is the solitary form of multiple myeloma.
✓ Masses are generally lytic, expansile, and involve flat bones.
✓ The margins are characteristically nonsclerotic.
✗ An assessment of the bony skeleton is fundamental in establishing true tumor burden.
✗ The detection of the "mini brain" appearance in spinal lesions has been thought to be sufficiently pathognomonic so as to obviate the need for biopsy.

Case 60

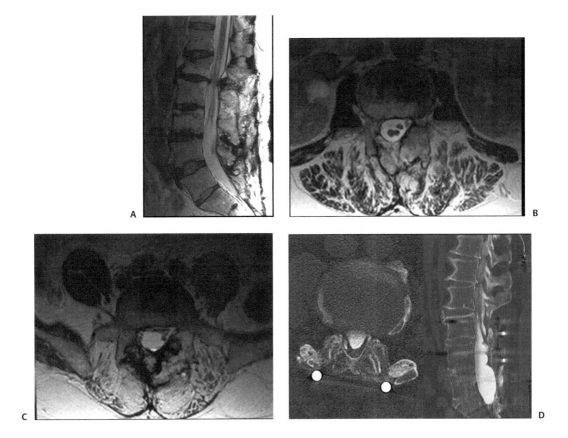

■ Clinical Presentation

A 76-year-old with a history of back surgery presents with pain and paresthesia in the lower extremities.

■ Imaging Findings

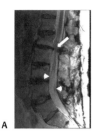
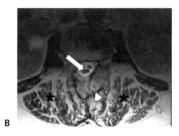
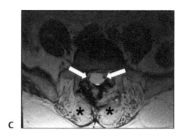
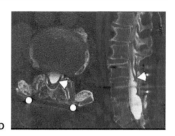

(A) Sagittal T2-weighted image (WI) demonstrates narrowing of the spinal canal at L1 with crowding of the roots of the cauda equina (*arrow*). There is an irregular distribution of the nerve roots more distally (*arrowheads*). **(B)** Axial T2WI at the level of L3 demonstrates thickened nerve roots (*arrow*). Postoperative changes in the posterior elements with fused bone grafts are noted (*arrowhead*). There is atrophy of the paraspinal muscles (*asterisks*). **(C)** Axial T2WI at the level of L5 demonstrates a peripheral distribution of the thickened nerve roots, which are adherent to the thecal sac (*arrows*). There is atrophy of the paraspinal muscles (*asterisks*). **(D)** Axial and sagittal images of a CT myelogram demonstrate changes of posterior decompression and fusion. Peripheral distribution of the nerve roots in the distal thecal sac (*arrowheads*) creates the so-called empty thecal sac appearance.

■ Differential Diagnosis

- ***Adhesive arachnoiditis:***
  - Postinflammatory changes in the cauda equina.
  - Thickening and clumping of nerve roots.
  - Adhesion of nerve roots to the peripheral dura ("empty sac" sign).
  - Soft tissue mass (pseudomass).
  - History of lumbar surgery, trauma, spinal meningitis, spinal anesthesia.
- *Failed back surgery syndrome:*
  - Clinical entity referring to the persistence or reappearance of pain after surgery on the spine.
  - This term encompasses both mechanical and nonmechanical causes.
  - Etiologies include stenosis, instability, pseudoarthrosis, recurrent herniation, fibrosis, and arachnoiditis.
- *Arachnoiditis ossificans:*
  - Ossification of the leptomeninges due to chronic inflammation of arachnoid cell clusters, most frequently located in the thoracic spine.
  - The ossification of the arachnoid has been classified into three different types: Type I has a semicircular or "bananalike" appearance most often along the dorsal aspect of the spinal cord, type II is more circular and circumferentially surrounds the thecal sac, and type III is characterized by a "honeycomb" pattern in which the thecal sac is traversed by the calcifications and may encase individual nerve roots.

■ Essential Facts

- The inflammation of the arachnoid mater may produce a fibrinous exudate around the roots that causes them to adhere to the dural sheath.
- Spinal cord tethering and cerebrospinal fluid (CSF) flow disturbance are two major features in the pathophysiology of spinal adhesive arachnoiditis.

■ Other Imaging Findings

- Small area of the thecal sac, which is filled by soft tissue consistent with clumped or matted nerve roots.
- Concentric contraction in the arachnoid and surrounding dura.
- Myelography:
  - Irregularity and narrowing of the subarachnoid space, obliteration of nerve root sleeves, apparent thickening of nerve roots, irregular distribution of introduced contrast medium with loculation and cyst formation, and impaired mobility of injected contrast.
  - Partial or complete CSF blockage.

✓ Pearls and ✗ Pitfalls

- ✓ Radiologic findings of adhesive arachnoiditis may be present without clinical symptoms.
- ✗ Other causes of thickened nerve roots with enhancement include carcinomatous meningitis (also known as leptomeningeal carcinomatosis), intradural metastases, and Guillain–Barré syndrome.
- ✗ Thickened nerve roots without adhesion or enhancement must raise the suspicion of Charcot–Marie–Tooth type I or Déjèrine–Sottas disease.

Case 61

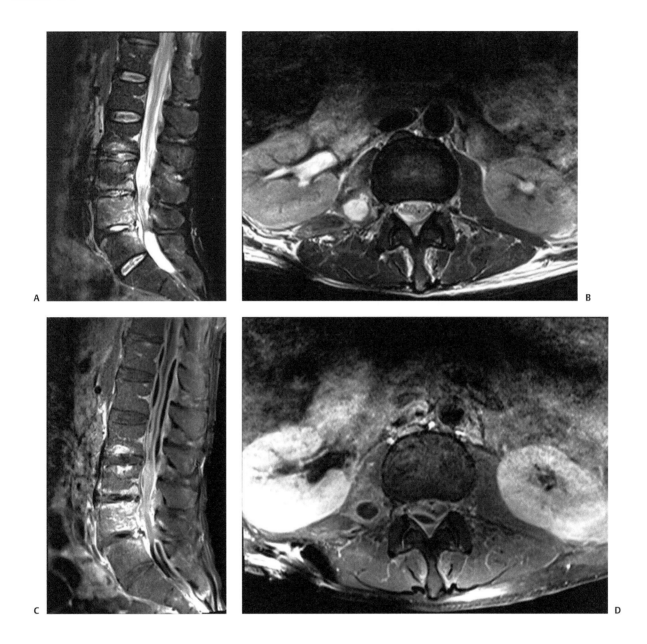

Clinical Presentation

A 60-year-old man presents with severe back pain and recent bladder dysfunction. The patient is currently undergoing treatment for spondylodiskitis.

■ Imaging Findings

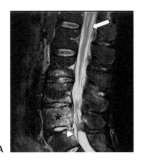
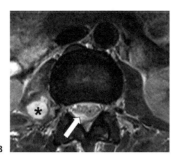
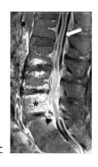
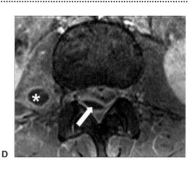

(A) Sagittal short T1 inversion recovery image of the lumbar spine shows increased signal in the L3–L5 vertebral bodies (*asterisk*). The spinal canal demonstrates irregular T2 hyperintensities anterior and posterior to the cauda equina (*arrow*). This T2 hyperintensity extends to the anterior epidural space and is contiguous with the L4/L5 intervertebral disk (*arrowhead*). **(B)** Axial T2-weighted image of the spine shows an anterior and posterolateral epidural fluid collection (*arrow*). An abscess is noted in the right psoas muscle (*asterisk*). **(C)** Fat-saturated sagittal T1 image with contrast shows enhancement of the L2–L5 vertebral bodies (*asterisk*). A phlegmon extends to the anterior epidural space adjacent to the L4/L5 intervertebral disk (*arrowhead*). An anterior and posterior epidural fluid collection with peripheral enhancement is noted throughout the lumbar spine (*arrow*). **(D)** Axial T1 image with contrast shows the anterior and posterior epidural fluid collections consistent with abscesses (*arrow*). An isolated abscess is noted on the right psoas muscle (*asterisk*).

■ Differential Diagnosis

• ***Spinal epidural abscess:***
  ○ Fluid collection inside of the spinal canal outside of the dura mater.
  ○ Narrows the spinal canal.
  ○ Increased T2 signal.
  ○ Can be associated with osteomyelitis or paraspinal infection.
  ○ Avid enhancement of the walls, thick capsule.
  ○ Extends along two to nine vertebral segments.
  ○ Diffuse abnormal T2 signal of the paraspinal soft tissues.
• *Epidural spinal hematoma:*
  ○ Intraspinal fluid collection outside of the dura mater.
  ○ Location is posterolateral or anterior.
  ○ Signal on MR image depends on age of hemorrhage.
  ○ It usually extends beyond three consecutive vertebral segments.
  ○ Can have marginal enhancement.
  ○ Most frequent cause is trauma.
• *Epidural lymphoma:*
  ○ Epidural lymphomas correspond to 9% of all the spinal epidural tumors. Primary spinal epidural lymphoma (PSEL) is a subset of lymphomas, in which there are no other recognizable sites of disease at the time of diagnosis.
  ○ Within the spinal canal, the location of the tumor is usually dorsal rather than ventral.
  ○ PSEL is usually isointense on T1-weighted image (WI) and iso- to hyperintense on T2WI, with marked contrast enhancement.
  ○ Occasionally, MRI demonstrates an extraforaminal component.

■ Essential Facts

• Spina epidural abscesses are a frequent complication of spondylodiskitis or osteomyelitis of the vertebral body.
• The primary source of infection is usually the vertebral body or disk, followed by the facet joint and the perivertebral soft tissues.
• The center of the abscess has fluid signal with thick peripheral enhancement.
• As many as 80% of epidural abscesses are anterior in location.
• *Staphylococcus aureus* and tuberculosis are the most frequent pathogens.

■ Other Imaging Findings

• MRI is the best diagnostic tool; it should include a T1WI with gadolinium and fat saturation.
• Abscesses are hyperintense on T2WI, may be hyperintense on diffusion-weighted image with low apparent diffusion coefficient signal.
• Fluid surrounded by thickened walls generate mass effect that can cause spinal cord or cauda equina nerve root compression.

✓ Pearls and ✗ Pitfalls

✓ Up to 30% of epidural abscesses are of unknown origin.
✓ The lack of early diagnosis may lead to a fatal outcome.
✓ Look for a lesion in the adjacent soft tissues, like the psoas abscess in the current case.
✗ Carefully explore the contours of the thecal sac if suspecting epidural abscess; the diagnosis is challenging in the noncontrasted images.
✗ There is an increased risk of epidural abscess in patients with indwelling catheters.
✗ CT imaging may not show the pathology.
✗ Epidural lesions are easily missed on CT image.

Case 62

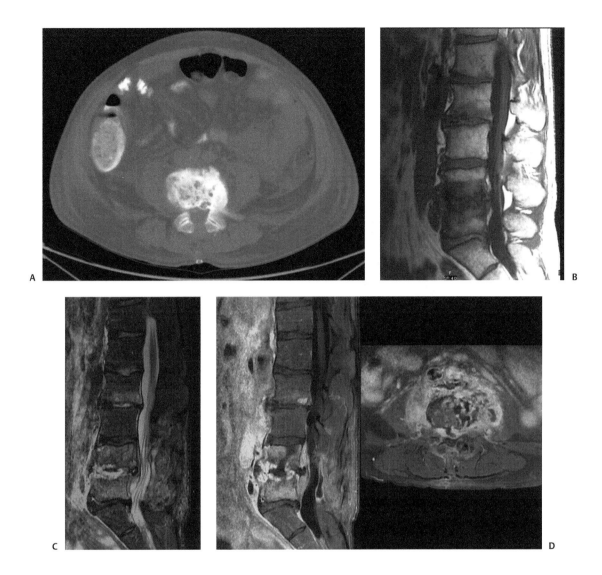

Clinical Presentation

A 52-year-old man presents with fever and back pain following lumbar spine surgery.

■ Imaging Findings

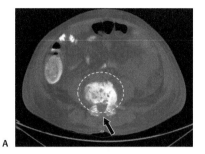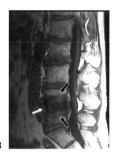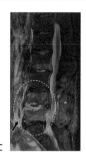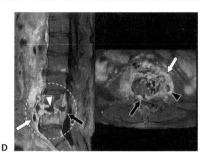

A   B   C   D

(A) Axial CT image through the abdomen, bone window, shows postoperative changes of bilateral laminectomies at the lower lumbar level (*black arrow*). There is collapse of the L4–L5 intervertebral disk with sclerosis of the L4 and L5 end plates (*circle*). **(B)** Sagittal T1 image demonstrates collapse of the L4–L5 intervertebral disk with end plate irregularity (*white arrow*). There is decreased signal at the end plates and the adjacent L4 and L5 vertebral bodies (*black arrows*). **(C)** Sagittal short tau inversion recovery image of the lumber spine shows edema involving the L4 and L5 vertebral bodies and L4–L5 disk (*oval*). There is heterogeneous prevertebral edema extending from L3 to the sacral spine and edema at the surgical site (*asterisk*). **(D)** Sagittal (*I*) and axial (*II*) T1 postcontrast images of the lumbar spine demonstrate enhancement of the L4 and L5 vertebral bodies and of the intervening disk (*circle*) with central hypointensity suggesting abscess formation (*white arrowhead*). There is ventral epidural enhancement causing moderate spinal canal stenosis (*black arrows*). Also, heterogeneous enhancement of the prevertebral soft tissues (*white arrows*) with small areas of lack of enhancement consistent with small abscesses (*black arrowhead*).

■ Differential Diagnosis

- **Bacterial spondylodiskitis:** Pyogenic disk space infection that attacks the end plate in adults and the disk edge in children. This process involves the disk and adjacent vertebral bodies, resulting in edema, enhancement, and inflammation that may extend to the perivertebral space and epidural compartment.
- *Tuberculous spondylitis (Pott disease):* Most common site of musculoskeletal involvement from tuberculosis (TB). The infection often spreads along the subligamentous compartment underlying the anterior longitudinal ligament and involves multiple levels. In general, it relatively spares the intervertebral disks in the early stages of the infection. There is irregularity that predominantly affects the anterior aspect of the vertebral body and end plate.
- *Degenerative spondylosis:* Degenerative disk disease may lead to collapse of disk height with edematous end plate changes (Modic type I) and even inflammatory enhancement. However, the extensive involvement of the prevertebral soft tissues and epidural space with small pockets of abscess formation make this diagnosis unlikely.

■ Essential Facts

- The lumbar spine is the most common site of involvement (50%), followed by the thoracic and then the cervical segments.
- Typically, only one level is affected, consisting of two vertebral bodies and their intervening disk.
- The most common causative organism is *Staphylococcus aureus*, accounting for 55 to 90% of cases.

- CT and radiographic images may be normal in early stages of the infection.
- Later in the course of the condition, CT and radiography can show end plate irregularity. Eventually, sclerosis of the affected bone may occur at 10 to 12 weeks.
- The involved level typically shows end plate irregularity with low signal intensity on T1 image, high signal intensity on T2 image, and variable enhancement, which may involve both the disk itself and the adjacent vertebral bone marrow.
- There can be phlegmon or abscess formation extending to the paravertebral soft tissues and to the epidural space.

■ Other Imaging Findings

- Restoration of normal fat signal in the bone marrow and reduction in the degree and extension of paravertebral enhancement are sensitive signs of treatment response.

✓ Pearls and ✗ Pitfalls

- ✓ In pyogenic spondylodiskitis, the disk space is involved early on in the course of the infection.
- ✓ The spread of disease occurs in a contiguous fashion.
- ✗ Clinical and imaging features may not always correlate. Although the patient may be clinically improving, vertebral and disk abnormalities can remain stable or even progress.
- ✗ Pyogenic infection from hematogenous seeding can affect solely the vertebral bodies with sparing of the intervertebral disk.

Case 63

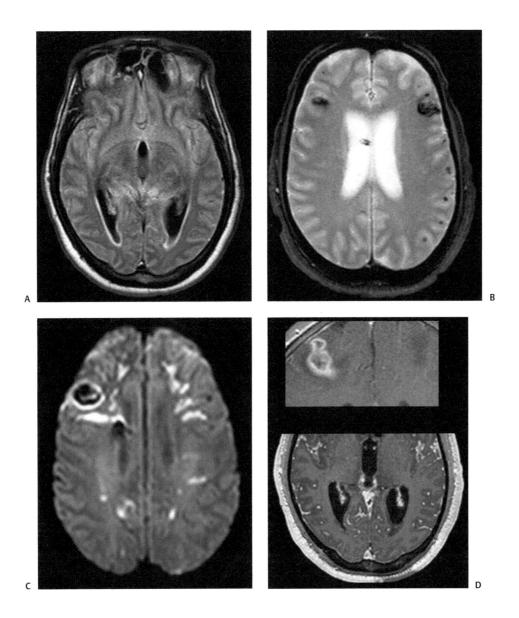

A 37-year-old immunosuppressed man presents in septic shock.

■ Imaging Findings

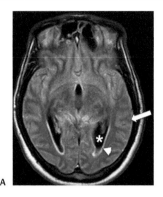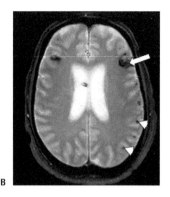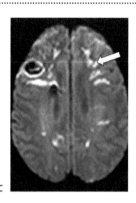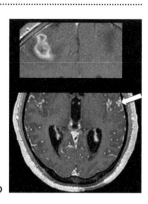

A   B   C   D

(A) Axial fluid-attenuated inversion recovery MR image shows effacement of the cerebral sulci with increased signal (*arrow*). The ventricles are dilated (*asterisk*), with periventricular white matter hyperintensity (*arrowhead*) consistent with hydrocephalus. **(B)** Axial gradient recalled image of the brain that shows multiple punctate areas of subcortical susceptibility (*arrowheads*) related to punctate hemorrhages. The lesions in the frontal lobes are larger (*arrow*). **(C)** Diffusion-weighted image shows multiple subcortical areas of restricted diffusion (*arrow*). **(D)** Axial T1-weighted image with contrast shows diffuse leptomeningeal enhancement (*arrow*). The *top image* shows irregular ring enhancement of one of the lesions related to septic emboli.

■ Differential Diagnosis

- ***Multiple cerebral septic emboli and meningitis:***
  - Hematogenous dissemination of septic emboli typically from cardiac valvular disease.
  - Multiple bilateral lesions in the territory of the middle cerebral artery involving terminal cortical branches.
  - Subcortical location.
  - Supratentorial more frequent than infratentorial.
  - Restricted diffusion due to ischemia.
  - Hemorrhage is common.
  - Nodular or ring enhancement.
  - Surrounding vasogenic edema.
- *Cerebral cryptococcosis:*
  - Diffuse meningeal involvement, with increased fluid-attenuated inversion recovery (FLAIR) signal, typically does not enhance.
  - Basal ganglia involvement with gelatinous pseudocysts.
  - Unusual in the subcortical white matter.
- *Cerebral lymphoma:*
  - Parenchymal disease that favors the basal ganglia presents as increased FLAIR signal and high cellularity seen as dark apparent diffusion coefficient maps.
  - Meningeal involvement, generally presenting as nodular enhancement, favors the basal cisterns.
  - Ependymal involvement is possible.

■ Essential Facts

- Septic emboli are common in patients with endocarditis.
- Doppler cardiac ultrasound is recommended.
- *Staphylococcus aureus* and *Streptococcus viridans* are the most common pathogens.
- In intravenous (IV) drug abusers, *Staphylococcus* and fungal septic emboli can occur.

■ Other Imaging Findings

- CT: Punctate areas of hypodensity. Hyperdense if hemorrhage is present.
- MRI:
  - T2: Vasogenic edema around a hyperintense lesion.
  - T1 with contrast: Nodular or ring enhancement.
  - FLAIR: Good for evaluating extension of vasogenic edema.
  - Diffusion-weighted image (DWI): Restricted diffusion in areas of ischemia and within abscesses.
  - Gradient echo (GRE): Susceptibility noted in areas of hemorrhage.

✓ Pearls and ✗ Pitfalls

- ✓ Hemorrhage is common in septic emboli.
- ✓ In IV drug abusers with intracranial hemorrhage, evaluation of the intracranial vasculature is warranted to exclude mycotic aneurysms.
- ✗ DWI and susceptibility-weighted imaging/GRE can help to differentiate between tumoral and nontumoral emboli to the brain.

Case 64

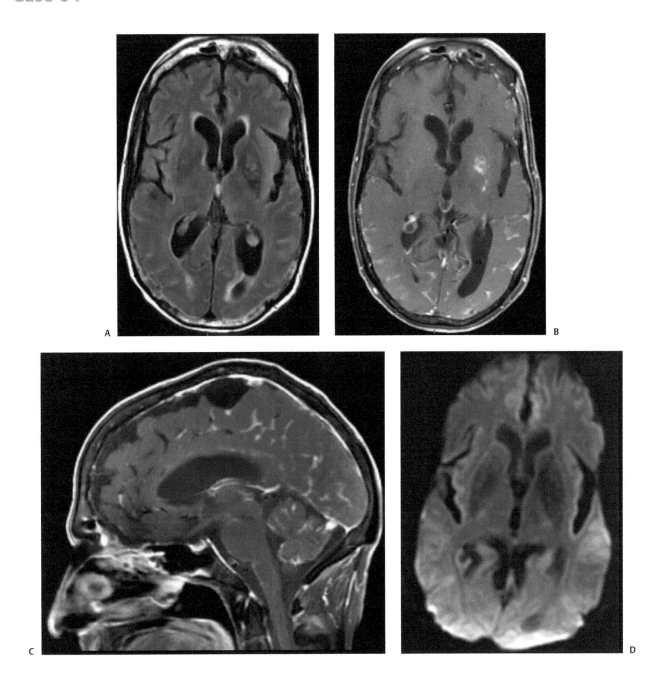

Clinical Presentation

A 54-year-old man presents with a history of chronic lymphoid leukemia.

■ Imaging Findings

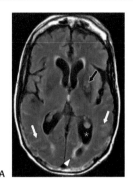 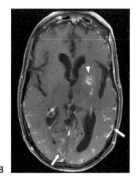 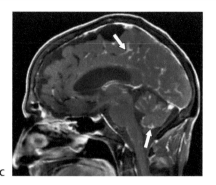 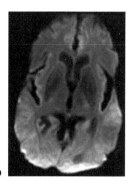

(A) Axial fluid-attenuated inversion recovery image shows diffusely increased signal intensity in the bilateral cerebral sulci, most pronounced in the temporal and occipital lobes (*white arrows*). There is an ill-defined focus of hyperintensity within the left lentiform nucleus (*black arrow*). The ventricles are diffusely prominent (*asterisk*) and there is transependymal flow of cerebrospinal fluid (*white arrowhead*). The diploic bone marrow shows hyperintensity in the occipital and parietal bones. **(B)** Axial T1 postcontrast image demonstrates thick nodular leptomeningeal enhancement predominantly in the posterior aspect of the bilateral cerebral hemispheres (*arrows*). There are small cystic lesions consistent with dilated perivascular spaces with peripheral enhancement in the left lentiform nucleus (*arrowhead*). **(C)** Sagittal T1 postcontrast image shows thick, nodular leptomeningeal enhancement involving the supra and infratentorial compartments (*arrows*). **(D)** Axial diffusion-weighted image shows no abnormal restricted diffusion.

■ Differential Diagnosis

- **Fungal meningitis:** Central nervous system (CNS) infection seen more commonly in the immunocompromised host. Caused by leptomeningeal infiltration of fungal pathogens with primary infectious foci generally in the lung or intestine. On imaging, the characteristic feature is thick, nodular leptomeningeal enhancement.
- *Leukemic infiltration of the meninges:* Invasion of the meninges due to leukemia may occur secondary to hematogenous spread or by direct invasion from adjacent affected bone marrow. This condition is more common in patients with acute forms of leukemia (acute myeloid leukemia and acute lymphoid leukemia). Diagnosis is determined by the detection of leukemic cells in cerebrospinal fluid (CSF). Radiographically, leptomeningeal involvement may be focal or diffuse and is generally multinodular in appearance.
- *Pyogenic meningitis:* Infectious disease of the CNS caused by bacterial pathogens and radiographically resulting in thin, linear leptomeningeal enhancement rather than thick, nodular enhancement. Diffusion-weighted imaging may demonstrate restricted diffusion in the cerebral sulci if purulent material has accumulated in the extra-axial space.

■ Essential Facts

- Fungi can be divided intro three categories: yeasts, molds, and dimorphic fungi.
- Yeast: *Cryptococcus* (most common fungal disease of CNS) and *Candida*.
- Molds: *Aspergillus* and *Mucorales*.
- Dimorphic fungi: *Blastomyces*, *Coccidioides*, and *Histoplasma*.
- Generally seen in patients with history of diabetes, AIDS, and/or organ transplantation.

- The most common pathogens in CNS fungal infections are *Cryptococcus*, followed by *Aspergillus* and *Candida*.
- CNS fungal infections that present primarily as meningitis include *Cryptococcus, Coccidioides, Blastomyces*, and *Histoplasma*.
- Meningitis is a single manifestation within a spectrum of manifestations seen in fungal CNS infections.
- In general, there may be parenchymal or meningeal involvement. Diagnosis is established by detection of fungi in CSF or by biopsy in the case of parenchymal masses.
- Thick, linear leptomeningeal enhancement tends to occur at the skull base.

■ Other Imaging Findings

- Obstruction of arachnoid granulations may result in hydrocephalus.
- Clusters of cysts in the basal ganglia and thalami due to accumulation of gelatinous material within perivascular spaces strongly suggests *Cryptococcus* as the causative agent.

✓ Pearls and ✗ Pitfalls

- ✓ Access to the CNS may be gained by hematogenous spread, CSF infection, or direct spread from sinonasal disease.
- ✓ Each pathogen demonstrates characteristic imaging features; however, microbiologic detection of the yeast or fungus is required for definite diagnosis.
- ✓ Some fungal meningitis processes are angiocentric and may present with multiple strokes.
- ✗ Due to the fact that patients are generally immunocompromised, imaging findings can show little to no inflammatory response.
- ✗ Cross-sectional imaging is not specific or sensitive in the detection of meningitis.

Case 65

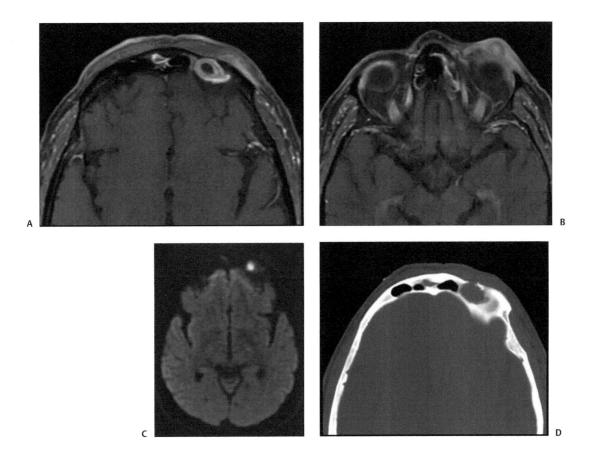

■ Clinical Presentation

An 18-year-old man presents with sinusitis for 1 year and an enlarged eyelid for 3 weeks.

■ Imaging Findings

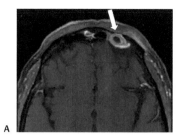 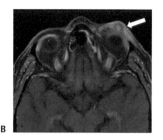 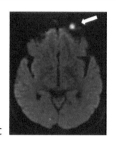 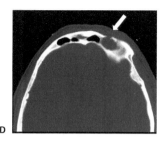

A   B   C   D

(A) Axial T1-weighted image (WI) with contrast demonstrates enhancing mucosal thickening in the left frontal sinus (*arrow*) causing thinning of the outer table and enhancement in the adjacent soft tissues. **(B)** Axial T1WI with contrast demonstrates an enhancing soft tissue collection on the left eyelid (*arrow*). **(C)** Axial diffusion-weighted image shows restricted diffusion in the center of the lesion in the left eyelid (*arrow*). **(D)** Axial CT image demonstrates complete opacification of the left frontal sinus, with bone erosion of the outer table and adjacent soft tissue swelling (*arrow*).

■ Differential Diagnosis

- **Pott's puffy tumor:** Pott's puffy tumor is a rare complication of frontal sinusitis, resulting in subperiosteal abscess of the frontal bone with underlying osteomyelitis.
- *Mucocele:*
  ○ Paranasal sinus mucoceles occur as a result of obstruction of the ostium of a sinus due to inflammation, trauma, mass lesion, among others, with resultant accumulation of mucus and eventual expansion of the sinus.
  ○ Frontal mucoceles may extend into the orbit and present as a mass.
- *Nasal glioma:*
  ○ Also known as nasal glial heterotopia.
  ○ Rare congenital lesion composed of dysplastic glial cells that have lost their intracranial connections and present as an extranasal or intranasal mass.
  ○ Clinically present in early infancy or childhood as a firm, red to bluish skin-covered mass.

■ Essential Facts

- Frontal osteomyelitis with associated subperiosteal abscess of the frontal bone.
- It is most commonly due to frontal sinusitis and may spread due to frontal sinus trauma, hematogenous spread of sinusitis, or retrograde thrombophlebitis via the diploic veins of Galen.
- It has also been described secondary to mastoiditis, insect bites, malignancy, and acupuncture.

■ Other Imaging Findings

- CT of the brain is the study of choice. It identifies intra- and extracranial complications associated with frontal sinusitis.
- MRI scan with gadolinium may help to further elucidate the intracranial extent of the disease.

✓ Pearls and ✗ Pitfalls

- ✓ The frontal sinuses develop from the ethmoid air cells and approach adult size between 12 and 13 years of age. The diploic veins are responsible for the venous drainage of the frontal sinus. Pott's puffy tumor tends to be a complication of frontal sinusitis in older children (preteen and teenage boys) because adolescence is the time when the vascularity of the diploic veins peaks.
- ✗ Pott's puffy tumor can spread inward, leading to intracranial or epidural abscess formation, cortical vein thrombosis, and subdural empyema. The intracranial structures need to be evaluated thoroughly.

Case 66

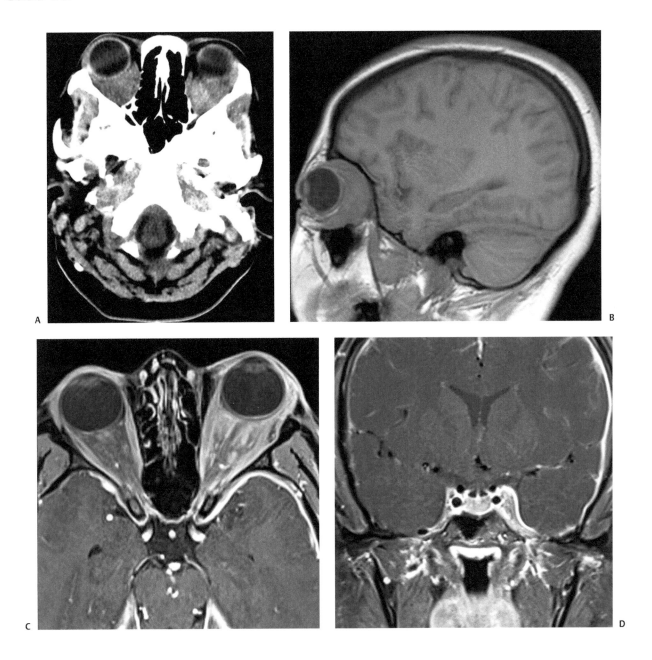

■ Clinical Presentation

A 31-year-old with antiphospholipid syndrome presents with left eye pain and proptosis.

■ Imaging Findings

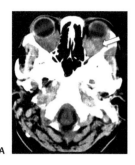 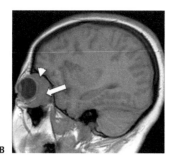 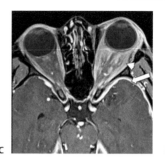 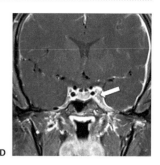

(A) Axial CT image without contrast shows increased density in the left intraconal space (*arrow*). (B) Sagittal T1-weighted image (WI) without contrast shows isointense lesion in the intraconal space (*arrow*) and the extraocular muscles (*arrowhead*) with expansile characteristics. (C) Axial T1 image with contrast demonstrates enhancement of the left orbit and of the extraocular muscles (*arrowhead*). The dura mater shows diffuse thick enhancement (*arrow*). (D) Coronal T1WI with contrast shows thickening and bulging of the lateral wall of the left cavernous sinus with enhancement (*arrow*).

■ Differential Diagnosis

• ***Idiopathic orbital inflammation (pseudotumor) and Tolosa–Hunt syndrome (THS):***
  ○ Ill-defined enhancing mass that can involve different spaces in the orbit.
  ○ Hypointense on T2-weighted image (WI) when associated with immunoglobulin G4 (IgG4).
  ○ Enhances with contrast.
  ○ THS consists of when it extends into the cavernous sinus and is associated with acute painful ophthalmoplegia.
  ○ Bilateral in 25% of cases.
• *Lymphoma:*
  ○ Mass with lobulated margins involving different structures of the orbit; the lacrimal gland is most frequently affected with diffuse enhancement.
  ○ Slightly hyperintense to muscle in T2WI.
  ○ Typically there is bilateral involvement.
  ○ Can be primary or secondary lymphoma, mostly non-Hodgkin type.
  ○ Clinical presentation is nonacute and painful.
• *Sarcoidosis:*
  ○ May affect multiple orbital structures favoring the optic nerve sheath and extending to the optic chiasm. Can present with uveitis.
  ○ Does not present as acute pain.
  ○ Intracranial disease favors the cisternal aspect of cranial nerves. Leptomeningeal disease follows the pia mater.
  ○ Basal ganglia involvement occurs through the perivascular spaces.

■ Essential Facts

• Chronic inflammatory disease of unknown origin.
• THS is defined as painful ophthalmoplegia combined with oculomotor palsies and sensory loss of the ophthalmic division of the trigeminal nerve.

■ Other Imaging Findings

• Pseudotumor can affect the orbit in multiple locations:
  ○ Diffuse orbital involvement.
  ○ Lacrimal gland.
  ○ Preseptal region.
  ○ Apical region with extension to the cavernous sinus.

✓ Pearls and ✗ Pitfalls

✓ THS is specific for patients with orbital pseudotumor extending to the cavernous sinus and presenting with acute painful ophthalmoplegia. Other diseases with similar clinical presentation include trauma, neoplasm, aneurysm, and inflammation.
✗ Orbital pseudotumor is a diagnosis of exclusion.
✗ THS can present with stenosis of the cavernous portion of the internal carotid artery.

Case 67

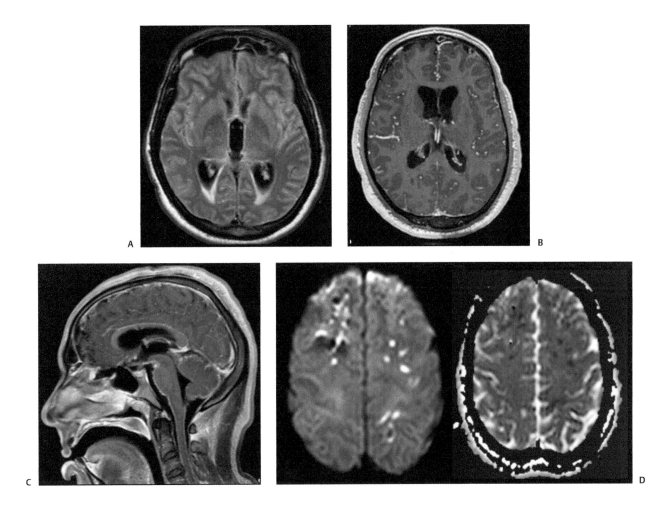

■ Clinical Presentation

A 38-year-old man with a history of HIV presents with septic shock.

■ Imaging Findings

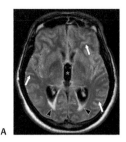 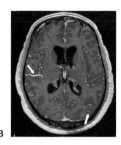 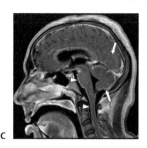 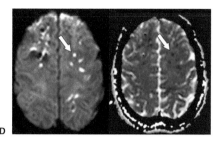

(A) Axial T2 fluid-attenuated inversion recovery image shows diffusely increased signal intensity in the cerebral sulci (*white arrows*). Additionally, there is dilatation of the third ventricle (*asterisk*) and lateral ventricles, with transependymal flow of cerebrospinal fluid (*black arrowheads*). **(B)** T1 postcontrast image demonstrates diffuse, extensive leptomeningeal enhancement (*arrows*). **(C)** Sagittal T1 postcontrast image shows diffuse leptomeningeal enhancement of both the supra- and infratentorial compartments (*arrows*) as well as lining the brainstem and superior cervical spine (*arrowheads*). **(D)** Diffusion-weighted image and corresponding apparent diffusion coefficient map show multiple focal areas of restricted diffusion in the centrum semiovale bilaterally (*arrows*).

■ Differential Diagnosis

- **Pyogenic meningitis:** Infectious disease of the central nervous system caused by bacterial pathogens and radiographically resulting in thin, linear leptomeningeal enhancement. This case demonstrates two described complications of bacterial meningitis: hydrocephalus and thrombosis with microinfarcts.
- *Leptomeningeal carcinomatosis:* Leptomeningeal carcinomatosis corresponds to the infiltration of the leptomeninges by malignant cells. Much like pyogenic meningitis, leptomeningeal carcinomatosis exhibits leptomeningeal enhancement. However, enhancement in leptomeningeal carcinomatosis tends to be thicker and more nodular in appearance.
- *Nonpyogenic infectious meningitis (i.e., viral, fungal, mycobacterial):* Viral, fungal, and mycobacterial pathogens can also spread to the meninges. Although viral and bacterial meningitis typically present as linear leptomeningeal enhancement, fungal meningitis is similar to leptomeningeal carcinomatosis in that it is more nodular/lumpier in appearance. Tuberculous meningitis shows enhancement centered near the basal cisterns and skull base.

■ Essential Facts

- Pyogenic meningitis can occur due to hematogenous spread of infection, from direct inoculation secondary to trauma or surgery, or from neighboring infections (e.g., sinusitis, orbital cellulitis).
- The most common causative agents are *Haemophilus influenzae*, *Streptococcus pneumoniae*, and *Neisseria meningitidis*.
- Clinically, patients present with fever, headache, neck rigidity, and altered mental status.
- Common complications include cerebritis, abscess formation, hydrocephalus, thrombosis, infarcts, ventriculitis, and extra-axial collections such as empyemas.
- This condition is more common in the immunocompromised host.

■ Other Imaging Findings

- The primary utility of imaging is to evaluate for associated complications.
- Noncontrast CT imaging can show early signs of hydrocephalus. This modality is also useful for determining whether any neighboring infection is present as a source of contiguous spread.
- When exudates accumulate in the extra-axial space, this may cause effacement of normal low-density cerebrospinal fluid (CSF) on CT image within the cerebral sulci.
- MRI is the imaging modality of choice.
- Typical features of pyogenic meningitis include increased T2 signal in fluid-attenuated inversion recovery (FLAIR) images in the cerebral sulci secondary to purulent exudates in the CSF.
- Thin, linear enhancement of the leptomeninges is seen. This can be associated with diffusion restriction.

✓ Pearls and ✗ Pitfalls

- ✓ Despite adequate diagnosis and treatment, pyogenic meningitis has significant morbidity and mortality rates.
- ✓ Although imaging can suggest a diagnosis and a possible causative agent if certain classic patterns are identified, lumbar puncture is required for establishing a definitive diagnosis and establishing optimal treatment.
- ✓ Imaging can be normal in patients with meningitis.
- ✗ Due to the possibility of herniation, CT is recommended before lumbar puncture in patients with suspected bacterial meningitis.

Case 68

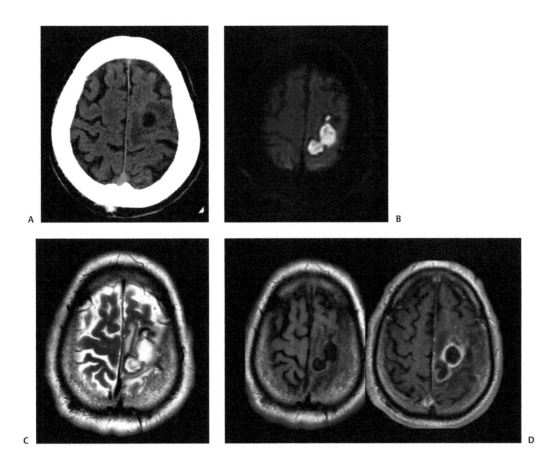

■ Clinical Presentation

A 67-year-old man with a past medical history of hypertension and type 2 diabetes mellitus presents with dysarthria and worsening right-sided weakness.

■ Imaging Findings

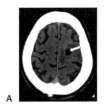 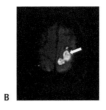 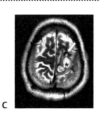 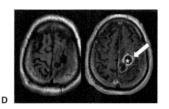

(A) Axial brain CT image shows a round hypoattenuating lesion with an isodense capsule in the left frontal lobe (*arrow*), surrounded by edema. (B) Axial diffusion-weighted image demonstrates restricted diffusion within the abscess cavity (*arrow*). Apparent diffusion coefficient (not shown) had corresponding signal dropout. (C) Axial T2-weighted image (WI) shows fluid signal in the center of the lesion (*asterisk*), whereas the peripheral capsule demonstrates low signal intensity (*arrow*). (D) Axial T1WI before and after contrast. Strong rim enhancement in the capsule of the lesion is noted (*arrow*). The necrotic center does not enhance (*asterisk*).

■ Differential Diagnosis

- ***Cerebral abscess:***
  - ○ Organized, late phase of brain infection.
  - ○ Bacterial infection is the most common cause.
  - ○ The most common location is the gray–white matter junction in the territory of the middle cerebral artery due to hematogenous spread.
  - ○ Ring enhancing lesion described as having smooth inner and outer margins.
  - ○ Surrounding edema.
  - ○ Restricted diffusion with apparent diffusion coefficient (ADC) correlation.
  - ○ Nodular or ring enhancement.
  - ○ Surrounding vasogenic edema.
- *Subacute hematoma:*
  - ○ The signal intensity of parenchymal hematomas evolves over time from the periphery to the center of the collection, with each phase of the degradation of blood products having a specific appearance in T1-weighted image (WI), T2WI, diffusion-weighted image (DWI), and gradient echo (GRE) T2* image.
  - ○ Oxyhemoglobin and extracellular methemoglobin molecules demonstrate increased signal on DWI with intermediate to low ADC signal. At these same two stages, T2* GRE images demonstrate intermediate signal intensity.
- *Metastasis:*
  - ○ Cortical or subcortical white matter.
  - ○ Multiple bilateral lesions in the territory of the middle cerebral artery.
  - ○ Surrounding vasogenic edema.
  - ○ Can have hemorrhage.
  - ○ Nodular or ring enhancement.
  - ○ Known primary.

■ Essential Facts

- Cerebral abscess occurs as a result of contiguous purulent spread (sinusitis, mastoiditis), hematogenous or metastatic spread (pulmonary infections and arteriovenous shunts, congenital heart disease and endocarditis, dental infections, and gastrointestinal infections), head trauma, neurosurgical procedure, and immunosuppression.

■ Other Imaging Findings

- CT: The capsule appears as an isodense rim around a hypodense center and with surrounding hypodense edema. The capsule enhances with contrast.
- MR: A smooth inner margin of the enhancing rim on contrast-enhanced images, the presence of satellite lesions, and a dark rim on T2WI are features that favor abscess over other rim-enhancing lesions.
- The dual rim sign favors abscess over necrotic glioblastomas:
  - ○ High-intensity ring on T2 representing granulation tissue surrounded by a ring of low signal corresponding to the abscess capsule.
  - ○ May be better appreciated on susceptibility-weighted image.
- MR spectroscopy findings: Absence of *N*-acetylaspartate, choline, and phosphocreatine:creatine ratio. Presence of cytosolic amino acids (leucine, isoleucine, and valine), lactate, acetate, succinate, and alanine, and occasionally lipids.

✓ Pearls and ✗ Pitfalls

- ✓ When DWI abnormalities are most pronounced along the periphery of a lesion (DWI ring lesions) the differential diagnosis should include progressive multifocal leukoencephalopathy, primary central nervous system lymphoma, cerebral toxoplasmosis, resolving cerebral hematoma, demyelinating lesions (multiple sclerosis, acute disseminated encephalomyelitis, Balo concentric sclerosis, and acute necrotizing encephalitis), and neoplastic lesions.
- ✗ In patients with recent brain surgery, the subacute blood products may appear similar to a cerebral abscess. Unexpected increase in the surrounding edema may be the first finding to raise suspicion of abscess formation.
- ✗ The presence of high-viscosity fluid and protein in the abscess conveys its typical appearance on DWI.

Case 69

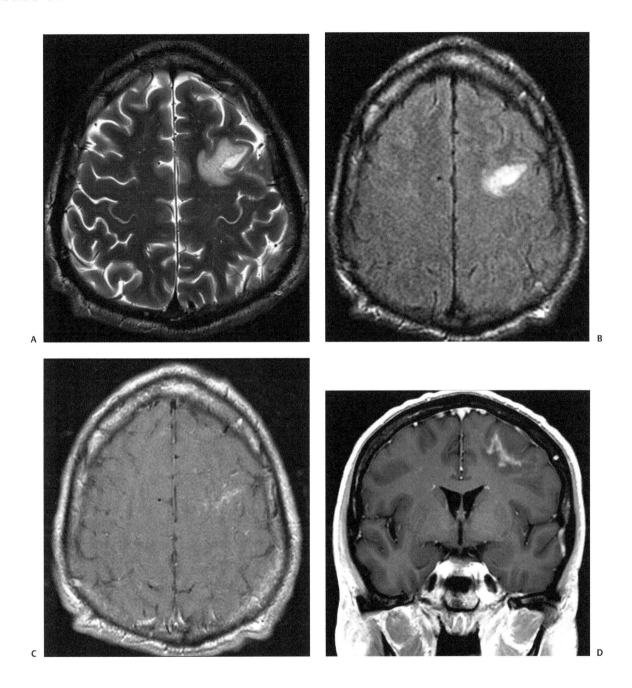

A 49-year-old patient who is HIV-positive, undergoing treatment with highly active antiretroviral therapy, now presents with cognitive decline.

■ Imaging Findings

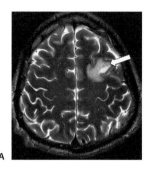
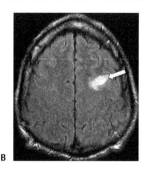
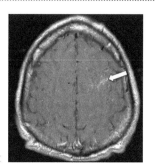
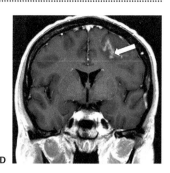

A   B   C   D

(A, B) Axial T2 **(A)** and fluid-attenuated inversion recovery **(B)** images of the brain demonstrate increased signal involving the subcortical white matter of the left frontal lobe (*arrows*). **(C, D)** Axial **(C)** and coronal **(D)** MR images of the brain with contrast show patchy enhancement of the left frontal lesion, more prominent in its medial aspect (*arrows*).

■ Differential Diagnosis

- ***Progressive multifocal leukoencephalopathy–immune reconstitution inflammatory syndrome (PML-IRIS):***
  - PML presents as patchy T2 and fluid-attenuated inversion recovery (FLAIR) image hyperintensities affecting mostly the subcortical white matter. It is bilateral and asymmetric.
  - The lesions rarely show faint enhancement in the periphery.
  - In some patients that recover immune function due to highly active antiretroviral therapy (HAART), lesions show a brisk inflammatory response known as IRIS. In this scenario, the lesions show patchy enhancement and mass effect.
- *Toxoplasmosis:*
  - Most common mass lesion in patients with AIDS.
  - Multiple ring enhancing lesions.
  - Location in the corticomedullary junction and basal ganglia.
  - Eccentric target sign enhancement.
  - Lesions do not extend to the ependymal surface.
  - Acute lesions can have vasogenic edema.
  - Occasional hemorrhage (helps differentiate from lymphoma).
- *Lymphoma:*
  - Basal ganglia and periventricular enhancing lesions.
  - Frequently affect the corpus callosum.
  - Can extend to the ependymal surface.
  - Vasogenic edema is less frequent.
  - No hemorrhage.

■ Essential Facts

- Demyelinating infection caused by the JC (John Cunningham) virus.
- The virus is activated in patients with cellular immunosuppression and infects oligodendrocytes.
- Can be seen in AIDS, in hematologic malignancies, or after the use of immunosuppressive drugs such as natalizumab.

■ Other Imaging Findings

- MRI is the best diagnostic tool for PML.
- Subcortical bilateral T2/FLAIR lesions without mass effect.
- Spares the cortex.
- Predilection for the supratentorial region (parietal and frontal lobes).
- Cortical atrophy (70%).
- Ventricular dilation (50%).
- Thalamic lesions (50%).
- No enhancement.
- Hypodense on CT.

✓ Pearls and ✗ Pitfalls

- ✓ The borders of the lesion may show a subtle rim of increased signal on diffusion-weighted imaging in the acute phases.
- ✓ The corpus callosum can be involved in some cases.
- ✗ Patients with HIV who develop PML-IRIS have a higher likelihood of surviving the PML than do HIV-positive patients who do not develop IRIS.

Case 70

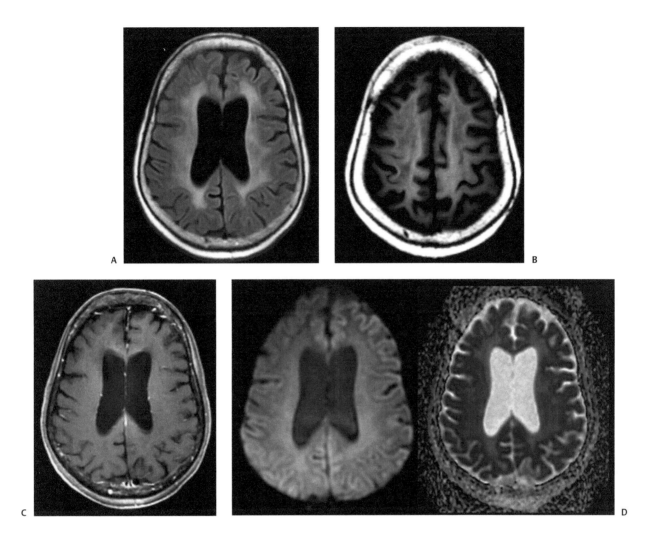

■ Clinical Presentation

A 47-year-old woman presents with a history of infection with HIV.

■ Imaging Findings

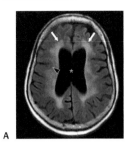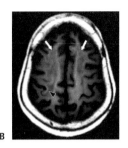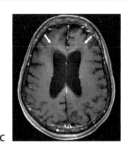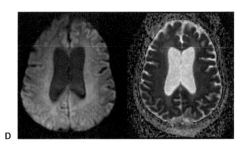

(A) Axial fluid-attenuated inversion recovery image shows symmetric, confluent areas of T2 hyperintensity involving the periventricular white matter (*white arrows*) and sparing the subcortical U fibers (*black arrowhead*). There is diffuse cerebral volume loss with prominence of the ventricles (*asterisk*) and cerebral sulci. **(B)** Axial T1-weighted image (WI) demonstrates areas of T1 prolongation within the white matter of the centrum semiovale with a predominance in the frontal lobes (*white arrows*). There is sparing of the subcortical U fibers (*black arrowhead*). **(C)** Axial T1 postcontrast image shows ill-defined areas of hypointensity in the periventricular white matter without mass effect or associated enhancement (*arrows*). **(D)** Diffusion-weighted image and corresponding apparent diffusion coefficient map do not demonstrate areas of abnormal restricted diffusion.

■ Differential Diagnosis

- **AIDS dementia complex:** AIDS dementia complex is a neurodegenerative condition seen in up to 15 to 20% of patients with AIDS. This syndrome is characterized by demyelination and gliosis of the white matter resulting in symmetric confluent periventricular T2 hyperintensities without mass effect or enhancement.
- *Chronic microangiopathic white matter changes:* Multifocal T2 hyperintense lesions usually seen in the subcortical and periventricular white matter and attributable to chronic small vessel ischemia. Initially, these lesions are punctate or nodular and can progress to confluent areas in advanced cases. Typically, this condition is seen in older patients with vascular risk factors such as hypertension and diabetes.
- *Radiation effects:* Delayed effects from whole-brain radiation can manifest as confluent areas of white matter T2 hyperintensity with variable volume loss secondary to gliosis. In patients with a history of HIV who develop central nervous system (CNS) lymphoma, radiation therapy is a common treatment and special attention must be paid to review the patient's chart for information regarding prior radiation.

■ Essential Facts

- Also known as HIV encephalitis, HIV encephalopathy, or HIV-associated dementia.
- Patients with AIDS dementia complex usually experience worsening cognitive and motor impairment.
- This condition represents one of the most common causes of morbidity in patients with AIDS in the United States.
- Occurs in the later stages of evolution of AIDS, especially in patients with CD4 counts < 200 cells/μL.

- Other risk factors include older age of seroconversion and prolonged duration of HIV infection.
- Histopathologically, disruption of the blood–brain barrier occurs due to monocyte proliferation. This allows the virus to infect microglial cells, which in turn activates an inflammatory response that leads to neural injury.
- Viral load within the CNS correlates with the severity of symptoms.

■ Other Imaging Findings

- CT demonstrates confluent periventricular areas of hypoattenuation.
- Typically, volume loss occurs that appears disproportionate to the patient's age.
- On MRI scan, these regions exhibit T1 and T2 prolongation.
- There is involvement of the deep and periventricular white matter with sparing of the subcortical white matter and of the posterior fossa.
- No mass effect or enhancement is identified.
- The frontal lobes are predominantly involved, and there can be extension to the genu of the corpus callosum.
- MR spectroscopy shows decreased *N*-acetylaspartate with increase in choline and myoinositol peaks.

✓ Pearls and ✗ Pitfalls

- ✓ If either mass effect or enhancement is identified, AIDS dementia complex is an unlikely diagnosis and another etiology should be considered.
- ✗ Highly active antiretroviral therapy may offer some improvement in white matter signal abnormality. Nevertheless, clinical and radiologic worsening may occur initially during treatment, prior to improvement.

Case 71

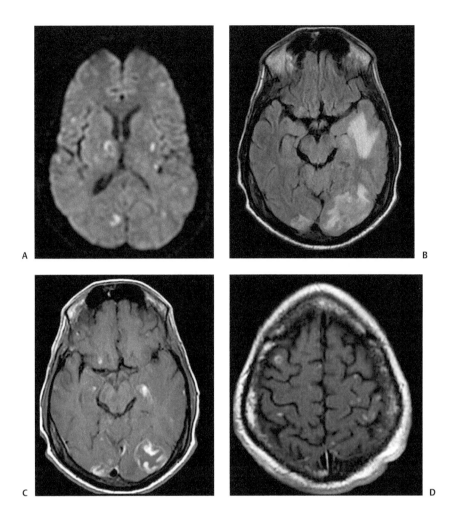

■ Clinical Presentation

A 48-year-old man presents with progressive headache, lethargy, and malaise over a period of 4 weeks.

■ Imaging Findings

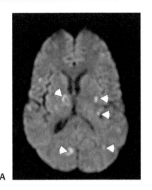 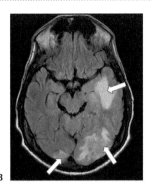 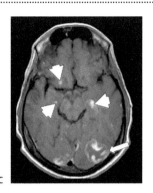 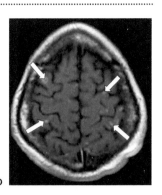

A   B   C   D

(A) Axial diffusion-weighted image (DWI) shows multiple foci of restricted diffusion in the right thalamus (*ring like*) and in the subcortical white matter in both cerebral hemispheres (*arrowheads*). **(B)** Axial fluid-attenuated inversion recovery image shows significant vasogenic edema around the lesions seen in the DWI sequence (*arrows*). **(C)** Axial T1-weighted image (WI) with contrast demonstrates peripheral enhancement in a lesion with central necrosis (*arrow*) and nodular enhancement in numerous other lesions (*arrowheads*). **(D)** Axial T1WI with contrast demonstrates multiple nodular enhancing in the cerebral cortex bilaterally (*arrows*).

■ Differential Diagnosis

- ***Cryptococcosis:***
  - Dilated perivascular spaces in deep gray nuclei of patients with AIDS, often without enhancement.
  - Miliary or leptomeningeal enhancing nodules and gelatinous pseudocysts.
  - Cryptococcoma: Ringlike or solid enhancement.
- *Toxoplasmosis:* The most common mass lesion in patients with AIDS. Multiple lesions with ring enhancement in the basal ganglia and corticomedullary junction. It does not extend to the ependymal surface.
- *Septic embolism:*
  - Infarcts in multiple arterial distributions from embolic source, often cardiac origin.
  - Frequently hemorrhagic.
  - May result in micro abscesses.

■ Essential Facts

- *Cryptococcus neoformans* is a fungus that causes opportunistic infection in HIV and other immunosuppressed patients.
- Cryptococci spread along the perivascular spaces and cause lesions in the basal ganglia, thalamus, brainstem, cerebellum, dentate nucleus, and periventricular white matter.
- The degree of enhancement depends on cell-mediated immunity of the host.

■ Other Imaging Findings

- Cortical and lacunar infarcts, often located in the small penetrating branches of the major cerebral arteries.
- Hydrocephalus.
- Elevated cerebrospinal fluid pressure is present in 50 to 75% of patients with cryptococcal meningitis.

✓ Pearls and ✗ Pitfalls

- ✓ The manifestations of cryptococcosis may vary depending on the treatment: patients not on antiretroviral therapy tend to show pseudocysts and lacunar ischemic lesions, whereas patients with immune reconstitution may show contrast-enhancing focal leptomeningeal and/or parenchymal lesions.
- ✓ In HIV-infected individuals, cryptococcal meningitis occurs in the setting of severe immune suppression, often with CD4+ cell counts of < 50 cells/mm³.
- ✗ Cryptococcal meningitis–induced inflammation and granulation at the sulci can mimic subarachnoid hemorrhage on CT and MRI scans.

Case 72

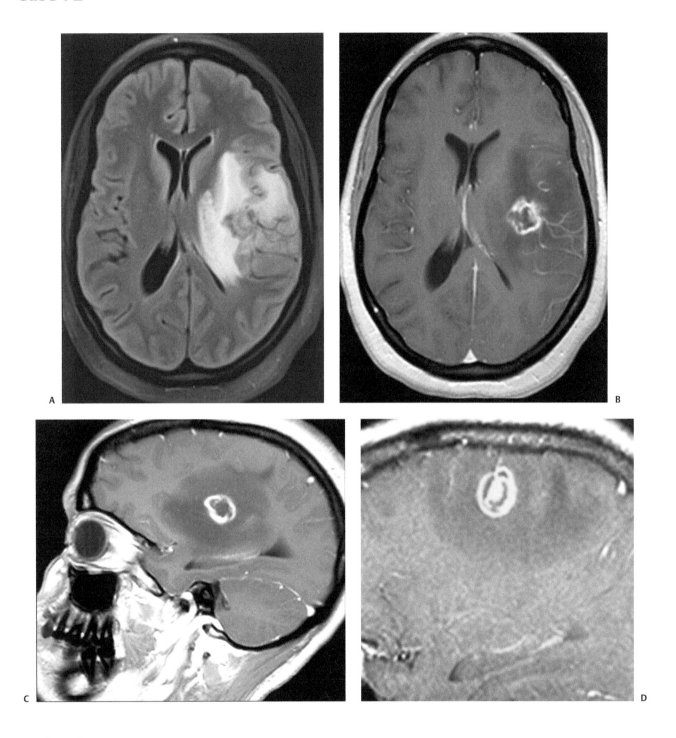

■ Clinical Presentation

A 34-year-old man presents positive for HIV with a CD4 count of 34.

■ Imaging Findings

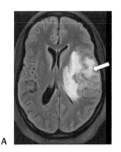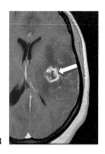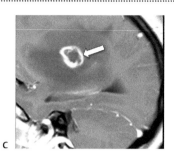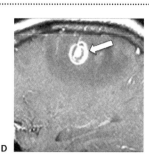

(A) Axial fluid-attenuated inversion recovery image shows increased signal with mass effect due to edema in the left frontal and parietal lobes (*arrow*). **(B, C)** Axial **(B)** and T1 **(C)** images with contrast show two irregular areas of ring enhancement (*arrow*). **(D)** Sagittal T1 image with contrast shows an "eccentric target sign" (*arrow*).

■ Differential Diagnosis

- *Toxoplasmosis:*
  ○ Most common mass lesion in patients with AIDS.
  ○ Multiple nodular or ring enhancing lesions.
  ○ Predilection for the corticomedullary junction and basal ganglia.
  ○ Eccentric target sign enhancement.
  ○ Does not show subependymal spread or ventricular enhancement.
  ○ Vasogenic edema is frequent.
  ○ Occasionally, treated lesions may hemorrhage (helps differentiate them from lymphoma).
- *Primary central nervous system lymphoma:*
  ○ Basal ganglia and periventricular enhancing lesions.
  ○ Frequently affects the corpus callosum.
  ○ Can extend to the ependymal surface.
  ○ Vasogenic edema is less frequent.
  ○ No posttreatment hemorrhage.
  ○ Lesions have lower apparent diffusion coefficient values than toxoplasma.
  ○ Lesions show increased cerebral blood flow (not a feature of toxoplasmosis).
- *Cerebral septic emboli:*
  ○ Hematogenous dissemination of septic emboli typically from cardiac valvular disease.
  ○ Multiple bilateral lesions in the territory of the middle cerebral artery involving terminal cortical branches.
  ○ Subcortical location.
  ○ Supratentorial more frequent than infratentorial.
  ○ Restricted diffusion due to ischemia.
  ○ Hemorrhage is common.
  ○ Nodular or ring enhancement.
  ○ Surrounding vasogenic edema.

■ Essential Facts

- Intracellular protozoan infection by *Toxoplasma gondii* found in cat feces and undercooked pork meat.
- Toxoplasma is the most common opportunistic central nervous system (CNS) infection in patients with AIDS (15–50%).

■ Other Imaging Findings

- One or more nodular or ring enhancing lesions with supratentorial distribution.
- Lesions have predilection for the basal ganglia and the corticomedullary junction.
- Some lesions form concentric irregular rings of enhancement known as the "eccentric target sign."

✓ Pearls and ✗ Pitfalls

✓ Controversy arises in trying to differentiate toxoplasmosis from primary CNS lymphoma.
✓ Polymerase chain reaction (PCR) testing is nearly 100% specific for active toxoplasma infection. CSF PCR for Epstein–Barr virus increases the likelihood for lymphoma.
✓ The presence of ependymal spread suggests CNS lymphoma. Toxoplasma lesions may hemorrhage after treatment, while CNS lymphoma does not.
✓ MRI perfusion studies have shown higher cerebral blood volume in lymphoma than in toxoplasmosis.
✓ Discrepant results have been obtained with MR spectroscopy (MRS).
✗ If no improvement is seen after empirical toxoplasmosis treatment, thallium-201 brain single-photon emission CT or positron emission tomography (both result in positive findings in lymphoma), or MRS can be used to reevaluate.

Case 73

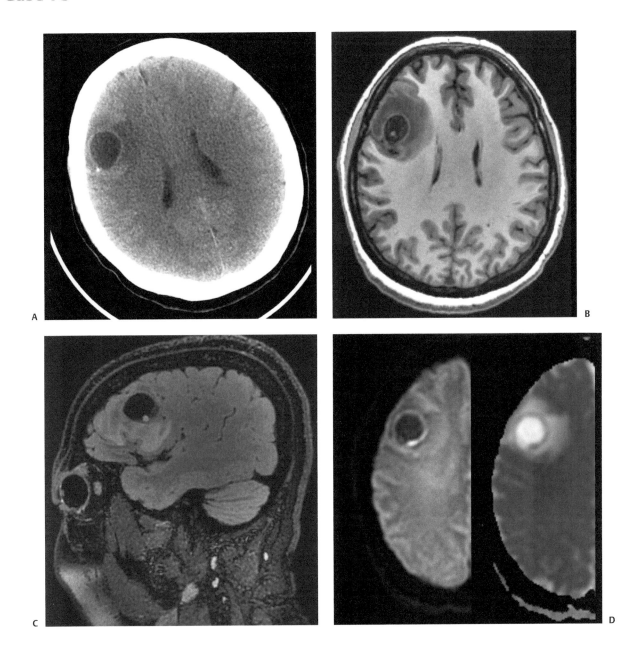

■ Clinical Presentation

A 39-year-old woman presents to the emergency department with seizures.

■ Imaging Findings

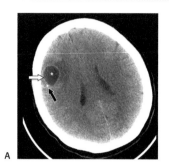
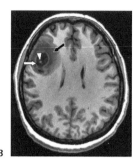
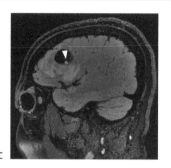
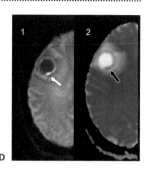

(A) Axial noncontrast CT image of the head demonstrates a well-defined, hypodense lesion (*asterisk*) with thin, hyperdense walls (*white arrow*) and a punc-tate calcification along its posterior margin (*black arrow*). **(B)** Axial T1-weighted image demonstrates a well-circumscribed, predominantly hypointense lesion in the right middle frontal gyrus, with a hyperintense border (*white arrow*), a small internal hyperintense nodule (*white arrowhead*), and significant surrounding vasogenic edema (*black arrow*). **(C)** Sagittal fluid-attenuated inversion recovery image shows low signal intensity within the lesion and in-creased signal intensity of the internal nodule along the inferior aspect of the mass (*arrowhead*). **(D)** Axial diffusion-weighted image (DWI) sequence (*1*) demonstrates increased signal along the borders of the lesion (*white arrow*) and no restricted diffusion internally. Apparent diffusion coefficient (ADC) map (*2*) image shows low ADC values along the periphery of the mass (*black arrow*), which corresponds with the area of increased DWI signal, consistent with restricted diffusion of the borders of the lesion.

■ Differential Diagnosis

- **Neurocysticercosis:** Highly endemic parasitic disease that presents as solitary or multiple cystic lesions with an eccentric, generally nonenhancing nodule representing the scolex (visible in ~50% of cases).
- *Pyogenic cerebral abscess:* Focal parenchymal infection that results in a central pus collection with a surrounding capsule composed of vascularized collagen. These lesions typically exhibit central restricted diffusion and an irregular or double rim enhancing margin.
- *Cerebral metastasis:* Cerebral metastases can be either solitary or multiple and tend to arise at the gray–white matter junction of the cerebral hemispheres. Extensive surrounding vasogenic edema is common and can be disproportionate to lesion size.

■ Essential Facts

- Most common parasitic infection of the CNS and most common cause of acquired epilepsy. Acquired from ingestion of water or food contaminated with human feces containing *T. solium* eggs.
- Classified according to location into subarachnoid-cisternal (most common), parenchymal, intraventricular, and spinal subtypes.
- Five stages of evolution have been described according to radiologic features: noncystic, vesicular, colloidal vesicular, granular nodular, calcified nodular.
- All are active forms except for the calcified nodular stage.

- Initially unapparent on imaging (noncystic stage), the infection evolves into a small cyst with a thin wall; little to no surrounding edema; and with a small, round, internal scolex representing the larval head (vesicular stage).
- As the associated inflammatory response ensues, surrounding edema and cyst wall thickness progresses (colloidal vesicular stage). During the granular nodular stage, the cyst walls are significantly thicker and there is more surrounding edema.
- Ultimately, the cyst involutes and calcifies, leaving behind nonenhancing nodules with no surrounding edema (calcified nodular stage).

■ Other Imaging Findings

- The cyst may be T1 and T2 hyperintense, if highly proteinaceous.
- Complications include vascular involvement, secondary obstruction, and inflammatory consequences.

✓ Pearls and ✗ Pitfalls

- ✓ Approximately half of patients exhibit signs of neurocysticercosis in various stages of evolution.
- ✗ Neurocysticercosis may be indistinguishable from other well-circumscribed lesions, especially during the colloidal vesicular and granular nodular stages.
- ✗ Increased relative cerebral volume in perfusion-weighted imaging indicates metastasis rather than neurocysticercosis.

Case 74

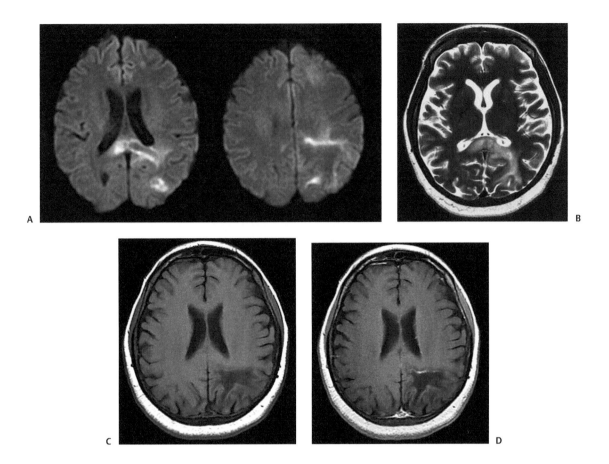

Clinical Presentation

A 36-year-old with a history of HIV infection, not on highly active antiretroviral therapy, presents with weakness and lethargy.

■ Imaging Findings

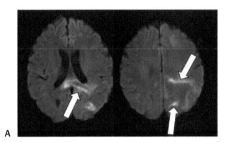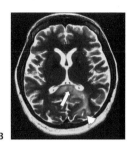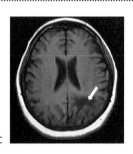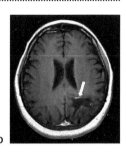

(A) Axial diffusion-weighted images demonstrate large lesions in the corpus callosum and left parietal white matter (WM) with restriction of diffusion at the edge (*arrows*). **(B)** Axial T2-weighted image (WI) demonstrates a large lesion in the corpus callosum and left parietal WM without significant mass effect (*arrows*). There is involvement of the subcortical "U fibers" (*arrowhead*). **(C)** Axial T1WI without contrast. The lesion in the left parietal deep WM shows low signal, without significant mass effect (*arrow*). **(D)** Axial T1WI with contrast. The lesion in the left parietal deep WM shows peripheral contrast enhancement that corresponds to the area of restricted diffusion (*arrow*).

■ Differential Diagnosis

- ***Progressive multifocal leukoencephalopathy (PML) non–immune reconstitution inflammatory syndrome (IRIS):***
  - Severe, often fatal opportunistic infection of the central nervous system caused by reactivation of the polyoma JC (John Cunningham) virus (JCV).
  - Typically characterized by multifocal asymmetric subcortical white matter (WM) lesions.
  - It may be monofocal and affect the cortical gray matter.
- *PML-IRIS:*
  - Immune reconstitution inflammatory syndrome, or IRIS, refers to atypical or worsening opportunistic infection that occurs in patients with HIV/AIDS following initiation of highly active antiretroviral therapy, or in patients with multiple sclerosis on monoclonal antibody therapy such as natalizumab.
  - The reconstitution of immunity causes abnormal immune response to infectious/noninfectious antigens, not a relapse/recurrence of preexisting disease.
  - Imaging: Worsening features of PML, including confluence and enlargement of the T2 hyperintensities, mass effect, and patchy atypical enhancement.
  - Patients with HIV who develop PML-IRIS have a higher likelihood of surviving the PML than do HIV-positive patients who do not develop IRIS.
- *Glioblastoma:*
  - Most common primary intracranial neoplasm.
  - Malignant astrocytic tumor characterized by necrosis and neovascularity.
  - World Health Organization grade IV.
  - Thick, irregularly enhancing ring of neoplastic tissue surrounding a necrotic core.
  - Frequently involves the corpus callosum.

■ Essential Facts

- PML most commonly occurs in patients with HIV infection (80% of cases), patients with lymphoid malignancies (13%), and transplant recipients taking immunosuppressants (5%).
- JCV is a ubiquitous human polyomavirus that is carried by 50 to 90% of the population. Initial JCV infection is asymptomatic, but in immunosuppressed patients the infection can reactivate, leading to PML.
- Reactivation typically takes place at a CD4+ cell count of < 100 cells/mm^3.

■ Other Imaging Findings

- MRI:
  - Poorly demarcated white matter hyperintensities on T2-weighted and fluid-attenuated inversion recovery images.
  - Moderate mass effect.
  - May or may not enhance.
  - May restrict diffusion.
  - One or more lesions can be present and may be located in different hemispheres.

✓ Pearls and ✗ Pitfalls

- ✓ Involvement of the subcortical U fibers is characteristic of PML.
- ✗ Mass effect is often absent in HIV-associated PML-IRIS, whereas in toxoplasmosis encephalitis and cryptococcal meningitis, focal mass lesions with mass effect can be present.

Case 75

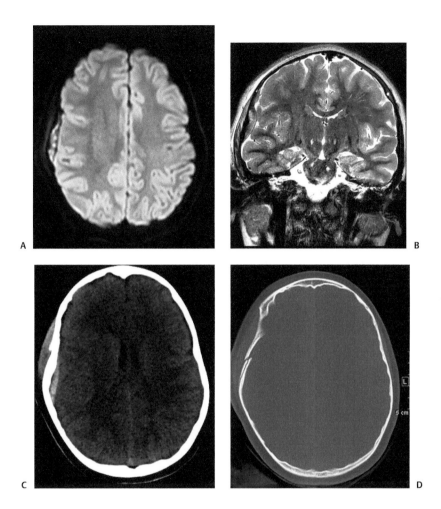

A

B

C

D

■ Clinical Presentation

A 42-year-old found lying on the sidewalk unconscious.

■ Imaging Findings

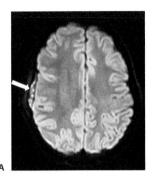
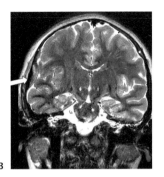
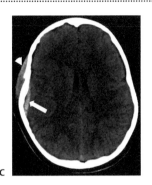
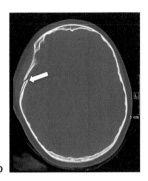

(A) Diffusion-weighted image shows an extra-axial fluid collection with a core of increased signal (*arrow*) and a hypointense periphery. **(B)** Coronal T2-weighted image (WI) shows an extra-axial fluid collection on the right (*arrow*), with heterogenous signal. **(C)** Axial CT image of the head shows an extra-axial hyperdense fluid collection (*arrow*) with a right temporal scalp hematoma *(arrowhead)*. **(D)** CT of the head in bone window shows a slightly displaced fracture on the right (*arrow*).

■ Differential Diagnosis

- ***Hyperacute epidural hematoma (EDH):***
  - ○ Extra-axial blood collection located between the inner skull and the dura mater.
  - ○ Biconvex or lentiform shape.
  - ○ 90% associated with skull fractures.
  - ○ On occasion, EDHs (and subdural hematomas) can be seen to contain alternating crescent-shaped regions of various densities, producing a "swirled" appearance, considered an indication of active hemorrhage.
  - ○ Supratentorial predominance (90%).
  - ○ EDHs do not cross sutures.
- *Empyema:*
  - ○ Pus accumulated in the epidural or subdural space.
  - ○ Restricted diffusion due to increased viscosity and protein content.
  - ○ 90% supratentorial.
  - ○ Prominent enhancement at the periphery.
  - ○ 70% are secondary to sinus or ear infections.
  - ○ Surgical emergency.
- *Meningioma:*
  - ○ Dural-based tumors that are isoattenuating to slightly hyperattenuating to the parenchyma.
  - ○ Homogeneous and intense enhancement after the injection of iodinated contrast material.
  - ○ Perilesional edema may be extensive.
  - ○ Hyperostosis and intratumoral calcifications may be present.

■ Essential Facts

- 95% are secondary to arterial bleeding due to shear injury of a meningeal artery branch.
- Fast growing if arterial in origin.
- Considered a surgical emergency if expanding rapidly.
- Usually located at the site of direct trauma, with associated scalp hematoma and skull fracture.

■ Other Imaging Findings

- CT: Acute lesions show increased density. Subacute lesions can be isodense to the cortex. Chronic hematomas are hypodense.
- MRI:
  - ○ Hyperacute and chronic epidural hematomas exhibit signal intensity similar to cerebrospinal fluid on T1- and T2-weighted images.
  - ○ The acute epidural hematoma is isointense on T1-weighted images and iso- to hypointense on T2-weighted images.
  - ○ Subacute and early chronic epidural hematomas are hyperintense on T1- and T2-weighted images.

✓ Pearls and ✗ Pitfalls

- ✓ Hyperacute hematomas (oxygenated hemoglobin) will show a core of increased signal on diffusion-weighted image. After the blood becomes deoxygenated hemoglobin, the core becomes dark.
- ✗ If a diastasis of a suture is present, the epidural hematoma may cross suture lines.

Case 76

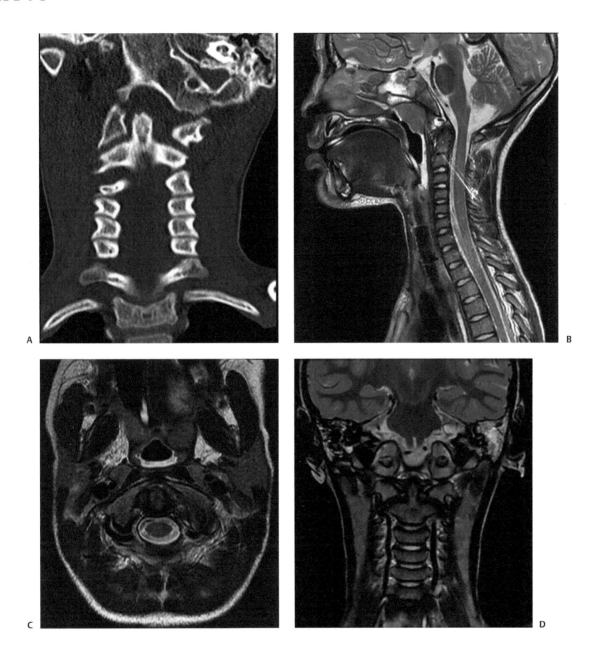

A

■ Clinical Presentation

An 11-year-old boy involved in a motor vehicle collision.

■ Imaging Findings

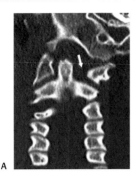 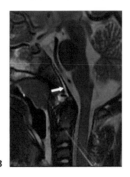 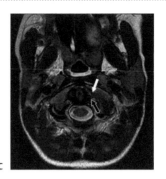 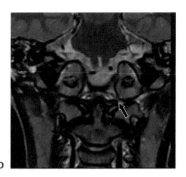

(A) Coronal CT image in bone window shows asymmetric positioning of the dens to the right with widening of the dens–left lateral mass of C1 interval (*arrow*). **(B)** Sagittal T2-weighted image (WI) demonstrates T2 hyperintense fluid accumulating between the tectorial membrane and posterior clivus (*arrow*) consistent with hematoma. **(C)** Axial T2WI demonstrates interruption of the fibers and increased T2 signal involving the left side of the transverse ligament (*black arrow*) and the left alar ligament (*white arrow*). **(D)** Coronal T2WI shows disruption of the alar ligament on the left (*arrow*).

■ Differential Diagnosis

- **Transverse and alar ligamentous injury:** Traumatic injury to stabilization ligaments in the upper cervical spine resulting in disruption of ligamentous fibers with increased signal on T2-weighted images.
- *Atlantoaxial laxity:* Asymmetric positioning of the dens with respect to the lateral masses of C1 can be seen in conditions resulting in increased ligamentous laxity, such as rheumatoid arthritis, Down syndrome, and Marfan syndrome.
- *Artifact:* Both asymmetric atlantoaxial alignment and increased ligamentous T2 signal intensity may be seen secondary to artifact resulting from image angle acquisition and patient positioning.

■ Essential Facts

- Ligamentous injury involving the atlantoaxial junction is typically seen in high-energy traumatic settings.
- Ligamentous injury is suspected when there is asymmetric widening of the atlantoaxial interval or increased basion–dens interval on conventional radiography or CT imaging.
- Occipital condyle avulsion fractures are associated with injury of the alar ligament. Alar ligament injury is generally caused by flexion and rotation forces resulting in traumatic rotatory subluxation. Rupture of the alar ligament in the setting of traumatic rotatory subluxation is more common in children.
- C1 burst and lateral mass fractures can be associated with tears of the transverse ligament, which are unstable.

■ Other Imaging Findings

- Transverse ligament rupture can occur with or without C1 fractures and are generally seen in conjunction with alar ligament injury.
- Transverse ligament ruptures may lead to instability resulting in dorsal displacement of the dens with possible compression on the thecal sac and upper cervical spinal cord.

✓ Pearls and ✗ Pitfalls

- ✓ Special scrutiny should be paid to additional traumatic findings in the head and neck, including intracranial hemorrhage, shear injury, vascular injury, and cervical spine fractures, among others.
- ✗ Absence of asymmetric widening of the atlantoaxial interval does not exclude alar ligament injury.
- ✗ Bilateral ligamentous injury is especially challenging for diagnosis because asymmetry is more often absent.

Case 77

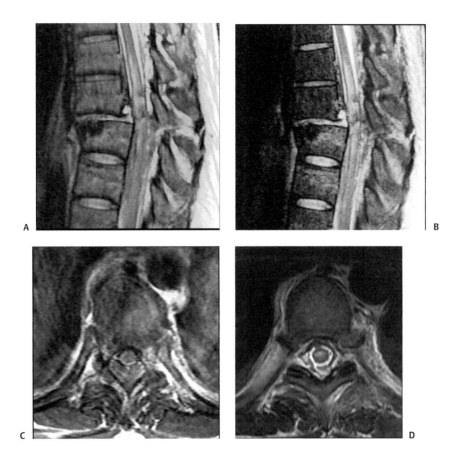

■ Clinical Presentation

A 42-year-old man involved in a motor vehicle collision.

■ Imaging Findings

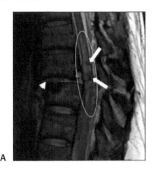
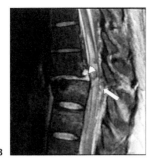
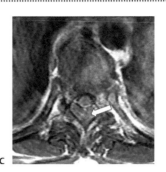
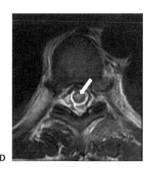

(A) Sagittal T2-weighted image (WI) shows a translation injury with anterior displacement of T9 over T10 (*arrowhead*) and fracture of the posterior elements. Notice the swelling (*oval*) and hemorrhage (*arrows*) of the cord. **(B)** Sagittal fat-suppressed T2WI shows a translation injury with anterior displacement of T9 over T10 and fracture of the posterior elements. Notice the swelling and hemorrhage of the cord. Disruption of the T9–T10 disk (*arrowhead*) and dorsal epidural hematoma (*arrow*) are also noted. **(C)** Axial T1WI shows intermediate to high signal in a dorsal epidural hematoma (*arrow*). **(D)** Axial T2WI demonstrates edema in the central cord (*arrow*).

■ Differential Diagnosis

- **Cord contusion:**
  - Traumatic spinal cord injury (SCI).
  - Most fractures with SCIs occur in the highly mobile cervical spine. Hyperflexion injuries tend to occur around the C5–C6 motion segment, whereas hyperextension injuries have a higher center of rotation.
- *Cord transection:* If the applied traumatic forces are sufficient, a complete disruption of the cord fibers results in transection.
- *Progressive posttraumatic myelomalacic myelopathy (PTMM):*
  - PTMM is a poorly understood entity described in the late subacute period, generally > 2 months postinjury.
  - It likely represents a presyrinx state following disruption of normal transparenchymal cerebrospinal fluid (CSF) transit. A contributory role for cord tethering by adhesions has also been proposed, which may be amenable to intraoperative lysis.

■ Essential Facts

- The functional consequences of an acute SCI are variable. Patients with incomplete SCI have a higher chance of some neurologic recovery as compared to patients with complete injuries.
- The spectrum of cord parenchymal injuries include edema (low T1 and high T2 signal), swelling (defined as a smooth enlargement of the cord contour), and hemorrhage.
- Spinal cord edema increases significantly during the early time period after injury, whereas intramedullary hemorrhage is comparatively static.

■ Other Imaging Findings

- Acute intramedullary hemorrhage is seen as a focus of T2 shortening (hypointensity).
- In the subacute stage, cord injuries evolve to myelomalacia, with areas of T2 hyperintensity and T1 signal intermediate between cord and CSF.
- Chronic posttraumatic cord cyst or syrinx is identified as an expansile structure that is isointense with CSF on all sequences and is more sharply marginated compared with myelomalacia.
- Cord atrophy is a common finding in patients imaged > 20 years after the initial trauma.

✓ Pearls and ✗ Pitfalls

✓ Cord symptoms can be secondary to extrinsic compression without damage to the cord itself. Fractures with bony retropulsion, disk extrusions, and epidural hematomas cause cord compression.

✓ Preexisting spondylosis and spinal stenosis will accentuate the vulnerability of the cord to extrinsic compression.

✓ Atrophy has been defined as an anterior posterior dimension of ≤ 7 mm in the cervical cord and ≤ 6 mm in the thoracic region.

✗ SCI without radiographic abnormality (SCIWORA) refers to the presence of neurologic deficit in the setting of normal X-rays and CT images.

✗ It includes cases with neural injuries seen on MRI scan and those with normal MRI findings. Children diagnosed with SCIWORA but with normal MRI findings have shown more favorable clinical outcomes than those with cervical cord abnormalities on MRI.

Case 78

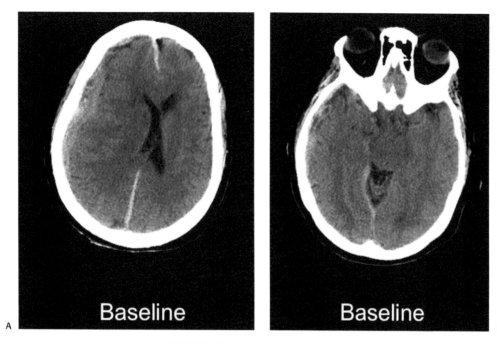

Baseline

Baseline

A

B

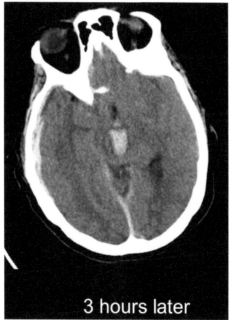

3 hours later

C

■ Clinical Presentation

A 46-year-old man is brought in following a motor vehicle collision and is found to have subdural hemorrhage. Follow-up CT exam is requested 3 hours later due to neurologic deterioration.

■ Imaging Findings

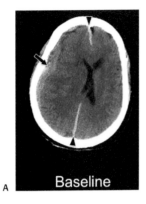 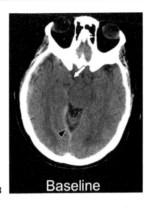 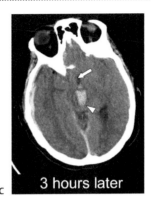

(A) Axial noncontrast CT image of the head shows subacute subdural hemorrhage along the right cerebral convexity (*black arrow*) and falx (*black arrowheads*), resulting in midline shift to the left. **(B)** Axial noncontrast CT image of the head shows subacute subdural hemorrhage along the tentorium (*black arrowhead*). There is effacement of the perimesencephalic cisterns, suggesting early uncal herniation (*white arrow*). **(C)** Axial noncontrast CT image shows uncal herniation (*white arrow*) with development of acute hemorrhage within the midbrain (*white arrowhead*).

■ Differential Diagnosis

- ***Duret hemorrhage:*** One or more foci of hemorrhage occurring within the brainstem as a result of downward transtentorial herniation.
- *Brainstem contusion:* Brainstem contusions may be indistinguishable from Duret hemorrhages. Unlike Duret hemorrhages, contusions tend to be smaller in size, are typically multiple, and generally occur along the dorsal brainstem.
- *Hypertensive brainstem hemorrhage:* The brainstem is a classic location for hypertensive hemorrhage, particularly the pons along with basal ganglia and thalami. The presence of downward transtentorial herniation is key when diagnosing Duret hemorrhages. However, when brainstem hemorrhage is present at the time of presentation, it is important to consider hypertensive hemorrhage as a possible cause of altered mental status that may have led to the cause of the accident.

■ Essential Facts

- Uncal herniation/downward transtentorial herniation leads to compression on the brainstem which in turn causes a reduction in the midbrain–pontine angle.
- As a result, small perforating vessels become compressed, leading to hemorrhagic infarction of the pons and midbrain.
- Although an arterial etiology is more commonly accepted, accompanying venous thrombosis may also play a role.

- Often, these hemorrhages are absent at initial presentation and develop as cerebral edema and herniation ensue.
- Clinical manifestations include oculomotor paresis, altered mental status, rigidity, and coma.

■ Other Imaging Findings

- Early manifestations of uncal herniation include effacement of the perimesencephalic cisterns.
- Duret hemorrhages more commonly develop in the ventral and paramedian aspects of the brainstem.

✓ Pearls and ✗ Pitfalls

- ✓ Follow-up imaging is warranted in patients with severe brain trauma if clinical deterioration occurs.
- ✓ Early signs of brain herniation syndromes should be reported so as to preemptively treat cerebral edema and avoid its potential complications.
- ✗ The main difference between Duret hemorrhages and direct brainstem injuries is the central location of Duret hemorrhages.

Case 79

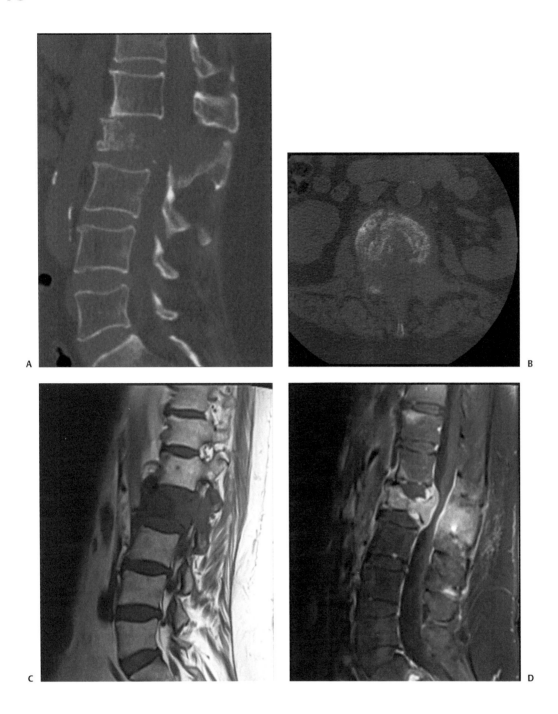

Clinical Presentation

A 74-year-old with a history of breast cancer presents with severe back pain following a fall.

■ Imaging Findings

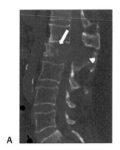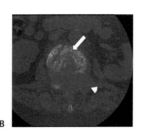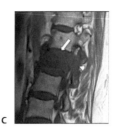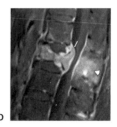

(A) Sagittal reformatted CT image shows biconcave deformity and loss of height of L2 (*arrow*), with loss of the normal bone trabeculae at the L2 vertebral body and posterior elements (*arrowhead*). **(B)** Axial CT image of the lumbar spine shows replacement of the trabeculae of L2 (*arrow*) with a soft tissue mass that extends to the left pedicle and paraspinal soft tissues (*arrowhead*). **(C)** Sagittal T1-weighted image (WI) of the lumbar spine shows loss of height and biconcave deformity of L2, with replacement of the normal bone marrow signal (*arrow*). There is involvement of the posterior elements (*arrowhead*). **(D)** Sagittal fat-suppressed postcontrast T1WI of the lumbar spine shows intense enhancement of the L2 vertebral body with convex posterior border expanding toward the spinal canal (*arrow*). There is involvement of the spinous process (*arrowhead*). These lesions cause narrowing of the spinal canal and compression of the cauda equina.

■ Differential Diagnosis

- *Pathologic fracture:*
  - Pathologic compression fractures of the spine more commonly show compression morphology, although burst morphology may occur.
  - The underlying mass may be obscured by fracture and hematoma.
  - CT and MRI may show trabecular and cortical destruction.
  - Identification of other tumor sites is helpful.
- *Insufficiency fracture:*
  - Fracture through osteoporotic/otherwise generally weak bone.
  - Usually no focal underlying lesion.
  - Frequently after minor trauma.
- *Brown tumor:*
  - Brown tumors seen in chronic renal disease result from rapid localized bone loss, with hemorrhage and reparative granulation tissue replacing the normal marrow contents. Hemosiderin imparts the brown color.
  - Other findings in hyperparathyroidism include: prominent primary trabeculae, resorption of secondary trabeculae, cortical thinning, and erosions at entheses, end plates, and sacroiliac joints.

■ Essential Facts

- A fracture is defined as pathologic when it arises in a bone tissue that has been modified and reshaped by a local or systemic pathologic process.
- The spine is a common site of involvement in patients with bone metastases.
- Spinal instability should be evaluated for surgical intervention.

■ Other Imaging Findings

- CT shows cortical destruction, tumor matrix, and associated soft tissue masses seen in relation to pathological fractures.
- MR findings:
  - Well-defined, masslike decreased T1 marrow.
  - Abnormal muscle signal and associated soft tissue masses seen in relation to pathological fractures.
  - Endosteal scalloping.
  - May see additional tumor deposits in metastatic disease or multiple myeloma.
- In-phase and out-of-phase T1WI may be useful in differentiating marrow edema from an infiltrative process:
  - Marrow edema: Signal dropout on out-of-phase images because marrow fat is retained.
  - Infiltrative process: No signal dropout because marrow fat is replaced.
  - Diffusion-weighted imaging: Tumor infiltration of marrow causes restricted diffusion.

✓ Pearls and ✗ Pitfalls

- ✓ MR imaging findings suggestive of metastatic compression fractures:
  - Convex posterior border of the vertebral body.
  - Abnormal signal intensity of the pedicle or posterior element.
  - Epidural mass or focal paraspinal mass.
  - Other spinal metastases.
- ✓ MR imaging findings suggestive of acute osteoporotic compression fractures:
  - Low-signal-intensity band on T1- and T2-weighted images across the vertebral body.
  - Spared normal bone marrow signal intensity of the vertebral body.
  - Retropulsion of a posterior bone fragment.
  - Multiple compression fractures.

Case 80

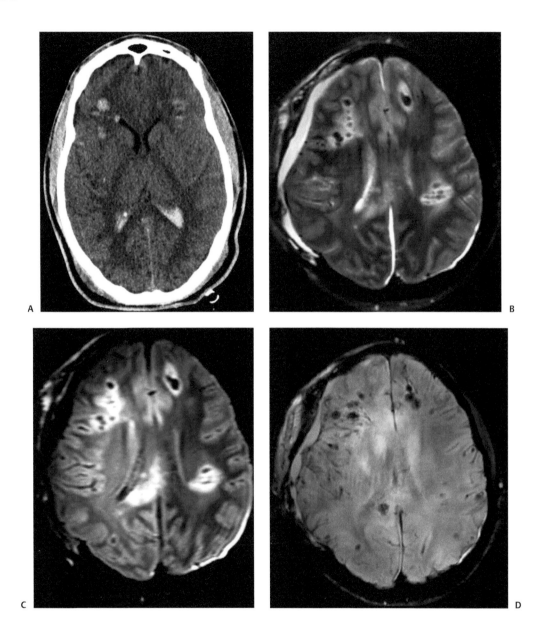

Clinical Presentation

A 38-year-old man presents with traumatic brain injury after a high-velocity motor vehicle collision.

■ Imaging Findings

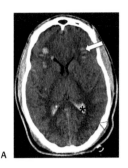 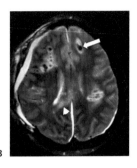 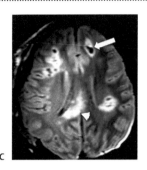 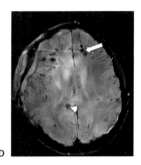

(A) CT image without contrast demonstrates diffuse effacement of the gyri (*arrowhead*) secondary to diffuse brain edema. Multiple subcortical white matter hemorrhages are present (*arrow*) and intraventricular blood is also seen (*asterisk*). (B, C) Axial T2-weighted fast spin echo image (B) and diffusion-weighted image (C) show the patient after decompressive craniectomy. The subcortical lesions show a center of hypointensity with surrounding vasogenic edema (*arrow*). Subdural fluid collections are noted bilaterally. The posterior aspect of the corpus callosum shows T2 hyperintensity and restricted diffusion (*arrowhead*). (D) Susceptibility-weighted image shows multiple small subcortical (*arrow*) and callosal (*arrowhead*) areas of microhemorrhage consistent with shear injuries.

■ Differential Diagnosis

- ***Diffuse axonal injury:***
  - Multiple petechial diffuse hemorrhages or linear microbleeds in the subcortical white matter best seen in gradient echo (GRE)/susceptibility-weighted image (SWI) sequences.
  - Predilection for the gray–white matter interface.
  - Injury in close proximity of dural folds occurs in the corpus callosum.
  - Secondary to disruption of the blood–brain barrier.
- *Brain parenchymal contusions:*
  - Brain parenchymal lesions secondary to direct impact of the brain with the adjacent skull.
  - More frequent in the frontal and temporal lobes.
  - Typically exhibit hemorrhage. Edema may precede hemorrhage by a few hours.
- *Cerebral amyloid angiopathy:*
  - Spontaneous cortical-subcortical intracranial hemorrhage (ICH) in the normotensive elderly.
  - ICH in cortical-subcortical distribution that generally spares the deep white matter, basal ganglia, and brainstem. May involve the cerebellum.
  - Cortical microhemorrhages, identified on T2*-weighted GRE, MRI, and SWI.
    - Focal or disseminated superficial siderosis.
  - Age ≥ 55 years.

■ Essential Facts

- Acceleration and deceleration forces associated with high-energy trauma give rise to shear injuries due to the differences in density of the gray and white matter, located in the subcortical white matter junction, which affect the axons (diffuse axonal injury [DAI]) and the vessels (microbleeds).
- Frequent cause of morbidity in patients with traumatic brain injuries, most commonly from high-speed motor vehicle accidents.

- Two thirds of DAI lesions occur at the gray–white matter junction. The corpus callosum, dorsolateral rostral brainstem, caudate nuclei, thalamus, tegmentum, and internal capsule are also affected.

■ Other Imaging Findings

- 50 to 80% demonstrate a normal CT scan upon presentation.
- One or more hemorrhages < 2 cm in diameter in the cerebral hemispheres or adjacent to the third ventricle.
- Intraventricular hemorrhage.
- Hemorrhage in the corpus callosum.
- Brainstem hemorrhage.
- MR can detect petechial hemorrhages that can persist after years.
- SWI is more sensitive to microbleeds than GRE sequences.
- DWI: Hyperintensities in areas of axonal injury.

✓ Pearls and ✗ Pitfalls

- ✓ DAI without microbleeds is infrequent but has been reported.
- ✓ Diffusion tensor imaging shows changes in the fractional anisotropy (lower values) in patients with DAI, which are related to poor outcome.
- ✓ MRS may show diffusely elevated lactate levels, even in normal appearing tissue on MRI, which correlates with poor clinical outcome.
- ✗ Cerebral fat embolism shares some of the imaging features of shearing injury: Scattered embolic ischemic foci on diffusion-weighted imaging and petechial hemorrhage on GRE or SWI can be seen in the acute stage. This condition occurs in the setting of long bone or pelvic fractures and presents with a clinical triad of respiratory changes, neurologic abnormalities, and petechial rash.

Case 81

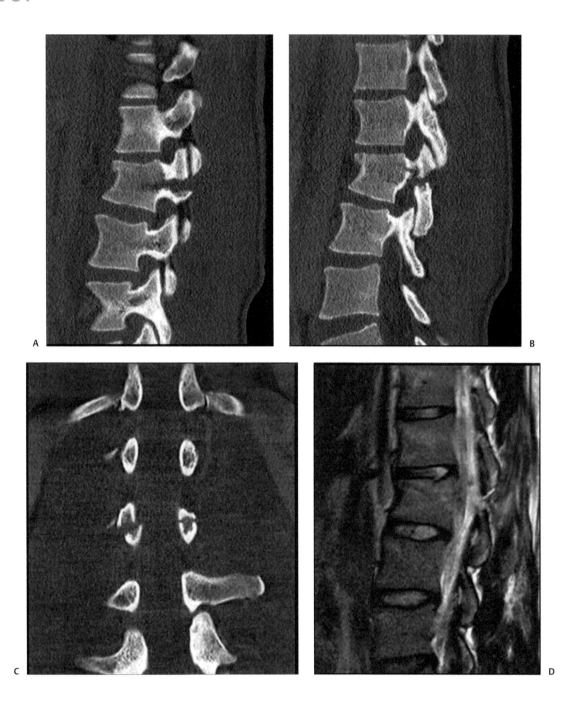

■ Clinical Presentation

A 15-year-old involved in a motor vehicle collision.

■ Imaging Findings

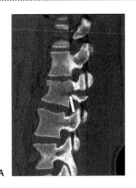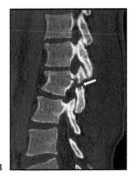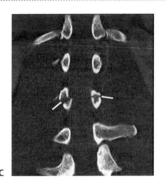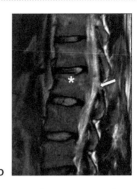

A B C D

(A) Left parasagittal reformatted CT image shows an axially oriented fracture of L1 extending through the pedicle (*arrow*). **(B)** Right parasagittal reformatted CT image shows an axially oriented fracture of L1 extending through the pedicle and pars interarticularis (*arrow*). **(C)** Coronal reformatted image demonstrates bilateral axially oriented pedicular fractures at L1 (*arrows*). **(D)** Sagittal T2-weighted image demonstrates a distraction morphology with widening if the interlaminar space, injury of the ligamentum flavum (*arrow*), and axially oriented fracture of the superior half of the T12 vertebral body (*asterisk*).

■ Differential Diagnosis

- *Chance fracture:*
  - These injuries belong to the broader category of flexion distraction injuries and are classified as B1 in the AOSpine Thoracolumbar Spine Injury Classification system.
  - Monosegmental osseous failure of the posterior tension band extending into the vertebral body.
- *Non-osseous disruption of the posterior ligamentous complex:* These injuries are part of the wider category of flexion distraction injuries and correspond to the B2 category in the AOSpine Thoracolumbar Spine Injury Classification system.
- *Distraction extension injury:*
  - It corresponds to type B3 injury in the AOSpine Thoracolumbar Spine Injury Classification system.
  - Disruption of the anterior longitudinal ligament that serves as the anterior tension band of the spine, preventing hyperextension. The injury may pass through either the intervertebral disk or through the vertebral body itself (particularly in the ankylosed spine), but there is an intact posterior element hinge preventing gross displacement.

■ Essential Facts

- In distraction injuries, one part of the spinal column is separated from the other, leaving a space in between. This can occur through disruption of anterior or posterior ligaments, through anterior or posterior bony elements, or a combination of both.
- Often very unstable injuries.
- Angulation is frequently seen in the sagittal and/or coronal planes across the fracture site.

- The distraction morphology is seen in flexion distraction injuries (as in a Chance fracture) and in distraction extension injuries (as in patients with diffuse idiopathic skeletal hyperostosis or ankylosing spondylitis).
- Flexion distraction mechanism and posterior ligamentous complex injury should be suspected if an inferior or superior posterior endplate fracture is seen because it reflects avulsion fracture from the comparatively strong annulus fibrosis of the vertebral disk.

■ Other Imaging Findings

- CT shows fracture through the pedicles extending to the vertebral body, and variable distraction of the posterior elements.
- MRI depicts extra-axial hemorrhages and cord injuries.
- MRI signs of posterior ligamentous complex (PLC) injury include disruption of the low signal intensity black stripe on sagittal T1- or T2-weighted images, indicative of supraspinatus ligament or ligamentum flavum tear, fluid in the facet joint capsules, and edema in the interspinous region.

✓ Pearls and ✗ Pitfalls

✓ Flexion distraction injuries may comprise up to 16% of spinal injuries and are most frequently encountered at the thoracolumbar junction between T11 and L1, although injuries have been reported in the literature between T5 and S1.

✗ Flexion distraction injuries are associated with intraabdominal injuries that may delay the treatment of the spine.

✗ Aortic vascular injuries, although infrequent, should not be overlooked.

Case 82

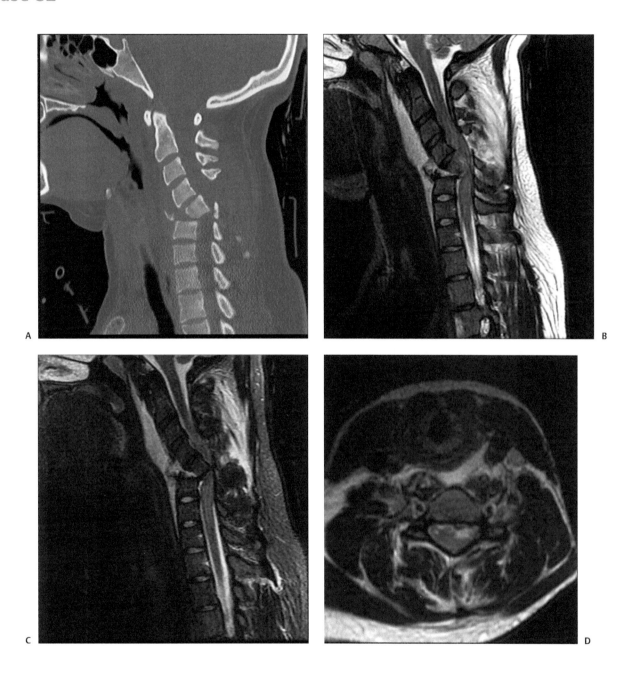

■ Clinical Presentation

A 35-year-old presents with severe neck pain and quadriplegia after a motor vehicle collision.

■ Imaging Findings

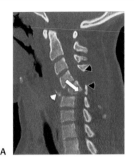 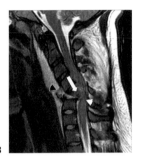 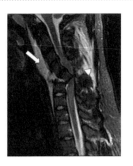 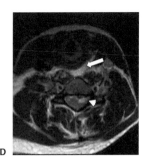

(A) Sagittal reformatted CT image of the cervical spine shows posterior translation of C5 (*arrow*); the vertebral body extends into the spinal canal. A fragment of the vertebral body is avulsed and seen ventrally (*white arrowhead*). There is widening of the interspinous space (*black arrowheads*). (B) Sagittal T2-weighted image (WI) of the cervical spine shows the body of C5 translated into the spinal canal (*arrow*) and compressing the spinal cord, which shows increased T2 signal (*white arrowhead*). The anterior longitudinal ligament is disrupted (*black arrowhead*). (C) Sagittal short TI inversion recovery image of the cervical spine shows a prominent prevertebral hematoma (*arrow*) with strain of the nuchal soft tissues (*arrowhead*). (D) Axial T2WI of the cervical spine shows prominent fluid in the prevertebral space (*arrow*) and the thecal sac being deformed by the presence of an epidural hematoma (*arrowhead*).

■ Differential Diagnosis

- ***Translation injury of the cervical spine and discoligamentous complex (DLC) disruption:***
  ○ Rotation/translation entails the horizontal displacement of part of the subaxial spine with respect to another.
  ○ Both the anterior and posterior columns have been damaged.
  ○ Most flexion-distraction and translation injuries occur at the C5–C6 and C6–C7 motion segments, where the fulcrum is located.
  ○ Traumatic spondylosis with disruption of the DLC.
  ○ Mechanism of injury can be hyperextension, hyperflexion, or rotation.
  ○ Associated with other ligamentous injuries and with bony fractures.
- *Distraction injury of the cervical spine:*
  ○ Dissociation of the vertical axis involving the DLC.
  ○ A gap between the vertebral bodies or posterior elements is seen, but there is no displacement in the horizontal plane.
  ○ Lesions may be circumferential and associated to facet dislocations.
  ○ No spondylosis is present.

■ Essential Facts

- The Subaxial Cervical Injury Classification (SLIC), proposed by Vaccaro in 2007, describes three morphologic patters of fracture:
  ○ Compression: visible loss of height of the vertebral body or disruption of the end plates.
  ○ Distraction: anatomic dissociation of the vertebral axis.
  ○ Translation/rotation: There is horizontal displacement between two segments of the cervical spine. These lesions imply disruption of both the anterior and posterior elements. Unilateral or bilateral joint facet dislocations or fractures, bilateral pedicle fractures, and separation of the lateral mass are typically seen in this category.

- Translation can occur in the sagittal plane, associated with pedicle fractures or joint facet fractures.
- Rotational injuries can also be present in addition to the axial translation.

■ Other Imaging Findings

- Multislice CT is the modality of choice for initial evaluation, and MR provides additional soft tissue detail.
- MR provides additional information of the status of the spinal cord, ligaments, and other soft tissue elements that could be missed in CT.

✓ Pearls and ✗ Pitfalls

✓ The DLC is composed of the intervertebral disk, the anterior and posterior longitudinal ligaments, the ligamentum flavum, the interspinous ligaments, and the facet joint capsules.
✓ Indirect signs of DLC injury include "fanning" of the spinous processes, facet joint dislocation, subluxation of the vertebral bodies, and a widened intervertebral disk space.
✓ Widening of the joint facet > 2 mm or apposition of the facet joints of < 50% and widening of the anterior disk space in neutral position or extension are considered absolute indications of DLC disruption.
✓ MR may provide other clues to DLC disruption, such as increased T2 signal seen horizontally in the intervertebral disk or increased signal in the intervertebral ligaments.
✗ Cerebrospinal fluid flow artifact is a challenge in the assessment of extra-axial hematomas in the spinal canal. Remodeling of the cord contour in the axial images is useful to distinguish between flow artifact and an extra-axial hematoma compressing the thecal sac.

Case 83

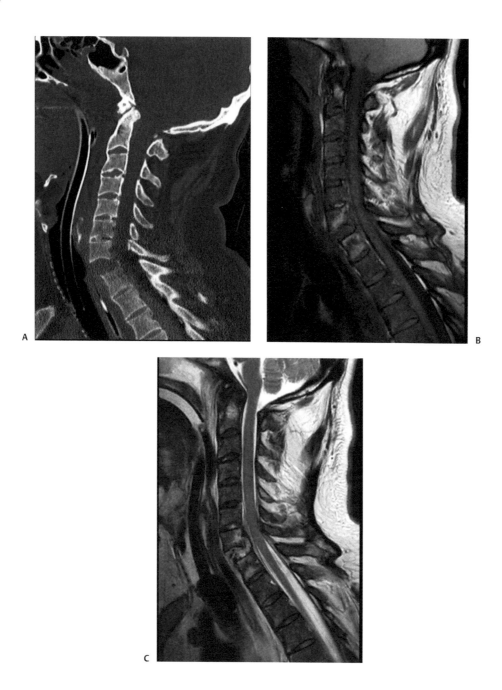

■ Clinical Presentation

A 50-year-old man found down and intoxicated.

■ Imaging Findings

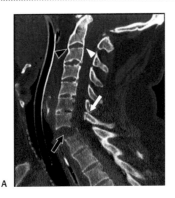 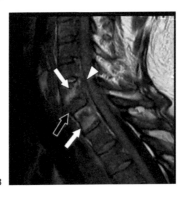 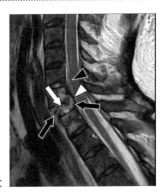

(A) Sagittal CT image of the cervical spine in bone window shows anterolisthesis of C7 on T1 with widening of the disk space (*black arrow*). A linear fracture through the base of the spinous process is vertically oriented (*white arrow*). Note preexisting calcification of the anterior (*black arrowhead*) and posterior longitudinal ligament (*white arrowhead*). **(B)** Sagittal T1-weighted image (WI) shows widening of the C7–T1 disk space with anterolisthesis and interruption of the anterior longitudinal ligament (ALL) and posterior longitudinal ligament (PLL) (*black arrow*). The C7 and T1 vertebral bodies demonstrate heterogeneous increased signal suggesting bone contusions (*white arrows*). There is isointense fluid in the ventral epidural space, consistent with epidural hematoma, resulting in effacement of the subarachnoid space (*white arrowhead*). **(C)** Sagittal T2WI demonstrates abnormally elevated T2 signal in the C7–T1 disk space (*white arrow*). There is anterolisthesis of C7 on T1 with interruption of the ALL and PLL (*black arrows*). A traumatic disk protrusion (*white arrowhead*) and a ventral epidural hematoma (*black arrowhead*) cause spinal canal stenosis with effacement of the subarachnoid space. Patchy increased T2 signal in the C7 and T1 vertebral bodies is likely due to bony contusions.

■ Differential Diagnosis

- **Hyperextension dislocation:** Severely unstable injury resulting from hyperextension forces resulting in major neurologic deficits. Ligamentous injury progresses from posterior to anterior with hyperextension dislocation representing the farthest along the spectrum. Classic findings include widening of the disk space, most pronounced at the anterior aspect, discoligamentous injury, and traumatic disk protrusion.
- *Hyperextension sprain:* The least severe along the spectrum of hyperextension injuries. This condition results from hyperextension forces leading to posterior ligament complex injury, which includes the ligamentum flavum, interspinous ligament, supraspinous ligament, and facet joint capsules. Unlike hyperextension dislocation, injury isolated to the posterior ligament complex is insufficient to result in instability.
- *Hyperextension with anterior subluxation:* More advanced than hyperextension sprain and less severe than hyperextension dislocation. This injury is characterized by disruption of the posterior ligament complex as well as of the PLL and posterior annulus. Findings generally include widening of the interspinous space, uncovering of the facets, and anterior subluxation.

■ Essential Facts

- Hyperextension dislocation generally involves the lower cervical spine.
- There is injury to the anterior longitudinal ligament (ALL), the anterior and posterior annulus fibrosus, the posterior longitudinal ligament (PLL), and the posterior ligament complex.

- Imaging findings can be subtle due to muscle spasm and immobilization devices masking the instability of the injury.
- On radiographs and CT images, hyperextension dislocation typically results in disk space widening and facet malalignment.
- MRI better reveals the degree of discoligamentous injury, which is characterized by increased T2 signal, widening of the disk space, and traumatic disk protrusion.
- There is typically soft tissue edema and cord injury.

■ Other Imaging Findings

- Hyperextension dislocation may be associated with avulsion fractures of the anteroinferior vertebral body. Unlike the teardrop fractures of hyperextension, avulsion fractures seen in hyperextension dislocation injury are more horizontally oriented rather than vertically oriented. Also, teardrop fractures occur more frequently in the upper cervical spine, whereas these are more common in the lower cervical spine.

✓ Pearls and ✗ Pitfalls

- ✓ Widening of the disk space may be more pronounced anteriorly and can be associated with vacuum phenomenon.
- ✓ Epidural hematoma and cord contusion are findings better depicted on MRI.
- ✗ Occasionally, the only imaging finding on radiograph to suggest hyperextension dislocation is severe prevertebral edema and neurologic deficit. This is an indication for CT and MR imaging.

Case 84

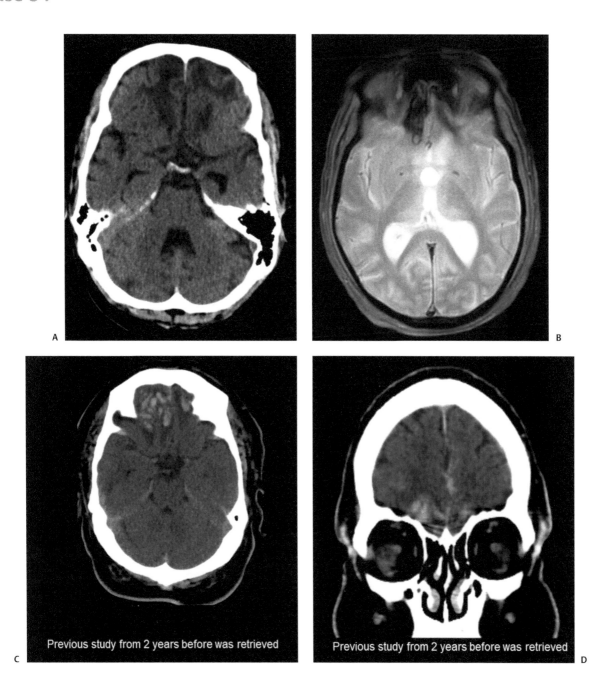

■ Clinical Presentation

History withheld.

■ Imaging Findings

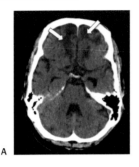 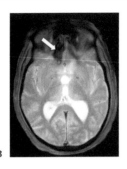 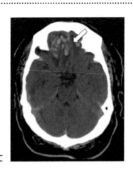 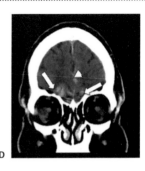

(A) CT image of the brain shows areas of low attenuation in the gyri recti and orbitofrontal gyri of both frontal lobes (*arrows*). (B) Axial gradient echo sequence demonstrates hemosiderin deposits in the anterior and inferior frontal lobes (*arrow*). (C) Axial CT image obtained 2 years before shows edema and hemorrhage in the anterior and inferior frontal lobes (*arrow*). (D) Coronal reformatted CT image obtained 2 years before shows edema and hemorrhage in the anterior and inferior frontal lobes (*arrows*). There is also subarachnoid hemorrhage in the interhemispheric region (*arrowhead*).

■ Differential Diagnosis

- ***Bifrontal contusion:***
  - Brain parenchymal lesions secondary to direct impact of the brain with the adjacent skull.
  - More frequent in the anterior temporal lobes and along the floor of the anterior cranial fossa and greater wing of the sphenoid, where the brain is in close proximity to the inner table of the skull.
  - Typically exhibit hemorrhage. Edema may precede hemorrhage by a few hours.
- *Amyloid angiopathy:* Cerebral amyloid angiopathy (CAA) refers to the deposition of β-amyloid in the media and adventitia of small and mid-sized arteries (and, less frequently, veins) of the cerebral cortex and the leptomeninges. CAA has been recognized as one of the morphologic hallmarks of Alzheimer disease (AD), but it is also often found in the brains of elderly patients who are neurologically healthy. CAA may lead to dementia, intracranial hemorrhage (ICH), or transient neurologic events. ICH is the most recognized result of CAA.
- *Pick disease:*
  - Pick disease (named after Arnold Pick) is a progressive dementia defined by clinical and pathologic criteria. It typically affects the frontal and/or anterolateral temporal lobes.
  - MRI: Frontal lobe atrophy out of proportion to atrophy in other brain regions, increased T2 signal in frontal lobe white matter, especially on fluid-attenuated inversion recovery sequences.

■ Essential Facts

- Stages of parenchymal contusion:
  - Acute: Less than 12 hours old. Intracellular oxyhemoglobin with the edematous brain undergoing necrosis. CT image shows low attenuation if hemorrhage is absent, and mixed or high attenuation if hemorrhage is present.
  - Subacute: A few days old. Liquefaction with development of vasogenic edema. May cause cerebral herniation.
  - Chronic: Neovascularization with removal of blood components and debris by macrophages. Clot resorption begins from the periphery inward, 1 to 6 weeks in duration. CT shows focal atrophy and cystic cavities surrounded by gliosis and hemosiderin scarring. Fibroglial scars may adhere dura to adjacent brain and cause seizures.

■ Other Imaging Findings

- CT angiography of the brain is used for suspected vascular trauma.
- Brain MRI is recommended in acute or subacute traumatic brain injury when initial or follow-up CT image is negative with unexplained neurologic findings.
- T2* and susceptibility-weighted imaging MRI sequences detect acute, early subacute, and chronic stages of diffuse axonal injury.

✓ Pearls and ✗ Pitfalls

- ✓ Coup and contrecoup cerebral injuries consist of parenchymal contusions and extra-axial hemorrhages adjacent to the site of injury and in the opposite side of the brain. The contralateral parenchymal injuries tend to be more severe.
- ✗ Subarachnoid hemorrhage in the olfactory sulcus can be easily missed in the baseline CT image due to volume averaging with the horizontal ethmoid plate, and it may become evident on follow-up exams when the swelling from the associated contusions ensues.

Case 85

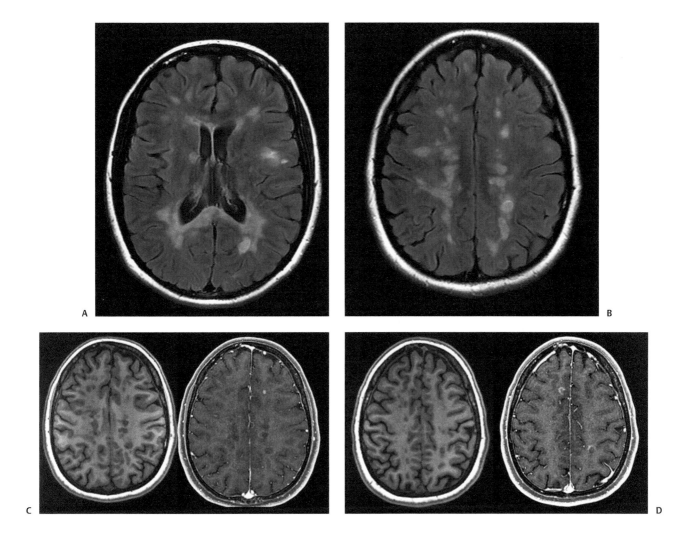

■ Clinical Presentation

A 21-year-old with sensory disturbance in upper and lower extremities.

■ Imaging Findings

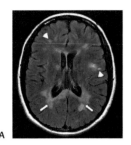
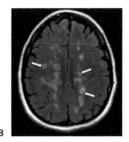
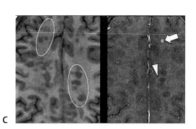
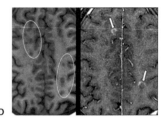

(A) Axial fluid-attenuated inversion recovery (FLAIR) image demonstrates numerous ovoid lesions in the periventricular (*arrows*) and juxtacortical white matter (*arrowheads*), more confluent near the atria of the lateral ventricles. **(B)** Axial FLAIR image shows numerous confluent ovoid lesions in the periventricular white matter (*arrows*). **(C)** Axial T1 pre- and postcontrast images demonstrate numerous white matter lesions with low T1 signal (*ovals*), some of which enhance in a solid (*arrow*) or incomplete ring (*arrowhead*) pattern. The simultaneous presence of T1 lesions with and without enhancement can be used to establish dissemination in time, in the absence of comparison exams. **(D)** Axial T1 pre- and postcontrast images demonstrate numerous white matter lesions with low T1 signal (*ovals*), some of which enhance in an incomplete ring pattern (*arrows*).

■ Differential Diagnosis

- ***Multiple sclerosis (MS):***
  - White matter lesions corresponding to acute and chronic demyelination.
  - Characteristic MS lesions are periventricular in location and ovoid in shape, > 3 mm (as opposed to being punctate), well circumscribed, and homogeneous in signal intensity, and they may or may not be associated with enhancement, which is often ring-like in morphology.
  - Juxtacortical, periventricular, infratentorial, and spinal cord lesions tend to be more specific for MS.
- *Leukoaraiosis:*
  - Also known as cerebral white matter disease and cerebral small vessel disease.
  - Increasing age and hypertension are the only accepted risk factors.
  - Lesions appear as low attenuation areas on CT and as areas with high signal on T2-weighted or fluid-attenuated inversion recovery (FLAIR) MRI scans.
  - Lesions typically spare the subcortical U-fibers.
  - In mild small-vessel disease, lesions are distinct from each other, but with increasing disease severity they become confluent and eventually diffusely involve an entire region.
- *Vasculitis:*
  - Cause of neurologic dysfunction and multiple focal (ischemic) lesions in the same age range as the MS-prone population.
  - The abnormalities of the corpus callosum, U-fibers, optic nerves, and spinal cord are not typical of vascular disease and may aid in the differentiation of MS from vascular disease.

■ Essential Facts

- MS is a chronic demyelinating disease of the central nervous system (CNS) that occurs primarily in young adults. Diagnosis of MS per 2010 McDonald criteria requires elimination of more likely diagnoses and demonstration of dissemination of lesions in space and time.

- Dissemination in space can be shown by involvement of at least two of five areas of the CNS (three or more periventricular lesions, one or more infratentorial lesions, one or more spinal cord lesions, one or more optic nerve lesions, one or more cortical or juxtacortical lesions).
- Dissemination in time can be established by the following: presence of at least one new T2 or gadolinium enhancing lesion on follow-up MRI scan, with reference to a baseline scan, irrespective of the timing of the baseline MRI scan; or the simultaneous presence of asymptomatic gadolinium enhancing and nonenhancing lesions at any time.

■ Other Imaging Findings

- MR spectroscopy can aid in the distinction between tumefactive demyelinating lesions and tumors.

✓ Pearls and ✗ Pitfalls

✓ Nonenhancing T1-hypointense lesions (black holes) are chronic lesions characterized by severe axonal damage. T1-hypointense lesion formation is more common in patients with long disease durations and progressive disease subtypes. For that reason, their presence in patients with a clinically isolated syndrome is indicative of an already-established MS disease process.

✗ The term *radiologically isolated syndrome* was first introduced in 2009 to define and characterize the group of individuals who are free of symptoms of CNS demyelination but who have visible features on brain MRI scans that appear to be consistent with MS and who appear to be at risk for future demyelinating events.

Case 86

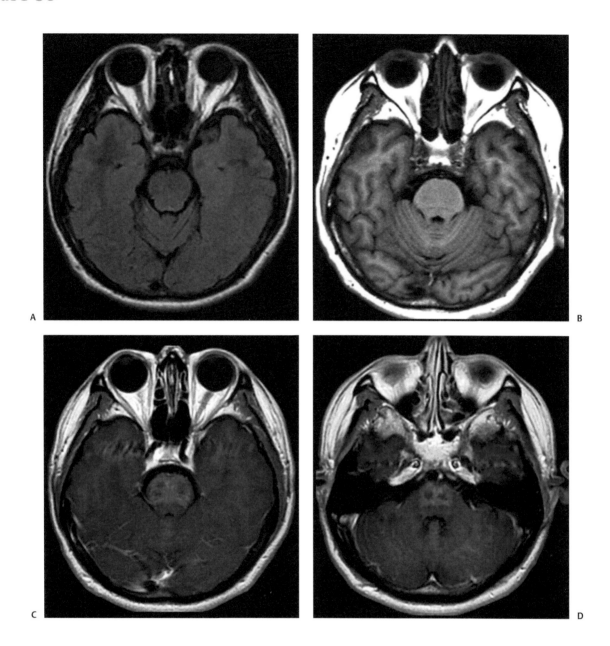

■ Clinical Presentation

A 41-year-old man presents with recent onset headache and chronic vertigo. Found to have elevated protein in cerebrospinal fluid.

■ Imaging Findings

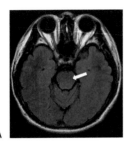 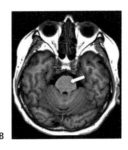 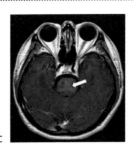 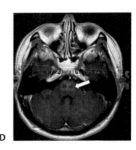

(A) Axial fluid-attenuated inversion recovery sequence shows normal signal intensity in the pons (*arrow*). **(B)** Axial precontrast T1-weighted image (WI) demonstrates normal signal intensity in the pons (*arrow*). **(C)** Axial postcontrast T1WI demonstrates confluent linear and punctate areas of enhancement in the pons (*arrow*). **(D)** Axial postcontrast T1WI demonstrates confluent linear and punctate areas of enhancement in the pons (*arrow*).

■ Differential Diagnosis

- ***Chronic lymphocytic inflammation with pontine perivascular enhancement responsive to steroids (CLIPPERS):***
  - Punctate and curvilinear gadolinium enhancement "peppering" the pons on MRI scans. A subtle radiating pattern can be seen.
  - Mainly involves the pons and the cerebellum but may extend to medulla and the midbrain, spinal cord, basal ganglia, or cerebral white matter.
  - Absence of restricted diffusion, marked hyperintensity on T2-weighted image, and of abnormalities on cerebral angiography.
- *Acute disseminated encephalomyelitis (ADEM):*
  - ADEM is a monophasic demyelinating disease of the central nervous system (CNS) that presents with numerous T2 hyperintense white and gray matter lesions.
  - The thalami and basal ganglia are frequently involved, typically in a symmetric fashion. The brainstem and posterior fossa can also be involved.
  - Contrast enhancement is infrequent.
  - Prior infectious episode or vaccination functions as a trigger to the inflammatory response.
  - Young and adolescent children are most affected.
  - It has a favorable prognosis.
- *Sarcoidosis:*
  - Multisystem inflammatory disease characterized by noncaseating epithelioid-cell granulomas.
  - Imaging manifestations include solitary or multifocal masses involving the dura, leptomeninges, subarachnoid and perivascular spaces, cranial nerves, brain parenchyma (hypothalamus, brainstem, cerebral hemispheres, cerebellum), and spine.

■ Essential Facts

- CLIPPERS is a chronic inflammatory disorder in the CNS characterized by white matter perivascular lymphohistiocytic infiltrate with or without parenchymal extension.
- Patients present clinically with subacute progressive ataxia, diplopia, and other clinical features referable to brainstem pathology.

- There is prompt and significant clinical and radiologic response to glucocorticosteroids.
- Differential diagnoses should be excluded: neurosarcoidosis, Sjögren syndrome, neuro-Behçet's disease, multiple sclerosis, ADEM, neuromyelitis optica, Bickerstaff encephalitis, other autoimmune encephalitides, CNS vasculitis, CNS infections, histiocytosis, lymphoma, glioma, paraneoplastic syndromes.

■ Other Imaging Findings

- The lesions usually cause no mass effect and minimal or no vasogenic edema.
- In some exceptional cases, brainstem mass effect in the form of pons or middle cerebellar peduncle swelling has been observed during relapses.
- Gadolinium enhancement decreases as the patient responds to immunosuppressive therapy.
- Pontocerebellar/cerebellar, spinal cord, and cerebral atrophy may be observed in the course of the disease.

✓ Pearls and ✗ Pitfalls

- ✓ An alternative diagnosis to CLIPPERS should be considered if:
  - There are unusual clinical findings such as fever, meningism, and systemic symptoms such as arthritis, uveitis, sicca syndrome, or lymphadenopathy.
  - MRI showing pontine lesions with necrosis may point to a primary CNS lymphoma.
  - MRI showing marked mass effect is suggestive of tumor.
  - Marked CSF pleocytosis ($> 100/\mu L$) or malignant cells should prompt reevaluation of the diagnosis.
- ✗ A biopsy from areas that are specifically involved radiologically may be necessary in selected situations such as:
  - Alternative etiologies remain a distinct possibility despite rigorous investigations.
  - Uncommon, atypical clinical or MRI findings are noticed (e.g., signs of systemic disease; MRI disclosing dominant brainstem mass effects or necrosis).
  - Resistance to glucocorticoid treatment.

Case 87

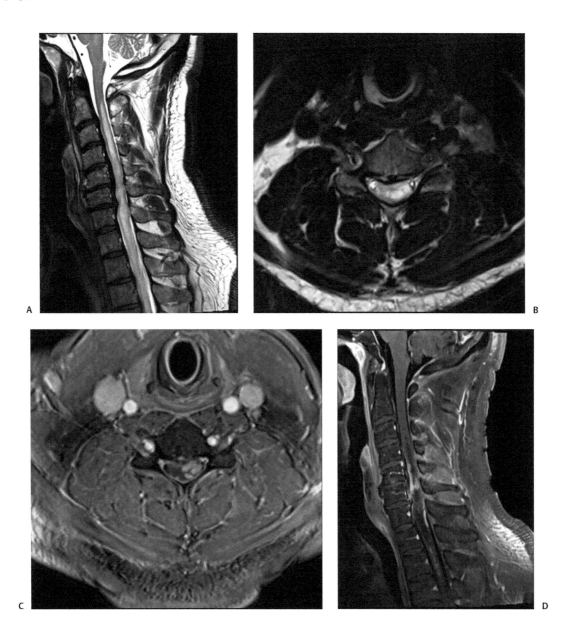

■ Clinical Presentation

A 37-year-old woman patient with progressive weakness in the superior and inferior extremities. Past medical history of recurrent optic neuritis.

■ Imaging Findings

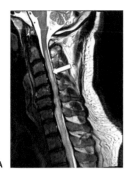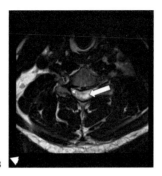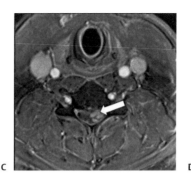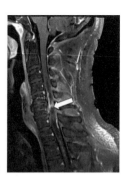

A   B   C   D

(A) Sagittal T2-weighted image (WI) shows diffuse thickening of the cervical and thoracic spinal cord with increased signal (*arrow*). **(B)** Axial T2WI shows bilateral increased T2 signal that involves more than two thirds of the cross-sectional area of the cord (*arrow*). **(C, D)** Axial **(C)** and sagittal **(D)** T1WI with contrast show areas of patchy enhancement in the spinal cord (*arrows*).

■ Differential Diagnosis

- ***Neuromyelitis optica (NMO):***
  - Longitudinally extensive T2 signal increases in the cord that involves more than three vertebral segments and affects > 50% of the cross-sectional area of the cord.
  - Patchy areas of enhancement in areas of relapse.
- *Multiple sclerosis (MS):*
  - Chronic inflammatory demyelinating disease affecting the brain and cord.
  - Peripherally located focal, asymmetric spinal cord lesions that extend less than two vertebral segments in length and occupy less than half the cross-sectional area of the cord.
  - In the axial images, lesions may have a wedge shape with their base at the cord surface, or a round shape if there is no contact with the cord surface.
- *Spinal cord astrocytoma:*
  - Eccentric infiltrative lesion of the spinal cord.
  - Hemorrhage is uncommon.
  - Can present with a cystic component.
  - Enhancement is common.
  - No increase in aquaporin levels.

■ Essential Facts

- Neuromyelitis optica is also known as Devic disease.
- Autoimmune disease.
- Elevated aquaporin-4.
- Characterized by bilateral visual disturbance and transverse myelopathy.
- Mono- or multiphasic course.
- Worse prognosis than MS.
- More frequent in females.
- In the brain, NMO presents with recurrent optic neuritis.

■ Other Imaging Findings

- Enhancement is noted during relapse and is smaller in extension than the T2 abnormalities in the spine.
- Brain lesions with morphology and location not typical for MS.

✓ Pearls and ✗ Pitfalls

- ✓ The value of fractional anisotropy is close to normal in NMO, whereas it tends to be lower than normal in MS.
- ✗ The presence of white matter lesions in the brain does not exclude NMO.
- ✗ NMO lesions are not associated with hemorrhage.

Case 88

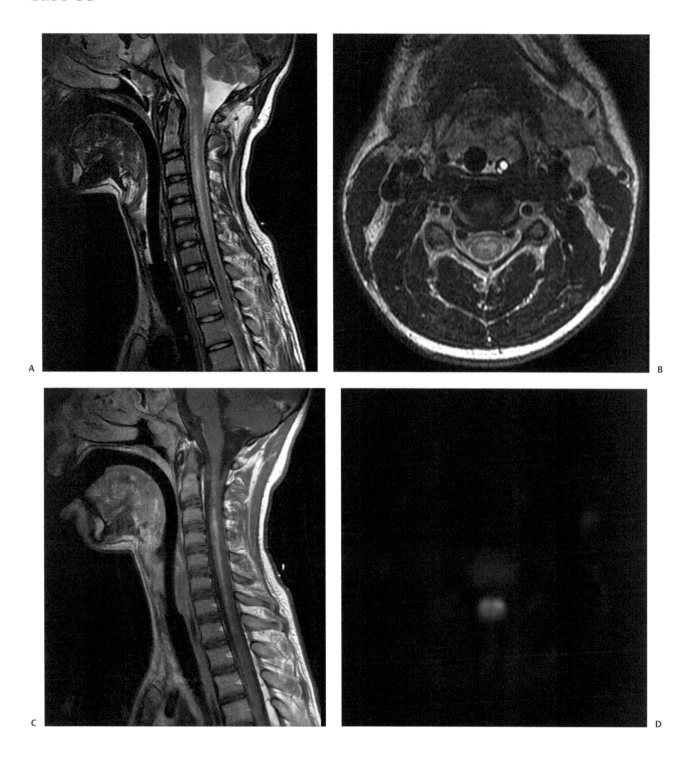

A

B

C

D

■ Clinical Presentation

A 13-year-old boy presents with back pain and bilateral arm numbness.

■ Imaging Findings

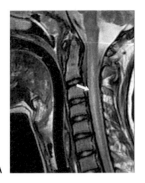
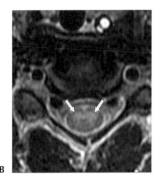
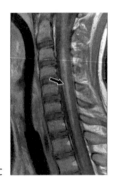
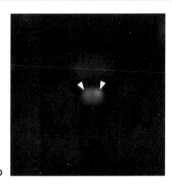

A   B   C   D

(A) Sagittal T2-weighted MR image of the cervical spine shows mildly expansile increased T2 signal along the ventral portion of the spinal cord extending from C2 to C7 (*white arrow*). **(B)** Axial T2-weighted MR of the cervical spine shows increased T2 signal involving the bilateral ventral horns of the cervical cord (*white arrows*). **(C)** Sagittal T1-weighted postcontrast image of the cervical spine shows ill-defined linear enhancement corresponding to the site of T2 signal abnormality of the ventral cord (*black arrow*). **(D)** Axial diffusion-weighted imaging at the cervical spine level demonstrates increased signal consistent with restricted diffusion in the ventral horns bilaterally (*white arrowheads*).

■ Differential Diagnosis

- **Spinal cord infarct:** Uncommon ischemic condition of acute presentation more commonly affecting the anterior cord and resulting in increased T2 signal that can be expansile in the acute/subacute stages secondary to edema. Diffusion-weighted imaging (DWI) sequences reveal restricted diffusion.
- *Transverse myelitis:* Inflammatory condition of the spinal cord resulting in acute motor, sensory, and autonomic dysfunction. MR imaging reveals long-segment increased T2 signal with variable enhancement. However, generally more than two thirds of the cross-sectional area of the cord is involved and no restricted diffusion is present.
- *Viral myelitis:* Viral myelitis secondary to entities such as enterovirus and poliovirus results in increased T2 signal and enlargement of the ventral horns of the spinal cord extending through long segments of the cord without associated restricted diffusion.

■ Essential Facts

- Blood supply to the spinal cord: Medullary arteries arising from radicular arteries, along with the anterior and posterior spinal arteries.
- The anterior spinal artery supplies the majority of the anterior two thirds of the cord, including the gray matter ventral horns and commissure, by giving off a sulcal artery.
- The outlining white matter receives its vascular supply from pial branches of the anastomotic circumferential plexus that also receives blood from paired posterior spinal arteries and medullary branches.
- Spinal cord ischemia can result from interruption of flow from a major branch, which typically results in either an anterior or posterior distribution, or in the case of severe hypoperfusion, there can be central spinal cord ischemia.

- Anterior cord infarcts are generally bilateral because of the single sulcal artery giving rise to the blood supply of the bilateral ventral horns.
- Posterior cord infarcts are typically unilateral because the posterior vertebral arteries are paired structures.

■ Other Imaging Findings

- T2 hyperintensity within the ventral horns bilaterally has been termed the "owl's eye sign" or "snake-eye sign" and is not pathognomonic of cord infarcts.
- There may be mild expansion of the cord secondary to edema in the subacute stage.
- The peripheral white matter is generally spared because it receives anastomotic blood supply from the posterior and radicular artery circulation.

✓ Pearls and ✗ Pitfalls

✓ Patients commonly present with acute back pain and urinary and bowel incontinence. However, clinical symptoms are highly variable depending on distribution and severity of ischemia.
✓ DWI reveals restricted diffusion and enhancement that may be present in the subacute stage.
✓ There is a wide range of causes ranging from idiopathic, traumatic, coagulopathic, and atherosclerotic, among others.
✗ DWI in the spinal canal is challenging because of flow artifact from pulsating cerebrospinal fluid and small cord size.
✗ MRI scan in cord ischemia may be normal during the first 1 to 2 days, after which T2 changes ensue and later enhancement may develop. Conversely, acute myelitis shows high T2 signal and enhancement in the acute phase, which may serve as a helpful way to differentiate these entities.

Case 89

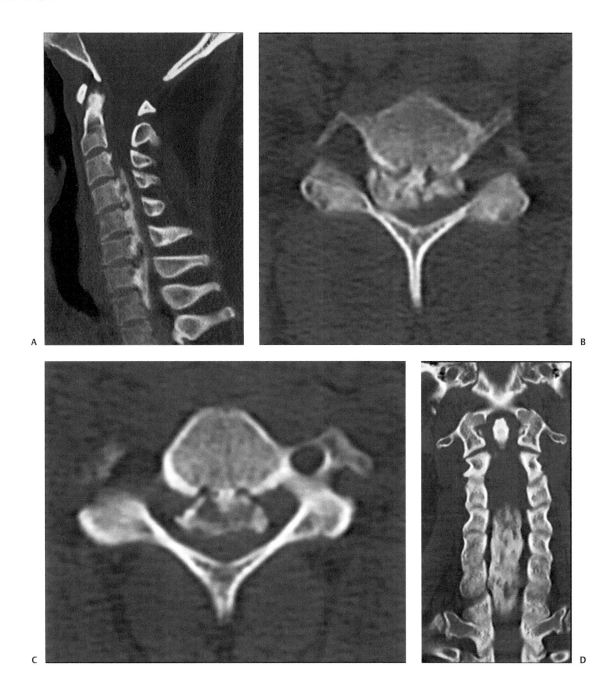

A

B

C

D

■ Clinical Presentation

A 65-year-old man presents with paresthesia in both upper extremities.

■ Imaging Findings

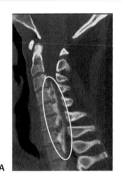
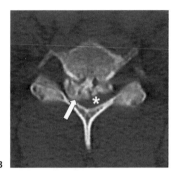
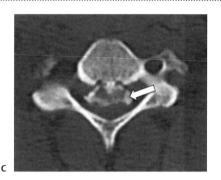
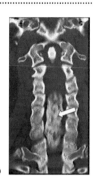

A   B   C   D

(A) Sagittal reformatted CT image of the spine shows continuous ossification of the posterior longitudinal ligament spanning from C4 to T1 (*oval*), leading to a narrow central spinal canal. **(B)** Axial CT image of the cervical spine demonstrates a large ossified posterior longitudinal ligament (*arrow*) occupying the majority of the spinal canal. The cord is presumably compressed in the small remaining space (*asterisk*). **(C)** Axial CT image of the cervical spine demonstrates a large ossified posterior longitudinal ligament (*arrow*) with a "mushroom" shape. **(D)** Coronal reformatted CT image of the spine shows continuous ossification of the posterior longitudinal ligament spanning from C4 to T1 (*arrow*).

■ Differential Diagnosis

- ***Ossification of the posterior longitudinal ligament (OPLL):***
  - Heterotopic ossification in the posterior longitudinal ligament, which can lead to abutment and/or compression of the cord.
  - In the axial images, it can be described as central or lateral, and the shape as square, mushroom, or hill-like.
  - In the sagittal images, the ossification can be continuous or discontinuous.
- *Diffuse idiopathic skeletal hyperostosis (DISH):*
  - Also known as Forestier disease.
  - Flowing anterior vertebral ossification spanning at least four contiguous vertebral bodies, with minimal degenerative disk disease or facet arthropathy.
  - More frequent in the thoracic spine.
  - Usually asymptomatic.
- *Ankylosing spondylitis (AS):*
  - Seronegative spondyloarthropathy characterized by fusion (ankylosis) of the spine and sacroiliac joints.
  - Imaging findings include:
    - Syndesmophyte formation, with paraspinous ligamentous or disk ossification bridging two adjacent vertebral bodies.
    - Sacroiliac joint erosive arthritis predominantly involving the lower one third of the joint.
    - Corner erosions of vertebral bodies.
    - Ossification of paraspinous ligaments and annulus fibrosus.
    - Inflammatory arthritis of synovial joints.
    - Atypical fractures through syndesmophytes, vertebral bodies, or end plates, and pseudoarthrosis may occur.

■ Essential Facts

- Familial inheritance and genetic factors have been implicated in the etiology of OPLL.
- The cervical spine is most commonly affected followed by the thoracic spine.

- The clinical manifestations range from asymptomatic to myelopathy or myeloradiculopathy.
- DISH can coexist with OPLL in ~ 25% of cases.
- Ossification of the ligamentum flavum can also be seen with OPLL, more commonly in the thoracic spine. The coexistence of both entities can exacerbate the degree of cord compression.

■ Other Imaging Findings

- CT can show OPLL type, thickness, length of involved segments, and associated diseases such as DISH.
- MRI can show degree of cord abutment, disk herniations, and signal changes in the cord, which have important prognostic implications.

✓ Pearls and ✗ Pitfalls

- ✓ The CT double-density or double-layer sign is seen on bone window axial CT as two separate ossified rims separated by a nonossified mass representing a hypertrophied PLL. It is thought to represent dural penetration or tight adherence of OPLL to the dura. This imaging finding is associated with a higher incidence of dural tear during anterior decompression.
- ✗ One of several OPLL classifications classifies them using sagittal images into bridge type (when the ossification is connected to the adjacent posterior margin of two or more vertebral levels) and non-bridge type. Distinguishing between bridge and non-bridge OPLL may be important because vertebral body segmental motion is lost where there is bridge-type OPLL and is increased adjacent to the bridge, perhaps leading to segmental instability.

Case 90

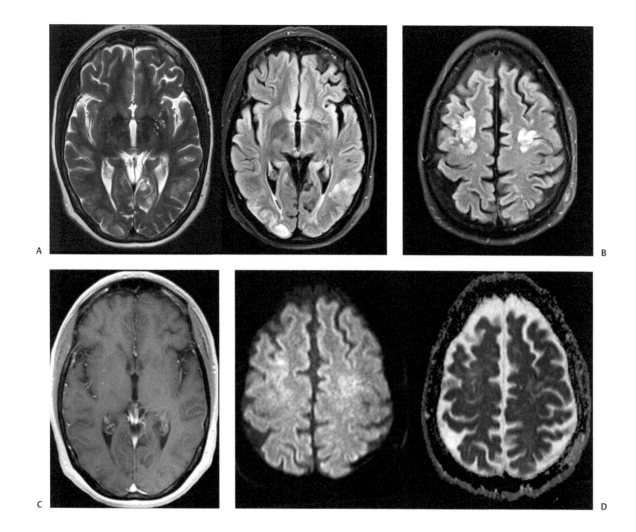

A

B

C

D

■ Clinical Presentation

A 28-year-old woman presents with visual disturbances after an episode of hypertension induced by pregnancy.

■ Imaging Findings

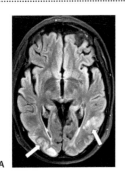 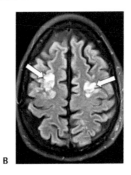 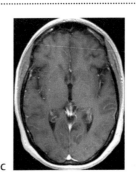 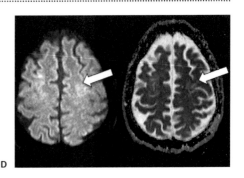

(A) Axial fluid-attenuated inversion recovery (FLAIR) image shows bilateral hyperintensities in the occipital and parietal lobes (*arrows*). **(B)** Axial FLAIR image shows increased signal in both frontal lobes in a "watershed" distribution (*arrows*). **(C)** Axial T1-weighted image with contrast, the lesions show no enhancement. **(D)** Diffusion-weighted image and apparent diffusion coefficient maps images show no restricted diffusion in the lesions (*arrows*).

■ Differential Diagnosis

- ***Posterior reversible encephalopathy syndrome (PRES):***
  - Also known as hypertensive encephalopathy.
  - Symmetric cortical-subcortical lesions favoring both parietal and occipital lobes.
  - Generally vasogenic, not cytotoxic, edema.
  - Decreased perfusion in affected areas.
  - Edema usually completely reverses.
  - Associated with high blood pressure (75%).
- *Venous infarcts:*
  - Sagittal sinus thrombosis can manifest as bilateral occipital venous infarcts.
  - Presence of the empty delta sign.
  - Cortical and subcortical petechial hemorrhages, with mixed hyperintense and hypointense T2 signal, typically not patchy like PRES.
  - Has both cytotoxic and vasogenic edema.
  - Lesions can be reversible.
  - Diffusion-weighted imaging (DWI) is positive if cytotoxic edema is present.
- *Watershed cerebral ischemia:*
  - Cytotoxic edema evident on DWI.
  - Involvement of the deep white matter (not subcortical) in a "string of pearls" pattern, or involvement of the cortex at the junction of the anterior-middle or middle-posterior cerebral artery junctions.

■ Essential Facts

- Disorder of the cerebrovascular autoregulation.
- Associated conditions include:
  - Toxemia of pregnancy (preeclampsia/eclampsia).
  - Posttransplantation.
  - Immune suppression (cyclosporine, tacrolimus).
  - Infection, sepsis, shock.
  - Autoimmune diseases.
  - Status post-cancer chemotherapy.

- Other conditions: dialysis/erythropoietin, triple-H therapy (combination of induced hypertension, hypervolemia, and hemodilution).

■ Other Imaging Findings

- Fluid-attenuated inversion recovery is the imaging of choice to recognize small abnormalities.
- DWI scan is usually normal but some patients may show restricted diffusion.
- Perfusion studies show low perfusion of the affected areas.
- Contrast: Patchy irregular enhancement.
- Angiography: Focal areas of vasodilatation, vasoconstriction, and "string of beads" have been described.

✓ Pearls and ✗ Pitfalls

- ✓ Hemorrhage (focal hematoma, isolated sulcal/subarachnoid blood) is seen in approximately 15% of patients.
- ✓ Holohemispheric watershed pattern: Linear involvement of the frontal, parietal and occipital lobes.
- ✓ Dominant parieto-occipital pattern: Typical posterior pattern affecting only the parietal and occipital lobes.
- ✗ Focal areas of restricted diffusion (likely representing infarction or tissue injury with cytotoxic edema) are uncommon (11–26%) and may be associated with an adverse outcome.
- ✗ Lesions tend to be more asymmetric when related to eclampsia and transplants. They are more symmetric when associated with hypertension, sepsis, and shock.

Case 91

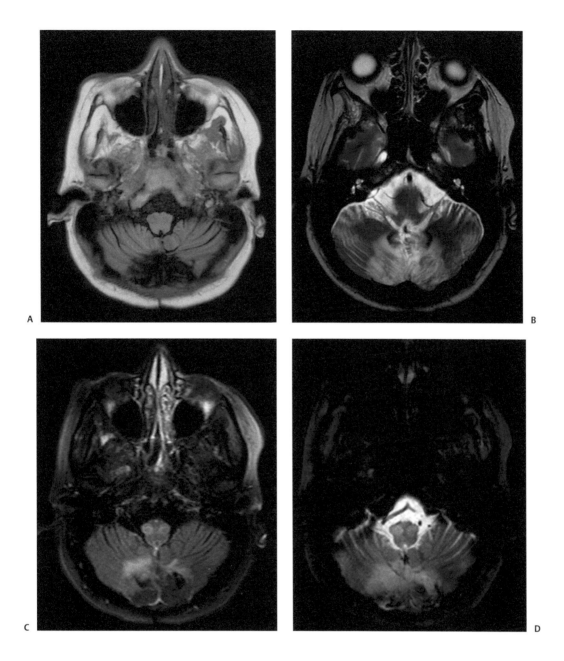

A

B

C

D

■ Clinical Presentation

A 37-year-old woman presents with history of posterior fossa astrocytoma resection.

■ Imaging Findings

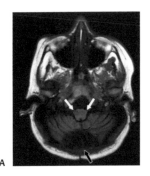 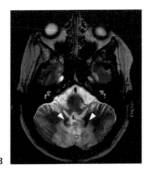 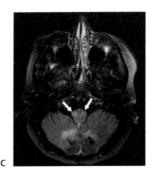 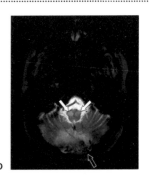

A   B   C   D

(A) Axial T1-weighted image (WI) of the brain. Postoperative changes are noted in the posterior fossa (*black arrow*) secondary to resection of astrocytoma. The inferior olivary nuclei are enlarged and demonstrate decreased signal bilaterally, right greater than left (*white arrows*). **(B)** Axial T2WI through the posterior fossa shows encephalomalacia and surrounding gliosis involving the medial cerebellar hemispheres (*asterisk*) and surrounding the dentate nuclei bilaterally, which in turn exhibit decreased T2 signal (*white arrowheads*). **(C)** Axial fluid-attenuated inversion recovery image better demonstrates the enlargement and increased T2 signal involving the bilateral inferior olivary nuclei (*white arrows*). **(D)** Axial gradient echo sequence shows areas of susceptibility artifact in the medial cerebellar hemispheres secondary to remote blood products (*black arrow*) from resection of posterior fossa mass. The inferior olivary nuclei are enlarged and well-demarcated (*white arrows*).

■ Differential Diagnosis

- **Hypertrophic olivary degeneration (HOD):** Caused by damage to the dentato-rubro-olivary pathway leading to degeneration of the inferior olivary nuclei, which become hypertrophic and characteristically exhibit increased T2 signal.
- *Infarction:* A focal infarction in the medulla may present as a small area of increased T2 signal with edema. Bilateral, symmetric foci due to ischemia are unlikely.
- *Demyelination:* Demyelinating plaques in the brainstem can have similar features. During an active phase, demyelination may show increased T2 signal, have a similar rounded morphology, and can show an expanded, edematous appearance. As with ischemia, the bilateral and symmetric appearance is unlikely in demyelinating conditions.

■ Essential Facts

- The Guillain-Mollaret triangle is a pathway composed of the ipsilateral red nucleus, ipsilateral inferior olivary nucleus, and the contralateral dentate nucleus. The communication between these three structures forms the dentato-rubro-olivary pathway.
- Damage to the dentato-rubro tract in the superior cerebellar peduncle or the central tegmental tract connecting the red nucleus to the inferior olivary nucleus may lead to HOD.
- Interestingly, the degeneration of the olive causes hypertrophy rather than atrophy with associated increased T2 signal.
- Common causes include neoplasms, surgery, trauma, ischemia, and hemorrhage.

■ Other Imaging Findings

- Increase in the T2 signal of the inferior olivary nuclei typically occurs 2 months following the insult, whereas hypertrophy appears at around 6 months and can last up to 3 to 4 years.
- Eventually, hypertrophy of the inferior olivary nuclei subsides and atrophy occurs. However, T2 hyperintensity can persist indefinitely.
- In the chronic stage, there can be contralateral cerebellar atrophy.

✓ Pearls and ✗ Pitfalls

- ✓ Evidence of interruption of the Guillain-Mollaret triangle.
- ✓ Unilateral or bilateral hypertrophy and increased T2 signal involving the inferior olivary nuclei.
- ✓ Delayed onset, occurs ~ 4 to 12 months following the insult.
- ✗ Perforating artery infarcts and demyelinating plaques may have similar appearance.
- ✗ HOD does not enhance, which may aid in differentiating it from acute demyelination.
- ✗ Perforating artery infarcts are rarely bilateral and symmetric.

Case 92

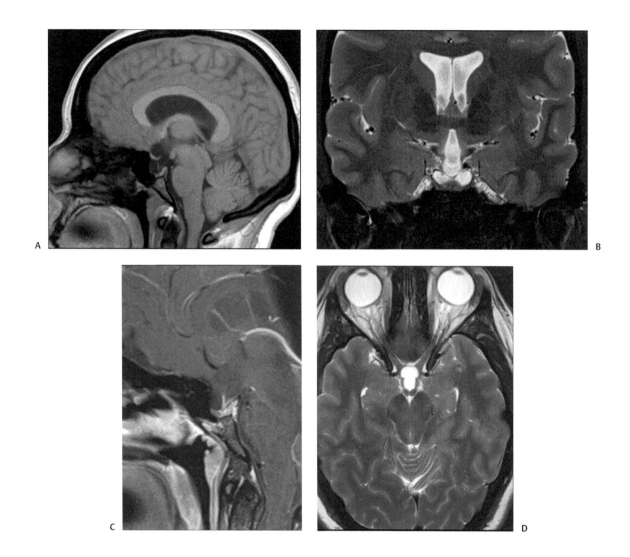

■ Clinical Presentation

History withheld.

■ Imaging Findings

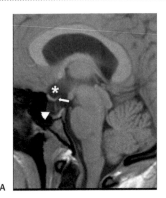 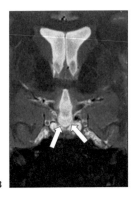 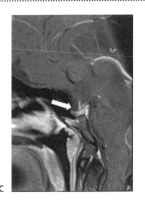 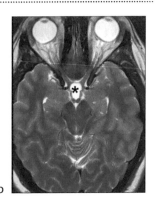

(A) Sagittal T1 without contrast shows prominence of the suprachiasmatic recess (*asterisk*) along with downward bowing of the optic chiasm (*arrow*) consistent with herniation into a partially empty sella turcica (*arrowhead*). (B) Coronal T2-weighted image (WI) shows a prominent third ventricle with downward bowing of the optic chiasm (*arrows*). (C) Sagittal T1 with contrast shows the prominence of the suprachiasmatic recess with no abnormal enhancement (*arrow*). (D) Axial T2WI shows prominence of the anterior recess of the third ventricle (*asterisk*).

■ Differential Diagnosis

- *Optic chiasm herniation:*
  - Herniation of the optic chiasm into a sella that demonstrates an empty or partially empty sella configuration.
  - Symptomatic herniation is more common in secondary empty sella configurations.
- *Septo-optic dysplasia:*
  - Congenital disease.
  - Small optic chiasm.
  - Small pituitary gland.
  - Absence of the septum pellucidum.
- *Kallmann syndrome:*
  - Aplasia or hypoplasia of the olfactory bulbs or tracts.
  - Hypoplastic anterior pituitary gland.
  - Hypoplastic optic chiasm and optic nerves.

■ Essential Facts

- Represented as a downward angulation of the optic chiasm into the sellar region. It can also be accompanied by herniation of the anterior and inferior third ventricle.
- Secondary signs include distention of the suprachiasmatic recess.
- Symptoms are rare and include upper bitemporal visual field defects and optic atrophy, and can progress to loss of vision.

■ Other Imaging Findings

- The patterns of herniation have been described as primary and secondary. Primary empty sella configuration has no known cause and may be secondary to pulsating arachnoidoceles. Secondary empty sella is due to a specific cause such as surgery, radiation, chemotherapy, or hemorrhage. The latter are associated with inflammation and adhesions.

✓ Pearls and ✗ Pitfalls

- ✓ It is crucial to evaluate for the possibility of herniation of the optic chiasm as a cause of visual field defects or delayed visual deterioration after pituitary interventions.
- ✓ Chiasmatic herniation is more frequent in secondary empty sella configurations.
- ✓ No correlation with the presence of herniation and pituitary gland hormonal disturbances has been identified.
- ✗ Look carefully for abnormal downward angulation of the optic chiasm in patients with visual field disturbances and empty sella configuration.
- ✗ Be sure not to confuse a hypoplastic optic chiasm with a herniation into the sella.

Case 93

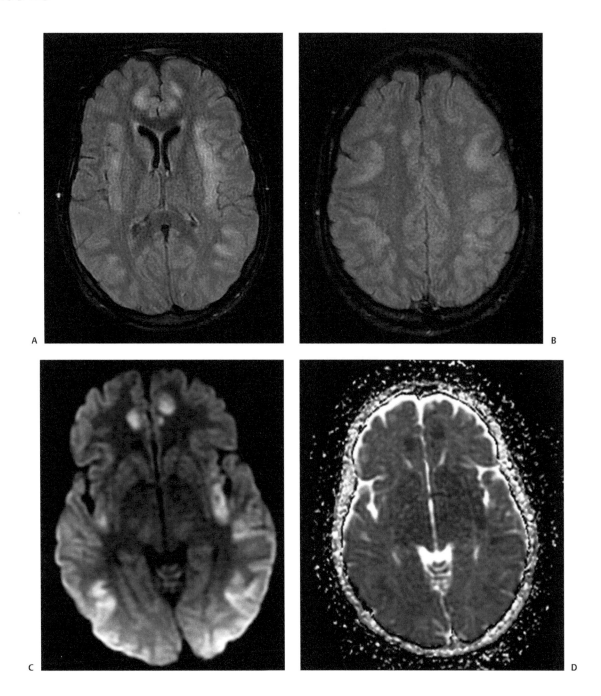

■ **Clinical Presentation**

A 23-year-old woman presents with altered mental status following induction chemotherapy for acute leukemia.

■ Imaging Findings

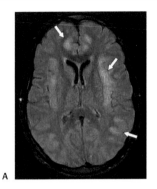 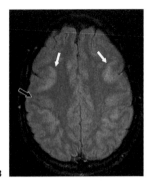 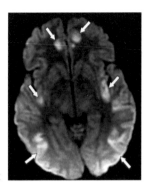 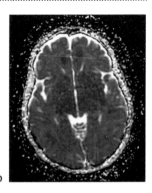

(A, B) Axial T2 fluid-attenuated inversion recovery images demonstrate hyperintensity involving the cortex and subcortical white matter of the medial frontal lobes, insulae, and parietal lobes bilaterally (*white arrows*). The perirolandic regions are relatively spared (*black arrow*). **(C, D)** Axial diffusion-weighted image (DWI) and corresponding apparent diffusion coefficient (ADC) map show increased DWI signal and low ADC values consistent with restricted diffusion at the site of increased T2 signal in the frontal lobes, temporooccipital regions, and insulae bilaterally (*white arrows*).

■ Differential Diagnosis

- **Hepatic encephalopathy (HE):** Neurologic condition resulting from increased ammonia and manganese levels that cause toxicity to astrocytes and neurons. This condition presents with bilateral increased T2 signal involving the insula, deep gray nuclei, cingulate gyrus, and internal capsule. Chemotherapeutic agents used in the treatment of acute myeloid leukemia have been linked with the development of HE, typically within the first 4 days of therapy.
- *Hypoxic-ischemic brain injury:* Decreased blood flow and/or blood oxygenation resulting in infarcts involving vulnerable sites including watershed regions, as well as deep and superficial gray matter structures with associated restricted diffusion, diffuse edema, and effacement of the subarachnoid spaces. Most commonly affected brain tissue includes watershed zones in mild-to-moderate insults, and gray matter structures in more severe injury.
- *Creutzfeldt–Jakob disease:* Prion-mediated spongiform encephalopathy that affects the basal ganglia, thalami, cortex, and white matter, with increased T2 signal and associated restricted diffusion. Signal abnormality of the dorsomedial thalamic nuclei results in the classic pulvinar sign or "hockey stick" sign. Patients are generally older than 60 years of age.

■ Essential Facts

- Also called acute hyperammonemic encephalopathy.
- HE may be further subclassified according to its course in either acute or chronic.
- Whereas acute HE can be rapidly fatal, chronic HE typically has a less severe course and carries a better prognosis.

- The most consistent finding includes increased T2 signal commonly with restricted diffusion affecting the insular cortices and cingulate gyri bilaterally.
- Cortical/subcortical involvement tends to be more variable and asymmetric.
- Generally, there is relative sparing of the occipital and perirolandic regions.

■ Other Imaging Findings

- MR spectroscopy: elevation of glutamine/glutamate (2.1–2.5 parts per million [ppm]) with a decrease in myoinositol (3.55 ppm) and choline (3.2 ppm).
- The degree of metabolic abnormalities is usually proportional to the severity of the hepatic encephalopathy and can be reversible with treatment.

✓ Pearls and ✗ Pitfalls

- ✓ Common causes of hyperammonemia include inborn errors of metabolism, liver and renal failure, chemotherapy, drugs, urinary tract infections, bone marrow and solid organ transplantation, septic shock, and parenteral nutrition, among others.
- ✓ Neurologic manifestations may range from subclinical deficits to death.
- ✗ Chronic brain exposure to increased ammonia levels may lead to an irreversible condition called *acquired hepatocerebral degeneration*. This condition is characterized by intrinsic T1 hyperintensity in the globus pallidus, subthalamic region, and substantia nigra.

Case 94

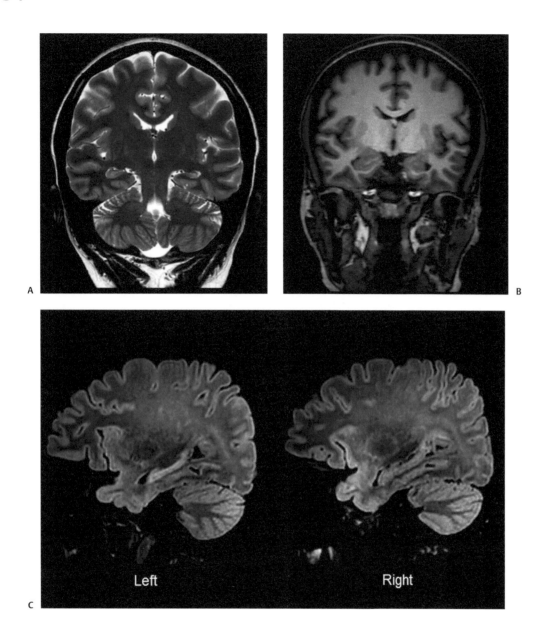

A

B

C

Left   Right

■ Clinical Presentation

A 37-year-old with complex partial seizures.

■ Imaging Findings

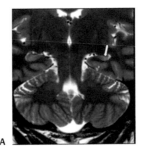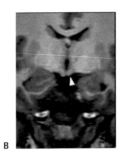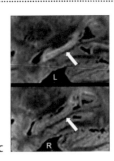

(A) Coronal high-resolution T2-weighted image (WI) of the brain shows decreased height and increased signal of the left hippocampal head (*arrow*). **(B)** Coronal reformatted three-dimensional T1WI of the brain shows asymmetry of the mammillary bodies, left smaller than right (*arrowhead*). **(C)** Sagittal three-dimensional T2 fluid-attenuated inversion recovery sequence of the left (*L*) and right (*R*) hippocampal formations demonstrates decreased height and increased signal intensity of the left hippocampus as compared to the right (*arrows*).

■ Differential Diagnosis

- *Mesial temporal sclerosis (MTS):*
  ○ Asymmetrically small or atrophic hippocampus ipsilateral to the seizure focus.
  ○ Increased T2 signal within the affected hippocampus.
  ○ Secondary intratemporal findings: Loss of internal architecture, loss of hippocampal head digitations, dilatation of the ipsilateral temporal horn, increased signal intensity of the amygdala, volume loss of the temporal lobe, and narrowed collateral white matter (between the hippocampus and the collateral sulcus).
  ○ Secondary extratemporal findings: Atrophy of ipsilateral mammillary body, fornix, thalamus, and cingulate gyrus, and contralateral cerebellar atrophy.
- *Autoimmune limbic encephalitis:*
  ○ Autoantibodies against various neuronal cell antigens may arise independently (nonparaneoplastic) or in association with cancer (paraneoplastic) and cause autoimmune damage to the limbic system.
  ○ MRI shows T2/fluid-attenuated inversion recovery (FLAIR) hyperintensity in the medial aspect of the temporal lobes. Other findings include cerebellar degeneration, striatal encephalitis, brainstem encephalitis, and leukoencephalopathy.
  ○ In general, antibodies against intracellular antigens are associated with underlying malignancies and poor prognosis, and structural abnormalities are not restricted to the limbic structures. Conversely, in restricted limbic encephalitis, neuronal cell-surface antigens are targeted, an associated malignancy is unusual, and its expected response to immunotherapy is superior.
- *Focal cortical dysplasia (FCD):*
  ○ Heterogeneous group of disorders of cortical formation.
  ○ Common cause of epilepsy.
  ○ MRI findings include cortical thickening, blurring of the gray–white matter junction with abnormal architecture of the subcortical layer, T2/FLAIR signal hyperintensity of white matter with or without the transmantle sign, T2/FLAIR signal hyperintensity of gray matter, abnormal sulcal or gyral pattern, and segmental and/or lobar hypoplasia/atrophy.
  ○ Blümcke type Ia FCD is usually confined to the temporal lobe.

■ Essential Facts

- Mesial temporal lobe epilepsy with hippocampal sclerosis (MTLE-HS) is a well-characterized disorder that associates electroclinical features suggestive of seizure onset in the mesial or limbic structures of the temporal lobe with hippocampal sclerosis.
- The most common pathologic finding in surgical specimens of patients with refractory partial seizures is hippocampal sclerosis.
- Surgical removal of this epileptogenic area may be curative or may provide significant reduction in seizure frequency in the majority of individuals.

■ Other Imaging Findings

- Quantitative MRI increases the detection rate and reliability for diagnosing HS, with reported sensitivities of 90 to 95%.
- Ictal single-photon emission CT in MTLE-HS shows typical perfusion patterns of ipsilateral temporal lobe hyperperfusion, as well as ipsilateral frontoparietal and contralateral cerebellar hypoperfusion.
- Interictal 18-fluoro-2-deoxyglucose positron emission tomography (PET) shows multiregional hypometabolism involving predominantly the ipsilateral temporal lobe.
- ^{11}C-flumazenil PET shows hippocampal decreases in central benzodiazepine receptor density.

✓ Pearls and ✗ Pitfalls

✓ An appreciation of forniceal atrophy may aid in assessment of MTS.

✓ MRI diagnosis of bilateral MTS is difficult. Hippocampal signal intensity increase on FLAIR and loss of visibility of the digitations of the head of the hippocampus are helpful in this situation.

✗ Dual pathology, the presence of another potentially epileptogenic extrahippocampal anomaly, is seen in 15 to 20% of MTS cases and is associated with poor postsurgical prognosis. Common types of such lesions include cortical dysgenesis and gliotic lesions acquired in early childhood.

Case 95

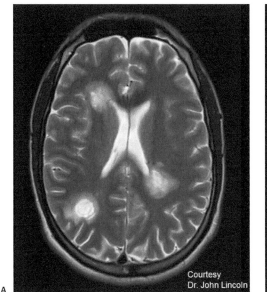

Courtesy
Dr. John Lincoln

A

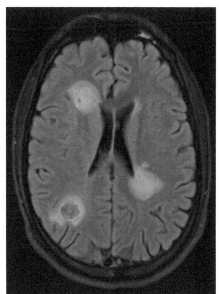

B

■ Clinical Presentation

History withheld.

■ Imaging Findings

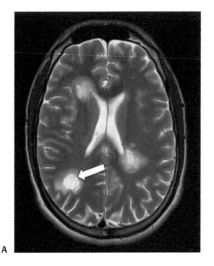 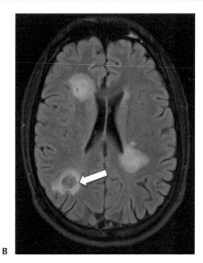

A   B

(A, B) Axial **(A)** T2 and fluid-attenuated inversion recovery **(B)** images show multiple T2 round hyperintensities on both hemispheres. The lesions demonstrate a concentric layered appearance (*arrows*).

■ Differential Diagnosis

- **Baló concentric sclerosis:**
  - Rare demyelinating disease.
  - Aggressive variant of multiple sclerosis (MS).
  - Lesions demonstrate concentric rings on T2-weighted imaging, resembling an "onion bulb."
  - Favors young adults.
- *Metastatic disease:*
  - Can be solitary or multicentric.
  - Favors the subcortical white matter and the posterior fossa.
  - Nodular or ring enhancing lesions.
  - Associated with vasogenic edema.
  - No evidence of "onion bulb" configuration.
- *Acute disseminated encephalomyelitis (ADEM):*
  - Monophasic, demyelinating autoimmune disease typically affecting children, usually following a viral infection.
  - Can mimic MS lesions.
  - Lesions can be symmetric, affect white matter more than gray matter.
  - Most lesions will show enhancement.
  - Not in a concentric ring presentation.
  - Spares the callososeptal interface.

■ Essential Facts

- Considered a variant of multiple sclerosis.
- Typically demonstrates a monophasic presentation, can be fulminant, progressive, or benign. Overall has better prognosis than tumefactive MS.
- MS variants:
  - Marburg disease (malignant).
  - Baló disease (concentric sclerosis).
  - Schilder disease (diffuse myelinoclastic sclerosis).
  - Tumefactive disease.

■ Other Imaging Findings

- Lamellar pattern of concentric rings seen on T2 and T1 contrasted images
- No surrounding vasogenic edema.
- The rings represent alternating areas of demyelination and remyelination.
- Can affect the cerebral hemispheres, cerebellum, brainstem, spinal cord, or optic nerves.
- The lesions typically enhance.

✓ Pearls and ✗ Pitfalls

✓ An overlap of other MS lesions, tumefactive MS, and Schilder disease can be seen at presentation.

Case 96

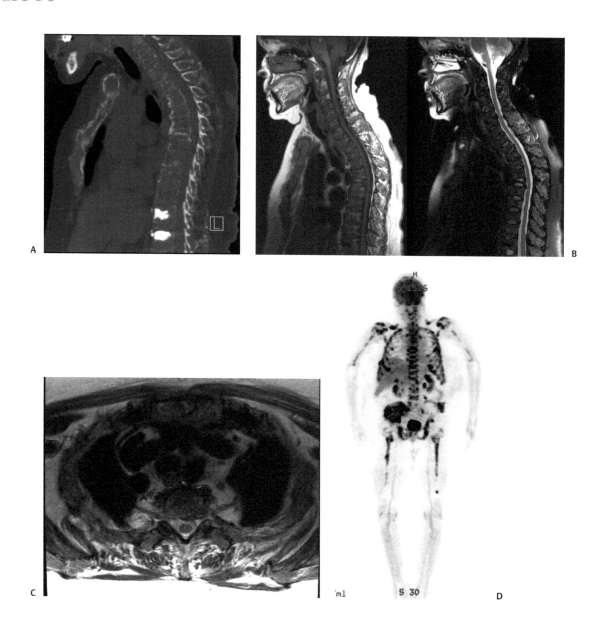

■ Clinical Presentation

A 69-year-old woman presents with diffuse back pain.

■ Imaging Findings

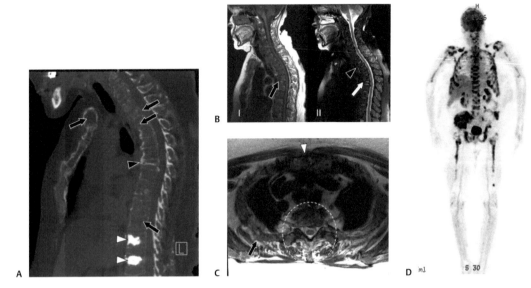

(A) Sagittal CT image of the chest, bone window, shows numerous relatively well-circumscribed "punched out" lucencies involving the imaged osseous structures superimposed on diffuse osteopenia (*black arrows*). Additionally, pathologic fractures are noted at multiple levels with a total collapse of vertebral height of a midthoracic vertebra (*black arrowhead*). Vertebroplasty changes are seen in the superior lumbar spine (*white arrowheads*). (B) Sagittal T1-weighted (*I*) and T2-weighted (*II*) sequences of the cervical and thoracic spine show diffuse permeative bone marrow lesions throughout the imaged osseous structures with low signal on T1 (*black arrow*) and high signal on T2 (*white arrow*). Again seen are multiple pathologic fractures of superior and midthoracic vertebrae (*black arrowhead*). (C) Axial T2 image through the thoracic spine again demonstrates the diffuse bone marrow signal heterogeneity involving both the anterior and posterior elements of the spine (*circle*), as well as the ribs (*black arrow*) and sternum (*white arrowhead*). (D) Fluorodeoxyglucose (FDG)-positron emission tomography shows innumerable FDG-avid skeletal lesions reflecting the sites of greater red marrow, including the vertebrae, ribs, skull, proximal humerus and femur, pelvis, and shoulder girdle.

■ Differential Diagnosis

- **Multiple myeloma (MM):** Diffuse punched-out lytic lesions predominantly involving the axial skeleton where there is greater concentration of red marrow. Typically, the lesions are T1 hypointense and T2 hyperintense, and regions of lysis show fluorodeoxyglucose uptake.
- *Diffuse osteolytic metastases:* Although MM has a greater affinity for the vertebral bodies, metastasis more frequently go to the posterior elements. The distribution within the skeleton is also similar since metastases have a greater tendency to affect red marrow, as does MM.
- *Langerhans cell histiocytosis (LCH):* LCH can have similar lytic/lucent osseous lesions with low T1 and high T2 signal. Also, LCH can be a cause of vertebra plana, especially in the thoracic spine. However, the distribution in the skeleton is slightly different with greater involvement of the skull, pelvis, and femur and usually less involvement of the spine.

■ Essential Facts

- Most common primary osseous malignancy.
- More frequently seen in males, typically between the ages of 40 and 80 years.
- Skeletal surveys can provide a general overview of myelomatous involvement. However, in patients with severe pain the numerous acquisitions can be intolerable. For this reason, low-dose CT can be considered.

- In general MRI, particularly T2 and short tau inversion recovery (STIR) images show high sensitivity for detecting lytic changes.
- Fat-suppression techniques allow for a better characterization of MM.
- Actively lytic lesions tend to enhance on postcontrast images, whereas treated lesions do not.
- Spinal compression fractures are seen in up to 70% of patients with MM.

■ Other Imaging Findings

- MM can also present as a single or as multiple expansile focal masses in the axial skeleton.
- MR is useful in assessing treatment response and can show a decreased extension or even complete resolution of disease burden.

✓ Pearls and ✗ Pitfalls

✓ Features that suggest MM rather than metastases include:
  - Lack of a known primary malignancy.
  - Diffuse marrow involvement, particularly at sites with high red marrow concentration.
  - Numerous compression fractures.
✗ Rarely, MM can progress as leptomeningeal spread and can further point the diagnosis toward metastatic disease.

Case 97

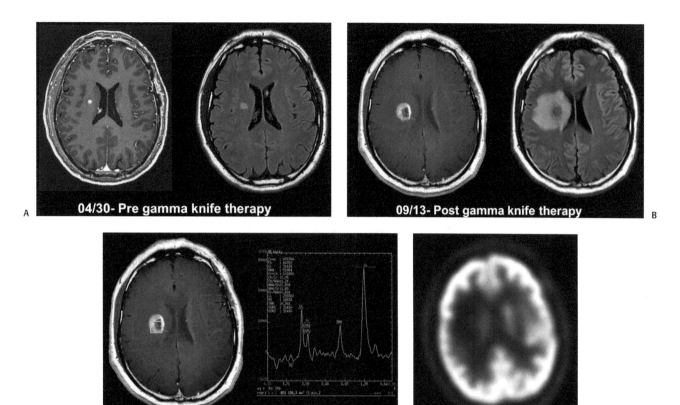

A **04/30- Pre gamma knife therapy**

B **09/13- Post gamma knife therapy**

C **09/13**

D **09/13**

■ Clinical Presentation

A 46-year-old man with history of non-small cell lung cancer with metastasis to the brain undergoes gamma knife therapy to a right frontal lobe lesion.

■ Imaging Findings

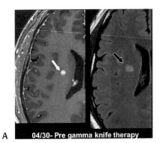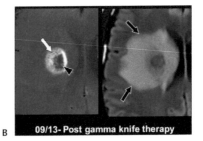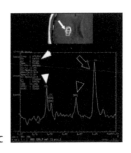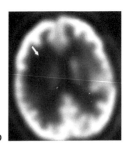

(A) Axial T1 postcontrast and axial T2 fluid-attenuated inversion recovery (FLAIR) images show a small nodular focus of enhancement (*white arrow*) in the right corona radiata with mild surrounding vasogenic edema (*black arrow*) consistent with a brain metastasis. **(B)** Axial T1 postcontrast and axial T2 FLAIR images following gamma knife therapy show interval enlargement of the lesion with central hypointensity (*black arrowhead*), peripheral "soap bubble" enhancement (*white arrow*), and marked progression in surrounding vasogenic edema (*black arrows*). **(C)** Axial T1 postcontrast image shows a single voxel MR spectroscopy box over the site of sampling (*white arrow*). The spectroscopy image shows inversion of the choline:creatine ratio with preservation of normal absolute choline values (*white arrowheads*), mild depression on *N*-acetylaspartate (*black arrowhead*), and a prominent lipid/lactate peak (*black arrow*) indicating a predominance of necrosis. **(D)** Fluorodeoxyglucose (FDG)-positron emission tomography image shows no significant increase in FDG uptake at the site of the enlarging treated lesion (*white arrow*).

■ Differential Diagnosis

- **Radiation necrosis:** Radiation necrosis occurs after radiation therapy to head and neck tumors in the vicinity of brain, radiation to a primary brain tumor, or following stereotactic radiosurgery for brain metastasis. This condition should be suspected when new or progressive enhancement occurs 3 to 12 months after treatment and develops within a lesion included in the radiation field.
- *Tumor recurrence/progression:* Unfortunately, radiation necrosis and tumor progression have overlapping imaging features and also occur at the same time period following therapy, making differentiation difficult. Much like radiation necrosis, tumor progression presents as enlargement of a treated lesion and increased surrounding edema. However, enhancement tends to be more solid and does not show a "soap bubble" appearance. Also, MR perfusion demonstrates increased cerebral blood volume and fluorodeoxyglucose (FDG)-positron emission tomography (PET) shows increased FDG uptake.

■ Essential Facts

- Following chemo and radiotherapy, the margins surrounding the treated lesion may undergo injury and breakdown of the blood–brain barrier.
- A central loss of enhancement within ringlike peripheral enhancement correlates with tumor regression within the year following treatment in ~ 60% of patients. Two to three months after radiation therapy.

- Enhancement in radiation necrosis has been termed "soap bubble" or "Swiss cheese" in appearance.
- Initially, there is an increase in surrounding edema followed by volume loss. The margins of a lesion with radiation necrosis have been described as feathery.

■ Other Imaging Findings

- Comparing the ratio of the size of enhancement on T1 postcontrast imaging to the size of the T2 hypointensity can aid in the diagnosis: The larger the T2 hypointensity and the closer the ratio is to 1, the greater the possibility of tumor progression.
- Relative cerebral blood volume is not increased in patients with radiation necrosis, whereas in tumor progression it is.
- Radiation necrosis is generally hypometabolic on FDG-PET.
- MR spectroscopy in radiation necrosis tends to show high lipid/lactate peak likely reflecting cellular debris. There is mild depression of *N*-acetylaspartate, with variable changes in choline and creatine.

✓ Pearls and ✗ Pitfalls

✓ In cases where radiation necrosis is difficult to differentiate from tumor progression, advanced brain tumor imaging with MR perfusion and spectroscopy, or FDG-PET may be performed for additional information.

✗ Often, lesions have a combination of treatment effects and recurrent/residual tumor, and no single diagnosis can be established.

Case 98

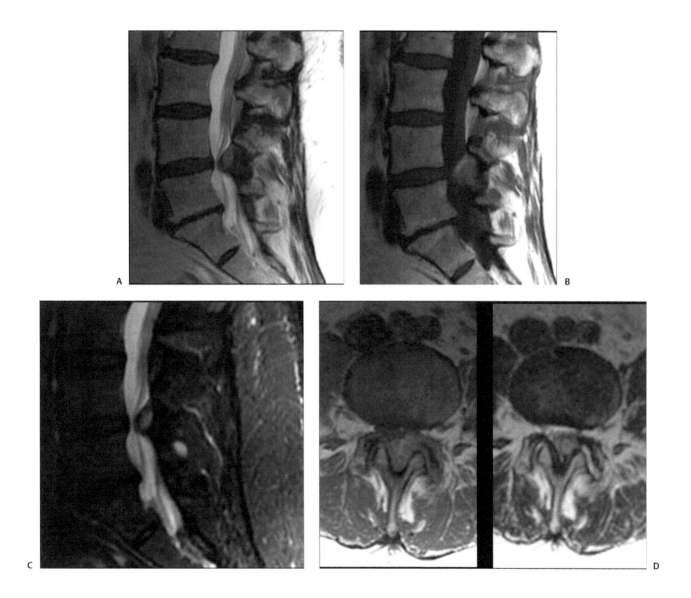

■ Clinical Presentation

A 68-year-old woman presents with a history of progressive back pain and claudication.

■ Imaging Findings

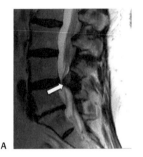 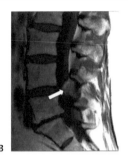 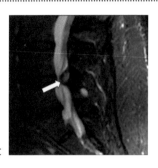 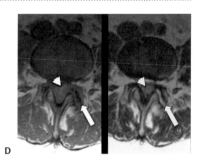

(A) Sagittal T2-weighted image (WI) of the spine shows a hyperintense lesion deforming the thecal sac from its posterior aspect (*arrow*). **(B)** Sagittal T1WI of the spine shows a hyperintense lesion deforming the thecal sac from its posterior aspect (*arrow*). **(C)** Sagittal short tau inversion recovery image of the spine shows hyperintense lesion deforming the thecal sac from its posterior aspect (*arrow*). **(D)** Axial T1 and T2WI of the spine show hypertrophy of the left facet joint (*arrows*) and a round lesion that projects into the spinal canal and connects with the facet joint (*arrowheads*), causing spinal canal stenosis.

■ Differential Diagnosis

- **Synovial cyst:**
  - Commonly seen in spondyloarthrosis of the facet joints, commonly affecting the lower lumbar levels. Typically show increased T2 and decreased T1 signal but can vary if high protein content or hemorrhage is present.
  - If projecting to the spinal canal, can cause spinal canal stenosis.
- *Sequestered disk:*
  - Disk herniation with disk material extending beyond the interspace and covering < 5% of the disk diameter.
  - Disk fragment separated from an extruded disk, more frequent in the lower lumbar spine. Can have peripheral enhancement.
- *Meningioma:* Intradural extramedullary masses with intense homogenous enhancement. Can cause spinal canal stenosis. Signal intensity typically follows that of the spinal cord but can be hypointense on T1 and hyperintense on T2-weighted image (WI).

■ Essential Facts

- Synovial cysts of the facet joints are bulges of the synovial lining that can project medially toward the spinal canal or laterally outside of the spine. Medial extension can compress the thecal sac or narrow the neural foramen.
- They are associated with ligamentum flavum hypertrophy and spondylosis.

■ Other Imaging Findings

- Most synovial cysts are bright on T2 and dark on T1. However, if increased protein content is present or hemorrhage has occurred, they can demonstrate increased signal in the T1WI.
- Hemorrhagic cysts can be fast growing and accompanied by fluid/fluid levels in the cyst.
- In an acute inflammatory phase, the cyst lining can enhance.

✓ Pearls and ✗ Pitfalls

- ✓ Most of the cysts can be treated with percutaneous intervention.
- ✓ Low signal intensity cysts on T2WI have shown to respond less favorably to percutaneous treatment.
- ✗ Extraforaminal synovial cysts can migrate in the soft tissues of the spine, posing a diagnostic challenge.
- ✗ Synovial cysts have a synovial lining, whereas ganglion cysts do not. Histologic analysis is necessary to tell the difference because it is not possible through imaging.

Case 99

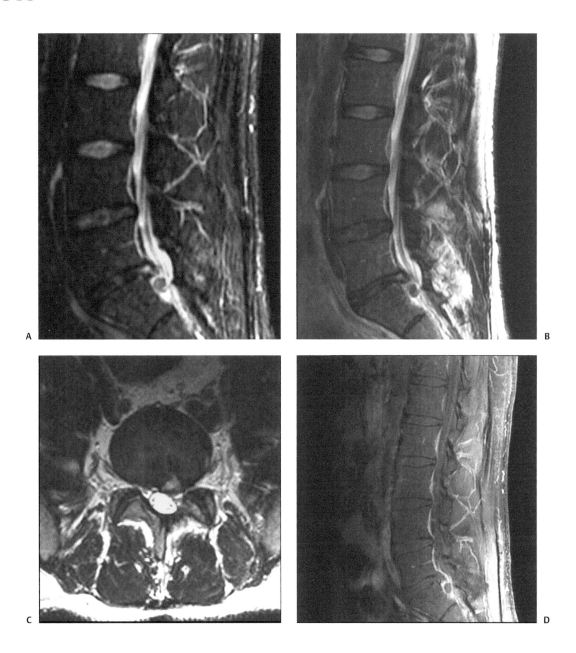

■ Clinical Presentation

A 43-year-old presents with leg weakness.

■ Imaging Findings

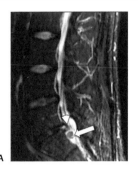 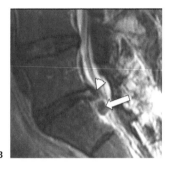 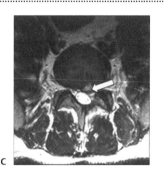 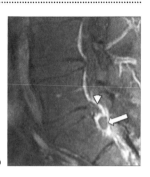

(A, B) Sagittal short tau inversion recovery **(A)** and T2-weighted image (WI) **(B)** sequence of the lumbar spine shows an annular fissure with an inferior extrusion in the L5/S1 disk (*arrowhead*). A free disk fragment is noted distal to the extrusion (*arrow*). **(C)** Axial T2WI shows a left annular fissure (*arrow*). **(D)** Sagittal T1WI with contrast shows the sequestered fragment with surrounding enhancement denoting inflammation (*arrow*). The disk extrusion is shown at L5/S1 (*arrowhead*).

■ Differential Diagnosis

• *Sequestered disk:*
  ○ Disk herniation is defined as disk material extending beyond the interspace covering < 5% of the disk diameter and may be classified as a disk extrusion or protrusion.
  ○ Disk herniation is defined as a localized or focal displacement of disk material beyond the limits of the intervertebral disk space. The disk material may be nucleus, cartilage, fragmented apophyseal bone, annular tissue, or any combination thereof.
  ○ Disk herniations include disk protrusion, disk extrusion, and sequestered disk fragments.
  ○ A sequestered disk is a disk fragment separated from the parent disk.
  ○ It appears as an extradural mass deforming the thecal sac.
  ○ Herniations are more frequent at the two lower lumbar levels.
  ○ Peripheral enhancement can be seen.
• *Facet synovial cyst:*
  ○ Frequently occupies the lateral recess and may extend to the central canal.
  ○ Cysts can contain synovial serous fluid, gelatinous material, air, or blood.
  ○ Continuous with the facet joint, but may abut the disk as well.
  ○ Peripheral enhancement can be seen if inflammation is present.
• *Spinal meningioma:*
  ○ Intradural extramedullary mass.
  ○ Isointense to spinal cord on both T1-weighted image (WI) and T2WI, but may be hypointense on T1WI and hyperintense on T2WI.
  ○ Homogeneous intense enhancement.

■ Essential Facts

• Disk herniation—morphological nomenclature:
  ○ Protrusion: If the greatest distance between the disk material presenting outside of the disk space is less than the distance between the edges.
  ○ Extrusion: In at least one plane, the diameter of the base of the herniated material is narrower than the diameter of the herniated material.
  ○ Sequestered fragment: Loss of continuity in which the disk fragment is separated from the parent disk.
• Disk migration is superior or inferior extension of the herniated material, independent of its attachment with the parent disk.

■ Other Imaging Findings

• CT:
  ○ Effacement of the epidural fat planes. Good for evaluation of bone, calcifications, and facet joints.
  ○ CT myelogram will show the deformity of the thecal sac but cannot show the continuity of the disk. It can be very useful in patients with contraindications for MRI.
• MR:
  ○ Herniated material follows the signal of the disk.
  ○ The sequestered fragment shows a gap separating it from the parent disk.
  ○ Peripheral enhancement is seen surrounding the disk herniation.

✓ Pearls and ✗ Pitfalls

✓ Sagittal views are better to evaluate disk continuity.
✗ Disk migrations can be missed in the axial images in scanning protocols that do localized axials through the disk spaces.

Case 100

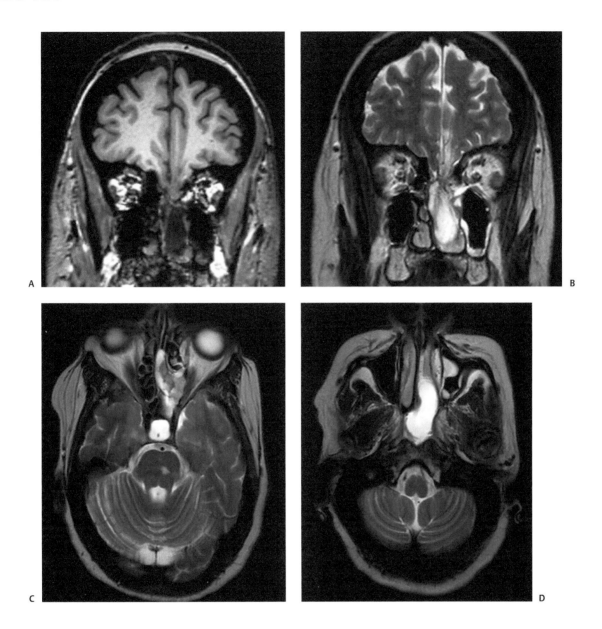

▪ Clinical Presentation

A 50-year-old man presents with nasal congestion and headaches.

■ Imaging Findings

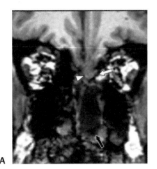
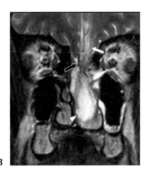
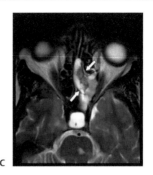
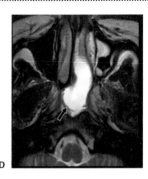

(A) Coronal T1-weighted image (WI) demonstrates a defect in the left cribriform plate and fovea ethmoidalis (*white arrow*) with herniation of cerebrospinal fluid (CSF)-filled meninges (*black arrow*) as well as of the inferomedial left frontal lobe (*white arrowhead*) to the nasal cavity and ethmoid. **(B)** Coronal T2WI shows herniation of brain and meninges (*white arrowhead*) to the nasoethmoidal region through a defect in the medial anterior skull base (*black arrow*). The gyrus rectus and orbital gyrus demonstrate a dysplastic appearance with increased T2 signal and loss of the gray–white matter interface (*white arrow*). **(C)** Axial T2WI shows isointense tissue corresponding to brain cortex and T2 hyperintense CSF in the left nasoethmoidal cavity (*white arrows*). **(D)** Axial T2WI demonstrates contained T2 hyperintense fluid corresponding to CSF within meninges occupying the posterior left nasal cavity and extending posteriorly to the nasopharynx (*arrow*).

■ Differential Diagnosis

- **Basal encephalocele-transethmoidal:** Basal encephaloceles are internal defects not generally visible externally. They occur more posteriorly than sincipital encephaloceles, either through the cribriform plate or through the sphenoid sinuses. They are characterized by cerebrospinal fluid (CSF)-filled meninges with or without brain parenchyma herniating through a skull base defect with persistent connection to the subarachnoid space.
- *Sincipital encephalocele—nasoethmoidal:* The most common of the sincipital encephaloceles. Characterized by herniation of brain parenchyma and meninges through a defect in the anterior cranial fossa to the nasoethmoidal cavity between the nasal bridge and above the nasal septum.
- *Nasal dermoid cyst:* Nasal dermoids arise from ectodermal elements persisting within suture sites. Classically, these cysts show a tract from the prenasal space to the foramen cecum and demonstrate heterogeneous signal intensity that is primarily hyperintense on T1 and hypointense on T2.

■ Essential Facts

- Encephaloceles are classified into three categories: occipital (75%), sincipital (15%), and basal (10%).
- All are characterized by a defect in the anterior skull base with herniation of meninges and CSF (meningocele) with or without brain parenchyma (meningoencephalocele).
- Basal encephaloceles may be further subdivided into transethmoidal, transsphenoidal, sphenoethmoidal, and frontosphenoidal.
- Unlike the sincipital encephaloceles, basal encephaloceles present as masses that may project as far back as the nasopharynx and oropharynx.

- The transethmoidal and transsphenoidal variants are the most common.
- The anterior skull base defect is present at the cribriform plate or posterior to it.

■ Other Imaging Findings

- CT is helpful to delineate bony anatomy.
- MR aids in characterizing the contents of the herniated tissue.
- The extent of brain parenchyma involvement and the connection to the intracranial compartment helps in presurgical planning and prognosis.
- MR venography can help show venous involvement of these lesions.

✓ Pearls and ✗ Pitfalls

- ✓ Encephaloceles have a known association with intracranial abnormalities including callosal defects, lipomas, schizencephaly, and cysts.
- ✓ Clinically, encephaloceles are characterized by masses that fluctuate with compression of the jugular veins or with crying.
- ✓ Treatment of choice is surgical resection.
- ✗ Biopsies of these lesions are contraindicated due to risk of CSF leak and infection.
- ✗ Diagnosis is highly reliant on imaging features.
- ✗ Intrathecal injection of contrast may aid in characterizing the connection to the subarachnoid space.

Case Questions and Answers

The questions and answers in the following section are numbered as cases 1 through 100. The questions correspond to the respectively numbered case reviews and are intended to be answered after working through the cases.

■ Case 1

1. Which of the following is a feature required for diagnosis of a Chiari I malformation?
   a) Small posterior fossa
   b) Cervical cord syrinx
   c) Myelomeningocele
   d) Cerebellar tonsils below the level of the foramen magnum

The correct answer is (**d**). Answers a and c are characteristics of Chiari II malformations. Although cervical cord syrinx is a common finding in Chiari I, it is not necessary to make the diagnosis.

2. Syringohydromyelia associated with Chiari I malformation typically begins at which level of the spinal cord?
   a) Cervical
   b) Thoracic
   c) Conus medullaris
   d) There is no predilection for a particular segment of spinal cord.

The correct answer is (**a**). Syringohydromyelia associated with Chiari I malformations generally begins between the C4 and C6 levels. However, the entire cord may be involved at the time of diagnosis. To our knowledge, no isolated involvement of the thoracic cord has been reported.

■ Case 2

1. Crowding of structures in the posterior fossa is seen in all except…
   a) Cerebellitis
   b) Cerebellar stroke
   c) Chiari II malformation
   d) Friedreich's ataxia

The correct answer is (**d**). This condition features cerebellar volume loss. In the other three conditions, there is crowding of the posterior fossa structures.

2. Which of the following conditions does *not* cause effacement of the fourth ventricle:
   a) Dandy–Walker malformation
   b) Chiari II malformation
   c) Medulloblastoma
   d) Pilocytic astrocytoma

The correct answer is (**a**). Dandy–Walker malformation presents with enlargement of the fourth ventricle, communicating with a posterior fossa cyst.

■ Case 3

1. Which of the following cystic malformations of the posterior fossa is not associated with hydrocephalus?
   a) Dandy–Walker malformation
   b) Blake pouch cyst
   c) Megacisterna magna
   d) Posterior fossa arachnoid cyst

The correct answer is (**c**). Dandy–Walker malformation and Blake pouch cyst are typically associated with hydrocephalus. Large posterior fossa arachnoid cysts can compress the fourth ventricle and result in hydrocephalus.

2. Which of the following posterior fossa cystic abnormalities is associated with a small vermian size?
   a) Dandy–Walker malformation
   b) Blake pouch cyst
   c) Megacisterna magna
   d) Posterior fossa arachnoid cyst

The correct answer is (**a**). Blake pouch cyst, megacisterna magna, and posterior fossa arachnoid cysts typically course with a normal cerebellar vermis.

■ Case 4

1. Which of the following is an abnormality associated with callosal agenesis?
   a) Gray matter heterotopia
   b) Holoprosencephaly
   c) Dandy–Walker complex
   d) Midline anomalies, including interhemispheric cysts and lipomas
   e) All of the above

The correct answer is (**e**). All of the malformations mentioned have been described in association with callosal agenesis.

2. The presence of Probst bundles is more common in patients with which of the following conditions?
   a) Agenesis of the corpus callosum
   b) Hypogenesis of the corpus callosum
   c) Probst bundles are normal structures found in patients with a completely formed corpus callosum.

The correct answer is (**a**). Probst bundles represent the white matter fibers that did not cross to form the corpus callosum. They are most commonly seen in complete agenesis of the corpus callosum, although they also can be seen in hypogenesis of the corpus callosum.

■ Case 5

1. A "Z"-shaped appearance of the brainstem in the sagittal view is typical of which condition?
   a) Joubert syndrome
   b) Walker–Warburg syndrome
   c) Pontocerebellar hypoplasia
   d) Dandy–Walker malformation

The correct answer is (**b**). A "Z"-shaped appearance of the brainstem in the sagittal view is typical of Walker–Warburg syndrome.

2. Which of the following is typical of Joubert syndrome?
   a) Normal decussation of the corticospinal tracts
   b) A large fourth ventricular cyst
   c) Elongated superior cerebellar peduncles
   d) Normal cerebellar vermis

The correct answer is (**c**). Joubert syndrome features lack of decussation of the both the corticospinal tracts and the superior cerebellar peduncles. Typical features also include elongated superior cerebellar peduncles and a small cerebellar vermis. A large fourth ventricular cyst is not a characteristic of Joubert syndrome.

■ Case 6

1. Which of the following leukodystrophies typically enhances?
   a) Canavan disease
   b) X-linked adrenoleukodystrophy
   c) Alexander disease
   d) Pelizaeus–Merzbacher disease

The correct answer is (**b**). X-linked adrenoleukodystrophy (ALD) is characterized by an intermediate zone that represents disruption of the blood–brain barrier that typically enhances. The other white matter diseases in the question do not enhance.

2. Which is a typical MR pattern of metachromatic leukodystrophy?
   a) Confluent symmetric white matter in a butterfly shape, no enhancement
   b) Symmetric frontal white matter with involvement of the subcortical "U" fibers, no enhancement
   c) Symmetric parieto-occipital white matter with sparing of the subcortical "U" fibers, enhancement
   d) Homogeneous white matter, globus pallidus and thalamus, increased *N*-acetylaspartate (NAA) peak

The correct answer is (**a**). Confluent symmetric white matter in a butterfly shape, no enhancement is typical of metachromatic leukodystrophy. The sparing of the perivenular white matter gives the tigroid pattern. Symmetric frontal white matter with involvement of the subcortical "U" fibers, no enhancement is typical of Alexander disease. Symmetric parieto-occipital white matter with sparing of the subcortical "U" fibers, enhancement is seen in ALD. Homogeneous white matter, globus pallidus and thalamus, increased NAA peak is characteristic of Canavan disease.

■ Case 7

1. Which of the following is true of porencephalic cysts?
   a) Occur only as a sequela of trauma
   b) Can increase in size
   c) Cause focal calvarial hyperostosis
   d) Cause effacement of the ventricle

The correct answer is (**b**). Porencephalic cysts may increase in size due to adhesions that serve as one-way valves. They may occur as a sequela of surgery, trauma, infarct, or various other etiologies. Porencephalic cysts may cause scalloping of the bone and enlargement of the adjacent ventricle.

2. What does gliosis surrounding a porencephalic cyst generally indicate?
   a) That the insult occurred in an early gestational period
   b) That the injury likely occurred in the postnatal period
   c) That the porencephalic cyst is a consequence of infection
   d) That the porencephalic cyst is the cause of ischemia

The correct answer is (**b**). Generally speaking, gliosis surrounding a porencephalic cyst indicates that the insult was not produced in the early gestational period but rather in later stages of development or in the postnatal period.

Case 8

1. The following pathologic conditions may feature a supratentorial midline cyst except...
    a) Alobar holoprosencephaly
    b) Agenesis of the corpus callosum
    c) Dandy–Walker malformation
    d) Cavum vergae

The correct answer is (**c**). In Dandy–Walker malformation, there is a midline cyst in the posterior fossa. In the other three entities, a midline cystic structure may be found in the supratentorial compartment.

2. The body of the corpus callosum may be absent in presence of a rostrum and splenium in all of the following except...
    a) Syntelencephaly
    b) Dysgenesis of the corpus callosum
    c) Epilepsy surgery
    d) Old anterior cerebral artery (ACA) infarct

The correct answer is (**b**). The development of the corpus callosum begins with the genu and then continues posteriorly along the body to the splenium. The rostrum is the last part to be formed. Presence of the rostrum confirms that the corpus callosum formation was completed. In destructive lesions of the corpus callosum (i.e., epilepsy surgery and ACA infarct) and in syntelencephaly, the body of the corpus callosum may be absent, whereas the rostrum and body are present.

Case 9

1. Which of the following is considered an open spinal dysraphism?
    a) Lipomyelocele
    b) Meningocele
    c) Myelomeningocele
    d) Lipomyelomeningocele

The correct answer is (**c**). Spinal dysraphisms are divided into open and closed spinal dysraphisms. In the open spinal dysraphisms, the central nervous system tissue is exposed with no skin covering it, and they include myelomeningocele, myelocele, hemimyelomeningocele, and hemimyelocele. The other options are part of the closed spinal dysraphisms.

2. Which is a characteristic of a meningocele?
    a) The defect is only lined by dura mater.
    b) It is an open spinal dysraphic state.
    c) The spinal cord protrudes through the defect.
    d) It is more common in the lumbosacral spine.

The correct answer is (**d**). Meningoceles are closed dysraphic states. These are lined with dura and arachnoid. By definition, the neural tube does not protrude through the defect. They are more frequent in the lumbosacral spine and are typically posterior. Anterior meningoceles can be seen in association with sacral agenesis.

Case 10

1. A characteristic of periventricular heterotopia is which of the following?
    a) It does not enhance with contrast.
    b) It is associated with subependymal giant cell astrocytoma.
    c) It is always symmetric.
    d) It undergoes calcification.

The correct answer is (**a**). Heterotopias are gray matter structures that do not enhance with contrast. They are frequently asymmetric. Subependymal giant cell astrocytoma and calcifications are features of tuberous sclerosis, not seen in heterotopias.

2. Which of the following is a malformation due to abnormal neuronal migration?
    a) Heterotopia
    b) Polymicrogyria
    c) Schizencephaly
    d) Hemimegalencephaly

The correct answer is (**a**). Heterotopias are malformations of cortical development secondary to abnormal neuronal migration. Polymicrogyria and schizencephaly are malformations secondary to abnormal postmigrational development. Hemimegalencephaly is a malformation secondary to abnormal neuronal and glial proliferation or apoptosis.

Case 11

1. Which of the following features is associated with the classic form of septo-optic dysplasia (SOD)?
    a) Hypoplasia of the olfactory nerves
    b) Large monoventricle
    c) Fusion of the thalami
    d) Lack of formation of the third ventricle

The correct answer is (**a**). Hypoplasia of the olfactory nerves is associated with the classic form of SOD. A large monoventricle with fusion of the thalami and lack of formation of the third ventricle are characteristics of lobar holoprosencephaly.

2. Which of the following statements is true about SOD?
   a) The pituitary gland is typically normal.
   b) The septum pellucidum is present.
   c) It is associated with schizencephaly.
   d) It is associated with pineal absence.

The correct answer is (**c**). One of the variants of SOD (SOD-plus) is associated with schizencephaly. The classic triad of SOD is optic nerve hypoplasia, pituitary hormone abnormalities, and brain midline defects.

■ Case 12
....

1. In which conditions may cerebrospinal fluid (CSF) lactate levels be elevated?
   a) Stroke
   b) Leigh syndrome
   c) Kearns–Sayre syndrome
   d) Central nervous system infection
   e) All of the above

The correct answer is (**e**). Increased CSF lactate is not pathognomonic for Leigh syndrome and may be found in a variety of mitochondrial disorders as well as various other conditions.

2. Which of the following mitochondrial disorders classically presents with cortical involvement?
   a) Leigh syndrome
   b) Myoclonus epilepsy with ragged red fibers (MERRF)
   c) Mitochondrial encephalopathy with lactic acidosis and strokelike lesions (MELAS)
   d) Kearns–Sayre syndrome

The correct answer is (**c**). MELAS is a mitochondrial disorder that presents with cortical and white matter involvement in a nonvascular distribution, mimicking stroke.

■ Case 13
....

1. In newborns with low APGAR score and suspected hypoxic-ischemic encephalopathy (HIE), when should MRI ideally be obtained?
   a) Immediately
   b) Delayed 24 to 48 hours
   c) After CT has ruled out hemorrhage
   d) Only if there is suspicion of hydrocephalus

The correct answer is (**b**). Conventional MR sequences typically appear normal in the first 48 hours post HIE. While diffusion-weighted imaging (DWI) and apparent diffusion coefficient (ADC) maps register the injury earlier, perhaps within the first 24 hours, it has been suggested that there may be a propensity at that early stage to underestimate the lesion severity or extent.

2. With regard to brain MRI interpretation in the setting of neonatal hypoxia, which statement is true?
   a) Absence of DWI/ADC map signal abnormalities rules out hypoxic-ischemic injury.
   b) The corrected gestational age of the newborn affects the appearance of the lesions, because the metabolically active areas vary with the maturation of the brain.
   c) The severity of the insult does not correlate with the onset of imaging findings.
   d) The unmyelinated areas of the brain are relatively protected from hypoxic-ischemic damage.

The correct answer is (**b**). The corrected gestational age of the newborn affects the appearance of the lesions, because the metabolically active areas vary with the maturation of the brain. Preferential areas of involvement in the premature brain and mature brain vary significantly.

■ Case 14
....

1. Which of the following congenital disorders courses with spinal canal stenosis?
   a) Mucopolysaccharidosis
   b) Alexander disease
   c) Mitochondrial encephalopathy with lactic acidosis and strokelike lesions (MELAS)
   d) Canavan disease
   e) Metachromatic leukodystrophy

The correct answer is (**a**). Mucopolysaccharidoses course with craniocervical junction abnormalities and with compromise of the central spinal canal and spinal cord with or without evidence of myelopathy.

2. Which of the following congenital anomalies presents with bullet-shaped vertebrae?
   a) Metachromatic leukodystrophy
   b) Lipomyelocele
   c) Achondroplasia
   d) Lipomyelomeningocele
   e) Alexander disease

The correct answer is (**c**). Achondroplasia as well as Hurler disease course with bullet-shaped vertebrae.

■ Case 15
....

1. Which is a benefit of MR over CT in the evaluation of diastematomyelia?
   a) Assessment of bony spurs separating the hemicords
   b) Evaluation of vertebral fusion abnormalities
   c) Evaluation of the level of the conus medullaris
   d) CT and MR are interchangeable in the evaluation of diastematomyelia.

The correct answer is (**c**). The evaluation of bony structures is better assessed with CT, whereas the contents of the thecal sac, including the level of the conus medullaris, is better seen on MR images.

2. Which of the following bony abnormalities is virtually pathognomonic for diastematomyelia?
   a) Butterfly vertebrae
   b) Scoliosis
   c) Hemivertebrae
   d) Intersegmental laminar fusion
   e) Klippel–Feil anomaly

The correct answer is (**d**). Intersegmental laminar fusion is pathognomic for diastematomyelia. The other anomalies are commonly seen in association but are not considered pathognomonic.

■ Case 16
....

1. Which of the following is true regarding hydranencephaly?
   a) The internal carotid arteries may be patent.
   b) The cerebral falx is typically absent.
   c) The thalami are fused.
   d) Deformity of the brainstem is present.

The correct answer is (**a**). Normal internal carotid arteries in hydranencephaly do not exclude their possible pathogenic role because the internal carotid artery might recanalize after having induced irreversible parenchymal damage. The brainstem is not affected in hydranencephaly. Absence of the cerebral falx and fusion of the thalami are features of holoprosencephaly.

2. Which of the following conditions may course with an abnormal posterior fossa due to compression?
   a) Hydranencephaly
   b) Congenital hydrocephalus
   c) Cortical heterotopia
   d) Lobar holoprosencephaly

The correct answer is (**c**). In hydranencephaly, the head size may be increased, normal, or microcephalic, depending on the distension of the sacs. In congenital hydrocephalus and lobar holoprosencephaly, the dilated cystic spaces may exert mass effect on the posterior fossa structures.

■ Case 17
....

1. Which of the following is always true with regard to focal cortical dysplasias (FCDs)?
   a) They are solitary lesions.
   b) They are visible on MRI scans.
   c) They have a variable appearance according to their subtype.
   d) They are associated with epilepsy.

The correct answer is (**c**). Of these statements, the only one that is always true is how variable FCDs are with regard to size, location, and appearance. FCDs can be solitary *or* multiple, they are not always visible on MRI, and they are not always associated with epilepsy.

2. Which of the FCDs most commonly occurs in the temporal lobes?
   a) FCD type I
   b) FCD type II
   c) FCD type IIIa
   d) Both a and c are correct.
   e) They all occur in equal rates in the temporal lobes.

The correct answer is (**d**). FCD type I and type IIIa more commonly occur in the temporal lobe as opposed to type II which occurs more frequently in the frontal lobes.

■ Case 18
....

1. Regarding tumors in patients with NF1, which statement is correct?
   a) Astrocytomas are less common in children with NF1 than in the general population.
   b) High-grade gliomas are more common than pilocytic astrocytomas in the NF1 population.
   c) The brainstem is infrequently involved with astrocytomas.
   d) Hamartomas of the hypothalamus have iso- or near-isointense T1 and T2 signals (compared to cortex), do not enhance, and remain stable on follow-up MR exams.

The correct answer is (**d**). Hamartomas of the hypothalamus have iso- or near-isointense T1 and T2 signals (compared to cortex), do not enhance, and remain stable on follow-up MR exams. Astrocytomas are more common in children with NF1 than in the general population. Pilocytic astrocytomas are more common than high-grade gliomas in the NF1 population. The brainstem is often involved with astrocytomas, especially the tectum and the medulla.

2. Regarding white matter T2 hyperintense lesions in NF1, which statement is true?
   a) Frequently located in the brainstem, middle cerebellar peduncles, cerebellar white matter, cerebral peduncles, basal ganglia (especially the globus pallidus), thalamus, and internal capsule
   b) Most common in children younger than 7 years, and become larger with advancing age
   c) Increased incidence of malignant transformation with age
   d) Do not demonstrate significant mass effect; however, enhance strongly with contrast

The correct answer is (**a**). White matter T2 hyperintense lesions in NF1 are frequently located in the brainstem, middle cerebellar peduncles, cerebellar white matter, cerebral peduncles, basal ganglia (especially the globus pallidus), thalamus, and internal capsule. These lesions are most common in children younger than 7 years and decrease in prominence with advancing age. They do not show increased incidence of malignant transformation with age. They do not demonstrate significant mass effect or contrast enhancement.

■ Case 19

1. Which of the following is considered a form of neurofibromatosis (NF)?
   a) Schwannomatosis
   b) Meningiomatosis
   c) von Hippel–Lindau disease
   d) Lhermitte–Duclos disease
   e) Sturge–Weber syndrome

The correct answer is (**a**). Schwannomatosis is considered the third type of NF. Meningiomatosis also occurs in chromosome 22 but is not considered an NF.

2. Which of the following is *not* a clinical feature of NF2?
   a) Vestibular schwannomas
   b) Facial schwannomas
   c) Cauda equina schwannomas
   d) Ventricular meningiomas
   e) Ependymomas

The answer is (**d**). Characteristic lesions of NF2 are multiple intracranial schwannomas, meningiomas, and ependymomas ("MISME"). The meningiomas are typically dural based.

■ Case 20

1. Which of the following characteristics is most concerning for the development of subependymal giant-cell astrocytoma (SEGA)?
   a) Calcification of a subependymal nodule
   b) Enhancement of a subependymal nodule
   c) Size of an subependymal nodule
   d) Growth of a subependymal nodule

The correct answer is (**d**). Growth of a subependymal nodule should raise concern for SEGA. Calcifications and enhancement are common findings. Size alone is not sufficient to raise concern.

2. Which finding is not characteristic of tuberous sclerosis (TS)?
   a) Cardiac rhabdomyomas
   b) Endolymphatic sac tumors
   c) Cortical tubers
   d) Renal angiomyolipomas

The correct answer is (**b**). Endolymphatic sac tumors are generally associated with von Hippel–Lindau syndrome. The remaining features are characteristic of TS.

■ Case 21

1. Which of the following is a manifestation of von Hippel–Lindau syndrome (VHL)?
   a) Endolymphatic sac tumor
   b) Vestibular aqueductal enlargement
   c) Infratentorial ependymomas
   d) Renal angiomyolipomas
   e) Pilocytic astrocytomas

The correct answer is (**a**). Endolymphatic sac tumors are associated with VHL, the other entities are not. VHL is associated with multiple brain hemangioblastomas, spinal cord hemangioblastoma, retinal hemangioblastomas, renal and pancreatic simple cysts, renal cell carcinoma, pheochromocytoma, islet cell tumor of the pancreas, and endolymphatic sac tumors.

2. Which of the following statements about hemangioblastomas is true?
   a) More than half of posterior fossa hemangioblastomas are associated with VHL.
   b) Almost 80% of spinal hemangioblastomas are associated with VHL.
   c) The walls of cystic hemangioblastomas show avid enhancement.
   d) One third of hemangioblastomas calcify.
   e) Hemangioblastomas are not seen on digital subtraction angiography (DSA) images.

The correct answer is (**b**). Almost 80% of spinal hemangioblastomas are associated with VHL; less than a third of cerebellar hemangioblastomas are. The walls of hemangioblastomas do not enhance, and these lesions are well seen on DSA images. They do not calcify.

■ Case 22

1. What is the most likely cause of mass effect of a cavernous malformation?
   a) Recent hemorrhage
   b) Spontaneous growth
   c) Venous thrombosis
   d) Immune reaction
   e) Ischemia

The correct answer is (**a**). Mass effect is rarely seen in diagnostic images around a cavernous malformation unless recent hemorrhage has occurred.

2. Which of the following can cause the development of cavernous malformations?
   a) Lung carcinoma
   b) Radiation therapy
   c) Steroid use
   d) Hypertension
   e) Amyloid deposits

The correct answer is (**b**). Cavernous malformations may be congenital or arise de novo in familial cases, after radiation, pregnancy, or brain biopsy.

■ Case 23

1. Which imaging modality is considered the gold standard for the evaluation of vasculitis?
   a) CT angiography
   b) MR angiography
   c) Digital subtraction angiography (DSA)
   d) Vessel wall MRI

The correct answer is (**c**). Although occasionally primary angiitis of the central nervous system (PACNS) is not seen on imaging, DSA is currently considered the gold standard for evaluation of PACNS due to its high spatial resolution.

2. What is the characteristic pattern of involvement in PACNS?
   a) Multifocal short-segment stenoses of small to medium-sized vessels without enhancement
   b) Long-segment uniform stenosis
   c) Multifocal short-segment stenoses of medium to large-sized vessels
   d) Multifocal short-segment stenoses of small to medium-sized vessels with enhancement

The correct answer is (**d**). Multifocal short-segment stenoses of small to medium-sized vessels with enhancement is characteristic of PACNS.

■ Case 24

1. Which of the following aneurysms involve all three vessel wall layers?
   a) Infectious aneurysm
   b) Blister aneurysm
   c) Dissecting aneurysm
   d) Berry (saccular) aneurysm

The correct answer is (**d**). Berry aneurysms involve all three vessel wall layers, whereas infectious aneurysms, blister aneurysms, and dissecting aneurysms typically do not.

2. Potential complications of dissecting aneurysms do not include which of the following?
   a) Subarachnoid hemorrhage
   b) Embolic ischemic infarct
   c) Septic embolism
   d) Vessel occlusion

The correct answer is (**c**). Dissecting aneurysms are not infectious in etiology and do not result in septic embolism. Subarachnoid hemorrhage, embolic ischemic infarct, and vessel occlusion are all potential complications of dissecting aneurysms.

■ Case 25

1. Which of the following statements is true in relation to traumatic carotid dissections?
   a) 40% associated with dissections of other vessels
   b) Occur at sites of atheromatous disease
   c) Are associated with cerebellar strokes
   d) Not associated with pseudoaneurysms
   e) Can present with Horner syndrome

The correct answer is (**e**). Clinical presentation includes stroke, Horner syndrome, face or neck pain, cranial neuropathy, pulsatile tinnitus. Fifteen percent are associated with dissections of other vessels. They do not occur at sites of atherosclerosis and are associated with cerebral strokes and with pseudoaneurysms.

2. Which of the following is associated with carotid artery dissection?
   a) Vitamin C deficiencies
   b) von Hippel–Lindau disease
   c) Maffucci syndrome
   d) Down syndrome
   e) Marfan syndrome

The correct answer is (**e**). Causes of carotid dissection include spontaneous external trauma, associated vasculopathy (fibromuscular dysplasia, other connective tissue diseases such as Ehlers–Danlos syndrome type IV, Marfan syndrome, autosomal-dominant adult polycystic kidney disease, osteogenesis imperfecta type I, and cystic medial necrosis).

■ Case 26
....

1. Which of the following vessels is part of the deep venous system?
   a) Vein of Trolard
   b) Vein of Labbé
   c) Rosenthal vein
   d) Sylvian vein

The correct answer is (**c**), Rosenthal vein; paired veins that course along the medial temporal lobes and drain into the vein of Galen.

2. Which of the following is a disadvantage of CT venography?
   a) Slow acquisition time
   b) Difficulty in reconstructing maximum intensity projection (MIP) images
   c) Less readily available than MRI
   d) Low-resolution images

The correct answer is (**b**). Reconstruction of MIP images involves bone subtraction, which can often erase portions of the adjacent venous sinus.

■ Case 27
....

1. Regarding moyamoya syndrome, which statement is true?
   a) It rarely presents with ischemic events.
   b) Digital subtraction angiography (DSA) imaging shows a beaded appearance of the anterior and middle cerebral artery branches.
   c) The venous congestion is responsible for the "puff of smoke" appearance on cerebral angiography.
   d) It can be seen in patients with neurofibromatosis type I (NF1).

The correct answer is (**d**). Moyamoya can be seen in patients with NF1, sickle cell anemia, Down syndrome, Fanconi anemia, brain radiation therapy, and familial occurrence. Moyamoya presents with ischemic and hemorrhagic events. The leptomeningeal collaterals are responsible for the "puff of smoke" appearance in cerebral angiography. A beaded appearance of the anterior and middle cerebral artery branches is a feature of vasculitides.

2. Regarding the imaging findings in moyamoya syndrome, all of the following are true except...
   a) The leptomeningeal collaterals can be observed on MRI T2-weighted images and on CT angiography (CTA) images.
   b) CT findings include recent and old ischemia and hemorrhagic lesions.
   c) MRI is helpful to differentiate acute from chronic ischemic lesions.
   d) DSA is the only imaging modality capable of visualizing the enlarged leptomeningeal collaterals.

The correct answer is (**d**); this statement is false. The leptomeningeal collaterals can be visualized on the CTA images and MRI scans, although a comprehensive depiction of the collateralization pathways is best achieved with DSA.

■ Case 28
....

1. Which expansile hemorrhagic lesion of the pons is associated with a developmental venous anomaly (DVA)?
   a) Metastatic disease
   b) Cavernous malformations
   c) Noncontrolled hypertension
   d) Primary glial tumors

The correct answer is (**b**). Cavernous malformations are the only lesions from the list that are associated with DVAs.

2. Which of the following hemorrhagic lesions of the pons demonstrate enhancement?
   a) Grade III infiltrating midline glioma
   b) Hyperacute hemorrhagic stroke
   c) Cavernous malformation
   d) Duret hemorrhage

The correct answer is (**a**). Grade III infiltrating gliomas typically enhance. Hypertensive hemorrhagic stroke enhances in the subacute phase.

■ Case 29
....

1. Which is the main difference between an arteriovenous malformation (AVM) and an arteriovenous fistula (AVF)?
   a) Size
   b) Clinical presentation
   c) Anatomic location
   d) The presence of a vascular nidus

The correct answer is (**d**), the presence of a vascular nidus. In both AVM and AVF, there is a shunting of the arterial and venous systems. In AVM, a vascular nidus is present between the arterial and venous systems, whereas in an AVF there is no nidus.

2. What does the Spetzler–Martin grade predict?
   a) Treatment and prognosis
   b) Risk of bleeding
   c) Risk of seizures
   d) Risk of thrombosis

The correct answer is (**a**). The Spetzler–Martin grading system determines treatment and prognosis of brain AVMs based on location, size, and venous drainage.

■ Case 30

1. Regarding spinal arteriovenous lesions, which statement is true?
   a) Neurologic injury can result from hemorrhage, mass effect, or vascular steal.
   b) The majority of arteriovenous lesions feature an arteriovenous nidus in the spinal cord parenchyma.
   c) The venous drainage can be to radicular, anterior spinal, and posterior spinal veins.
   d) The fistulous connections are intradural.

The correct answer is (**a**). Neurologic injury can result from hemorrhage, mass effect, or vascular steal. The majority of arteriovenous lesions feature an arteriovenous nidus in the dura, not in the cord parenchyma. The arterial feeders are radicular, anterior spinal, and posterior spinal arteries. The fistulous connections can occur in the epidural space, intradural space, or cord/conus medullaris.

2. Regarding the imaging of spinal arteriovenous lesions, which statement is true?
   a) CT with contrast allows evaluation of cord edema and infarction.
   b) MRI with contrast is useful to localize the feeders prior to angiography.
   c) Digital subtraction angiography (DSA) characterizes the arterial feeders and venous drainage.
   d) MR angiography (MRA) without contrast can be used to localize the feeders prior to angiography.

The correct answer is (**c**). DSA characterizes the arterial feeders and venous drainage. CT with contrast is not sensitive enough to evaluate features of the cord in spinal arteriovenous lesions. MRI with contrast and MRA without contrast do not clearly depict vascular structures for evaluation of vascular malformations.

■ Case 31

1. Which of the following lesions can show increased T1 signal in the sellar region?
   a) Pituitary microadenoma
   b) Pituitary macroadenoma
   c) Rathke cleft cyst
   d) Hamartoma of the tuber cinereum

The correct answer is (**c**). Rathke cleft cyst, pituitary apoplexy, sellar aneurysms, and hemorrhagic sellar metastasis can typically demonstrate increased T1 signal.

2. Which of the following conditions arises from tissue of Rathke's pouch?
   a) Cystic pituitary adenoma
   b) Pituitary microadenoma
   c) Hamartoma of the tuber cinereum
   d) Craniopharyngioma
   e) Pituitary apoplexy

The correct answer is (**d**). Rathke cleft cyst and craniopharyngiomas are part of a continuum that arises from embryonic remnants of Rathke's pouch, which should regress by the 12th gestational week.

■ Case 32

1. Which is typically the first site of involvement in hypoxic-ischemic injury (HII) with mild to moderate insult?
   a) Cerebellum
   b) Brainstem
   c) Watershed zones
   d) Deep gray nuclei

The correct answer is (**c**). In mild to moderate insults, watershed zones are more commonly affected. In severe injury, gray matter structures are typically involved.

2. Which cortex is more vulnerable to HII?
   a) Frontal
   b) Cerebellar
   c) Temporal
   d) Perirolandic

The correct answer is (**d**). The perirolandic and occipital cortices are more vulnerable to HII.

■ Case 33

1. Regarding postictal MR changes, which statement is false?
   a) Restricted diffusion indicates irreversible cytotoxic edema.
   b) Contrast enhancement may be present.
   c) Abnormalities can be uni- or bilateral.
   d) The abnormalities can be located in cortical/subcortical areas, basal ganglia, white matter, corpus callosum, cerebellum, and hippocampus.

The correct answer is (**a**). This statement is false. Very frequently, postictal diffusion-weighted image changes are reversible. Contrast enhancement, uni- or bilateral abnormalities, and signal abnormalities located in cortical/subcortical areas, basal ganglia, white matter, corpus callosum, cerebellum, and hippocampus are all possible features on MRI scans in postictal states.

2. Identification of focal cortical T2 hyperintensity in a patient with seizures may indicate all of the following except...
   a) Seizure-induced cytotoxic edema
   b) Focal cortical dysplasia
   c) Tumor
   d) Gliosis from prior insult
   e) Cavernous angioma

The correct answer is (**e**). Cavernous angioma has mixed high and low T2 signal. All of the other pathologies demonstrate high T2 signal.

■ Case 34

1. Which is an uncommon manifestation of cerebral amyloid angiopathy (CAA)?
   a) Lobar hemorrhage
   b) Disseminated superficial siderosis
   c) Deep gray matter hemorrhage
   d) Corticosubcortical hemorrhage

The correct answer is (**c**). CAA is not significantly associated with deep white matter hemorrhage because sporadic Aβ-type CAA is commonly found in the meningeal and cortical vessels of cerebral and cerebellar cortices and rarely in those of the deep gray matter, including basal ganglia, thalamus, and brainstem.

2. Causes of intracranial hemorrhage (ICH) include all except...
   a) Factor V Leiden deficiency
   b) Arteriovenous malformation (AVM)
   c) CAA
   d) Hypertension
   e) Supratherapeutic anticoagulation

The correct answer is (**a**). Factor V Leiden mutation causes thrombophilia and predisposes patients to pregnancy complications, deep vein thrombosis, and pulmonary embolism. AVM, CAA, hypertension, and supratherapeutic anticoagulation are common causes of ICH.

■ Case 35

1. Which is not a characteristic of superficial siderosis?
   a) History of trauma or surgery
   b) Leptomeningeal enhancement
   c) Susceptibility artifact along the surfaces of the posterior fossa
   d) Hearing loss and ataxia

The correct answer is (**b**). Leptomeningeal enhancement is not common in siderosis. It is more frequently seen in meningioangiomatosis and neurocutaneous melanosis.

2. In which condition is there signal abnormality of the underlying parenchyma?
   a) Superficial siderosis
   b) Neurocutaneous melanosis
   c) Meningioangiomatosis
   d) None of the above

The correct answer is (**c**). Meningioangiomatosis shows serpentine enhancement along the surface of the gyri and sulci, as well as gliosis and/or edema of the underlying parenchyma.

■ Case 36

1. Regarding evaluation of leptomeningeal collaterals in the setting of acute stroke, which statement is true?
   a) Intra-arterial recanalization within the first 6 hours of stroke symptom onset improves prognosis regardless of the status of the distal circulation.
   b) CT angiography (CTA) obtained in an early arterial phase may underestimate the status of the collateral circulation.
   c) Digital subtraction angiography (DSA) is recommended for collateral evaluation in all patients with stroke.
   d) In middle cerebral artery (MCA) occlusion, no significant leptomeningeal collateralization is provided by the anterior and posterior cerebral arteries.

The correct answer is (**b**). This statement is true. Intra-arterial recanalization in patients with poor collateral circulation does not improve prognosis. DSA is reserved for patients in which intra-arterial recanalization is strongly considered or the diagnosis of stroke etiology is not clear. In MCA occlusion, the main sources of leptomeningeal collateralization are the anterior and posterior cerebral arteries.

2. Information regarding the status of the collateral circulation cannot be obtained from which of the following studies?
   a) Conventional angiography
   b) Single-phase CTA
   c) Multiphasic CTA
   d) Diffusion-weighted imaging (DWI)
   e) Fluid-attenuated inversion recovery (FLAIR)

The correct answer is (**d**). DWI delineates the core of the infarct but does not provide information regarding the status of the collateral circulation. Conventional angiography, single-phase CTA, multiphasic CTA, and FLAIR provide direct or indirect information regarding the leptomeningeal collateral circulation.

■ Case 37

....

1. Which of the following pontine lesions is typically asymptomatic?
   a) Pontine stroke
   b) Multiple sclerosis
   c) Capillary telangiectasia
   d) Central pontine myelinolysis
   e) Chronic lymphocytic inflammation with pontine perivascular enhancement responsive to steroids (CLIPPERS)

The correct answer is (**c**). Capillary telangiectasia is a vascular lesion that is usually found incidentally. Pontine stroke, multiple sclerosis, central pontine myelinolysis, and CLIPPERS usually present acutely, although some of the symptoms may improve.

2. For what reason is MRI indicated in cases of a suspected brainstem lesion?
   a) Normal structures may mimic pathology.
   b) Beam hardening on CT limits evaluation.
   c) Most brainstem lesions are normal on CT.
   d) Cerebrospinal fluid pulsation affects CT interpretation.

The correct answer is (**b**). Beam hardening artifact typically affects the correct evaluation of the brainstem on CT.

■ Case 38

....

1. With which carotid-vertebrobasilar anastomosis can there be mass effect on the pituitary gland?
   a) Persistent hypoglossal artery
   b) Persistent otic artery
   c) Persistent trigeminal artery (PTA): medial variant
   d) PTA: lateral variant

The correct answer is (**c**). The medial variant of the PTA courses near the pituitary gland and can even compress it.

2. Which is true with regard to the PTA?
   a) It may be associated with other vascular malformations.
   b) It may pose a risk for transfrontal surgeries.
   c) It is a variant of posterior communicating artery anatomy.
   d) It is seen approximately at the level of the third cranial nerve.

The correct answer is (**a**). PTA may be associated with other vascular malformations. PTA poses a risk for transsphenoidal surgeries, it is classified as a carotid-vertebrobasilar anastomosis, and it is seen at the level of the fifth cranial nerve.

■ Case 39

....

1. Common causes of parenchymal hemorrhage in the elderly do not include which of the following?
   a) Hypertension
   b) Amyloid angiopathy
   c) Anticoagulation
   d) Arteriovenous malformation (AVM)

The correct answer is (**d**). One third of AVMs that are diagnosed due to hemorrhage are identified before the age of 20 years. Overall, AVMs are diagnosed at a mean age of 31 years. Hypertension, amyloid angiopathy, and anticoagulation are frequent etiologies for intracranial hemorrhage in the elderly.

2. Which of the following is a characteristic of the spot sign?
   a) Enhancement continuous with normal vasculature adjacent to the hemorrhage
   b) Enhancement continuous with abnormal vasculature adjacent to the hemorrhage
   c) Focus of contrast pooling within the intraparenchymal hemorrhage
   d) Attenuation < 120 Hounsfield units

The correct answer is (**c**), focus of contrast pooling within the intraparenchymal hemorrhage. Enhancement discontinuous with normal or abnormal vasculature adjacent to the hemorrhage and attenuation > 120 Hounsfield units are characteristics of the spot sign.

■ Case 40

1. Which of the following techniques is *not* considered a perfusion technique?
   a) Arterial spin labeling (ASL)
   b) Time of flight
   c) Dynamic contrast enhanced (DCE)
   d) Dynamic susceptibility contrast (DSC)

The correct answer is (**b**). Time of flight is not a perfusion technique. ASL is a perfusion technique that tags red blood cells and does not need exogenous contrast agents. DSC uses T2* effects of gadolinium contrast to estimate cerebral perfusion. DCE uses the T1 shortening effect of gadolinium-based contrast to estimate cerebral perfusion; the most common parameter is K^{trans}.

2. A new nodular area of enhancement is noted in a tumor surgical site between 3 and 6 months after chemo-radiotherapy. The perfusion study shows a low cerebral blood volume and the MR spectroscopy sequence demonstrates low *N*-acetylaspartate and low choline peaks. The lesion slightly decreases in size in a 4-week follow-up; no steroid treatment was given. The likely diagnosis is which of the following?
   a) Pseudoresponse
   b) Pseudoprogression
   c) Progression
   d) Radiation necrosis
   e) Acute leukoencephalopathy

The correct answer is (**b**). This is a typical example of pseudoprogression. Although imaging cannot completely exclude tumor progression, the advanced imaging findings and the reduction of size over time favor the diagnosis.

■ Case 41

1. The most common location of intramedullary ependymoma is which of the following?
   a) Cervical cord
   b) Thoracic cord
   c) Conus medullaris
   d) All locations are equal in prevalence.

The correct answer is (**a**). The cervical cord is the most common location for intramedullary ependymomas.

2. Which of the following masses generally presents with a complete peripheral ring of hemosiderin deposition?
   a) Ependymoma
   b) Astrocytoma
   c) Cavernous malformation
   d) Myxopapillary ependymoma

The correct answer is (**c**). Cavernous malformations typically demonstrate a complete ring of hemosiderin. Ependymomas, on the other hand, present with hemosiderin caps at the poles of the tumor. Myxopapillary ependymoma and astrocytomas do not commonly present with hemorrhagic products.

■ Case 42

1. Which of the following features favors medulloblastoma (MB) over ependymoma?
   a) Increased apparent diffusion coefficient (ADC) value
   b) Extension through the foramina of Luschka and Magendie
   c) Arising from the superior medullary velum (roof of fourth ventricle)
   d) Arising from the cerebellar vermis

The correct answer is (**c**). Arising from the superior medullary velum (roof of fourth ventricle) is a feature of MBs. MBs tend to have lower ADC values than the other posterior fossa tumors in children. Extension through the foramina of Luschka and Magendie is typically associated with ependymomas. Pilocytic astrocytomas arise from the cerebellar vermis.

2. Regarding extension of a fourth ventricular tumor through the foramina of Luschka, which statement is false?
   a) It is typical for ependymomas but has also been reported in medulloblastomas.
   b) Must be differentiated from the normal enhancement of the choroid plexus in the foramina of Luschka.
   c) It is frequently seen in pilocytic astrocytomas.
   d) Cerebrospinal fluid (CSF) seeding of a primary MB can mimic extension of the solid tumor through the foramina of Luschka.

The correct answer is (**c**). Pilocytic astrocytomas do not typically extend through the foramina of Luschka. This feature is most characteristic of ependymomas, although it has been described in MBs. Direct foraminal extension must be differentiated from the normal enhancement of the choroid plexus in the foramina of Luschka and from CSF seeding of a primary MB.

Case 43

1. Which of the following temporal lobe lesions is located within the cortex and has a "bubbly" appearance?
   a) Ganglioglioma
   b) Dysembryoplastic neuroepithelial tumor (DNET)
   c) Embryonal tumor with multilayered rosettes (formerly *primitive neuroectodermal tumor*)
   d) Pilocytic xanthoastrocytoma
   e) Oligodendroglioma

The correct answer is (**b**). DNETs present as cortically based lesions with a multicystic "bubbly" appearance.

2. Which of the following temporal lobe lesions typically present as a cystic mass with an enhancing nodule?
   a) Supratentorial ependymoma
   b) Central neurocytoma
   c) Ganglioglioma
   d) DNET
   e) Embryonal tumor with multilayered rosettes

The correct answer is (**c**). Gangliogliomas present as cystic masses in the temporal lobe with a mural nodule. Supratentorial ependymomas tend to be extraventricular and show a heterogenous appearance, such as embryonal tumors with multilayered rosettes.

Case 44

1. Which of the following is not a tumor of pineal parenchymal origin?
   a) Pineocytoma
   b) Pineoblastoma
   c) Papillary tumor of the pineal region
   d) Primary parenchymal tumor of intermediate differentiation (PPTID)

The correct answer is (**c**). Papillary tumors of the pineal region are uncommon neuroepithelial tumors that occur in children and are not classified as a tumor of pineal parenchymal origin. The remaining three (pineocytoma, pineoblastoma, and PPTID) are the tumors of pineal parenchymal origin.

2. The presence of macroscopic fat within a pineal region tumor mass should indicate which diagnosis?
   a) Pineoblastoma
   b) Teratoma
   c) Pineocytoma
   d) Trilateral retinoblastoma

The correct answer is (**b**). Teratomas in the pineal region are well-circumscribed, heterogeneous masses with fat signal.

Case 45

1. Regarding choroid plexus papilloma (CPP), which statement is true?
   a) It is more common in adults.
   b) Hydrocephalus is not common.
   c) It is highly lobulated and vividly enhancing.
   d) It is typically located in the trigone in adults and in the fourth ventricle in children.

The correct answer is (**c**). CPP is highly lobulated and vividly enhancing. CPP is more common in children than adults, frequently causes hydrocephalus, and is typically located in the trigone in children and in the fourth ventricle in adults.

2. Regarding intraventricular tumors, which statement is false?
   a) Central neurocytoma and subependymal giant-cell astrocytoma (SEGA) are more frequent in the frontal horn.
   b) Glioma and primitive neuroectodermal tumor (PNET) arise from the ventricular wall.
   c) Choroid plexus carcinoma arises from the ventricular wall.
   d) Choroid plexus papilloma is more frequent in the trigone in children and in the fourth ventricle in adults.

The correct answer is (**c**). Choroid plexus carcinoma arises from the choroid plexus, not from the ventricular wall. Central neurocytoma and SEGA are more frequent in the frontal horn. Glioma and PNET arise from the ventricular wall. CPP is more frequent in the trigone in children and in the fourth ventricle in adults.

Case 46

1. Which of the following statements about craniopharyngiomas is true?
   a) Their origin is neuroectodermal.
   b) Calcifications are rare in the pediatric population.
   c) There is a high incidence in the 3rd decade of life.
   d) Malignant transformation is common.
   e) Superior extension can compress the third ventricle.

The correct answer is (**e**). Superior extension of craniopharyngiomas can compress the third ventricle. Craniopharyngiomas originate from epithelium from Rathke's pouch, calcifications are common in the pediatric population, and they have a bimodal presentation with the peak incidence in children at 5 to 14 years and in adults at 65 to 74 years of age.

2. A dark rim is noted on susceptibility images in a cystic lesion of the sella/suprasellar region. Which of the following is the most likely diagnosis?
   a) Chronic pituitary apoplexy
   b) Rathke cleft cyst
   c) Suprasellar meningioma
   d) Papillary craniopharyngioma
   e) Cystic degeneration of a pituitary adenoma

The correct answer is (**a**). Chronic pituitary apoplexy will present as a cystic lesion with a hemosiderin rim better seen on the susceptibility sensitive images. None of the other options would present like this. Adamantinomatous craniopharyngiomas are more frequently seen in the pediatric population and tend to calcify.

■ Case 47

1. Which is the most common histopathologic diagnosis associated with resected tectal gliomas?
   a) Pilocytic astrocytoma
   b) Anaplastic astrocytoma
   c) Glioblastoma
   d) Medulloblastoma

The correct answer is (**a**). The most common pathology for resected tectal gliomas is pilocytic astrocytoma.

2. Which is a characteristic feature of tectal gliomas?
   a) Obstruction at the level of the foramen of Monro
   b) Intense homogeneous enhancement
   c) Tectal atrophy
   d) High T2 signal

The correct answer is (**d**). These tumors generally have low T1 signal and increased T2 signal. Tectal gliomas cause obstruction at the level of the cerebral aqueduct, not the foramen of Monro; they expand the tectum and show little to no enhancement.

■ Case 48

1. Common tumors that present as a cyst with a mural nodule include all of the following except…
   a) Glioblastoma
   b) Hemangioblastoma
   c) Pilocytic astrocytoma
   d) Ganglioglioma
   e) Pleomorphic xanthoastrocytoma (PXA)

The correct answer is (**a**). Glioblastoma presents as a solid tumor with necrosis but not as a cyst with a mural nodule.

2. Common characteristics of PXA include all of the following except…
   a) Patients may present with longstanding epilepsy.
   b) Peak incidence in the 4th decade of life
   c) Low apparent diffusion coefficient values in the solid portion
   d) Frequent in childhood and young adulthood
   e) Predominantly supratentorial, more frequent in the temporal lobe

The correct answer is (**b**). Peak incidence in the 4th decade of life is false. PXA presents in children and young adults, usually before age 18.

■ Case 49

1. Which of the following genetic features must be present in order to call a mass an oligodendroglioma?
   a) IDH-mutant and 1p/19q codeletion
   b) IDH wildtype and 1p/19q codeletion
   c) IDH-mutant and 1p19q intact
   d) IDH-wildtype and 1p19q intact
   e) ATRX-mutant

The correct answer is (**a**). IDH-mutant and 1p/19q codeletion.

2. Which of the following statements about oligodendrogliomas is true?
   a) The most frequent location is the temporal lobe.
   b) Calcifications are rarely seen.
   c) They are neuroepithelial in origin.
   d) Enhancement is seen in 80%.
   e) Vasogenic edema is uncommon.

The correct answer is (**e**). Vasogenic edema is uncommon. The most frequent location for oligodendroglioma is the frontal lobe, its origin is glial, and enhancement is seen in ~20% of cases.

■ Case 50

1. Which is true regarding the new World Health Organization classification of glioblastomas?
   a) IDH-mutant is the most common variant.
   b) IDH-wildtype tumors generally develop from lower grade gliomas.
   c) The term *glioblastoma NOS* is reserved for tumors whose IDH status is not established.
   d) IDH-mutant tumors generally develop in older patients.

The correct answer is (**c**). Glioblastoma NOS is reserved for tumors whose IDH status is not established. NOS stands for *not otherwise specified* and is used to classify tumors whose IDH status is unknown. IDH-wildtype tumors are more common and tend to occur de novo in older patients. IDH-mutant tumors develop in younger patients and may arise from lower grade gliomas.

2. Which is true regarding advanced brain tumor imaging for glioblastoma?
   a) Decreased tumor permeability (K^{trans})
   b) Reduction in relative cerebral blood volume (CBV) as compared to normal brain
   c) Inversion of the choline:creatine ratio
   d) Elevation of *N*-acetylaspartate (NAA)

The correct answer is (**c**). Glioblastomas demonstrate depression of NAA with elevation of choline and inversion of the choline:creatine ratio. MR perfusion shows elevated cerebral blood flow, CBV, and K^{trans}.

▪ Case 51

1. The following are examples of tissues with intrinsic T1 hyperintensity except…
   a) Melanin
   b) Hemosiderin
   c) Methemoglobin
   d) Manganese
   e) Inspissated protein

The correct answer is (**b**), hemosiderin. Blood molecules with high T1 signal are intra- and extracellular methemoglobin. Intracellular oxyhemoglobin and deoxyhemoglobin demonstrate intermediate to low T1 signal intensity. Hemosiderin demonstrates low T1 signal.

2. Regarding melanoma metastasis, which statement is true?
   a) Due to intrinsic T1 hyperintensity of melanoma, postcontrast images are unnecessary.
   b) Amelanotic melanomas do not present with intrinsic T1 hyperintensity.
   c) Melanoma metastases occur early in the course of the disease and have good response to therapy.
   d) On unenhanced brain CT examination, melanoma metastases tend to be hypodense.

The correct answer is (**b**). Amelanotic melanomas do not present with intrinsic T1 hyperintensity. T1 with contrast is more sensitive than nonenhanced MRI for detection of melanoma metastasis. Melanoma metastases occur late in the course of the disease and have poor prognosis. On unenhanced brain CT examination, melanoma metastases tend to be hyperdense.

▪ Case 52

1. Which of the following statements is true about multiple meningiomas?
   a) Seen in one third of patients with meningiomas
   b) More common in males
   c) Higher grade than solitary meningiomas
   d) May be associated with a mutation of chromosome 22
   e) If syndromic, associated with NF1

The correct answer is (**d**). Multiple meningiomas are associated to mutations of chromosome 22 in almost 50% of the cases. They are seen in < 10% of patients with meningiomas and are more frequent in the female population. If syndromic, it is associated to NF2.

2. Which of the following findings would favor the diagnosis of dural metastasis over multiple meningiomas?
   a) The presence of dural lentiform enhancing masses
   b) Diffusion-weighted image showing increased cellularity
   c) The presence of calcification
   d) Hemorrhage within the lesions

The correct answer is (**d**). Hemorrhage is rarely seen in multiple meningiomas.

▪ Case 53

1. Which characteristic is more common in patients with optic nerve glioma (ONG) not associated with neurofibromatosis (NF) as compared to those with NF?
   a) Optic chiasm involvement with cystic degeneration
   b) Tendency to remain stable over time
   c) Bilateral optic nerve involvement
   d) Less symptomatic at the time of diagnosis

The correct answer is (**a**). In non-NF patients with optic chiasm involvement, ONG is more masslike, with cystic degeneration and extension to structures outside the optic pathway. These patients have a tendency for progression and they are generally more symptomatic at the time of involvement. Bilateral optic nerve involvement is more common in NF patients.

2. Intense enhancement of an enlarged optic nerve sheath with a nonenhancing nerve is a classic appearance of which condition?
   a) Optic neuritis
   b) Optic nerve meningioma
   c) ONG
   d) None of the above

The correct answer is (**b**). Intense enhancement of an enlarged optic nerve sheath with a nonenhancing nerve is termed the "tram-track sign" and is described in optic nerve meningioma.

■ Case 54

1. Regarding subependymomas, which is true?
   a) They are aggressive tumors, usually World Health Organization (WHO) grade III.
   b) They are more common in the fourth (60%) and lateral ventricles in middle-aged or elderly patients.
   c) Subependymomas tend to be large at the time of diagnosis, usually > 2 cm.
   d) They frequently cause hydrocephalus.

The correct answer is (**b**). The majority of subependymomas occur within the fourth (60%) and lateral ventricles in middle-aged or elderly patients. Subependymomas are benign (WHO grade I) tumors, typically < 2 cm and asymptomatic.

2. Which of the following lesions is *not* typically located in the fourth ventricle?
   a) Ependymoma
   b) Hemangioblastoma
   c) Subependymoma
   d) Choroid plexus papilloma/carcinoma
   e) Epidermoid cyst

The correct answer is (**b**). Hemangioblastomas are common in the cerebellar hemisphere, not in the fourth ventricle. Common masses in the fourth ventricle include ependymoma, subependymoma, choroid plexus papilloma/carcinoma, epidermoid cyst, neurocysticercosis, and rosette-forming glioneuronal tumor.

■ Case 55

1. Which of the following diseases involving the meninges can present with no enhancement?
   a) Cryptococcal meningitis
   b) Meningeal carcinomatosis
   c) Bacterial meningitis
   d) Tuberculous meningitis

The correct answer is (**a**). Meningitis from *Cryptococcus* can present with no enhancement, due to a lack of inflammatory response. The exudates are better seen on fluid-attenuated inversion recovery sequences.

2. The presence of restricted diffusion in the extra-axial spaces favors which of the following?
   a) Meningeal carcinomatosis
   b) Pott's puffy tumor
   c) Viral meningitis
   d) Cryptococcal meningitis
   e) Chronic subdural hematoma

The correct answer is (**b**). Pott's puffy tumor is a nonneoplastic subperiosteal abscess secondary to infectious sinusitis and osteomyelitis. The abscess can show restricted diffusion. Meningeal carcinomatosis, viral meningitis, cryptococcal meningitis, and chronic subdural hematomas do not demonstrate restricted diffusion.

■ Case 56

1. Which is a characteristic feature of clival chordoma?
   a) Homogeneous enhancement
   b) Low T2 signal
   c) Off-midline origin
   d) Bone destruction on CT image

The correct answer is (**d**). CT image shows a slightly hyperdense, well-circumscribed mass arising from the midline with bone destruction. Clival chordomas generally present with heterogeneous, "honeycomb" pattern of enhancement and they have characteristically high T2 signal.

2. Which is the most common location for chordomas?
   a) Petrous apex
   b) Sacrum
   c) Clivus
   d) Cervical spine

The correct answer is (**b**). The most frequent site is the sacrum in 50% of cases, followed by the clivus in 35%, and then the remainder of the spine. Chordomas rarely arise from the petrous apex.

■ Case 57

1. In the differentiation of epidermoid cysts from arachnoid cysts, which of the following is helpful?
   a) Epidermoid cysts have high T1 signal, whereas arachnoid cysts have low T1 signal.
   b) Epidermoid cysts enhance and arachnoid cysts do not enhance.
   c) Epidermoid cysts have low T2 signal and arachnoid cysts have high T2 signal.
   d) Epidermoid cysts have mixed iso- to hypersignal intensity on fluid-attenuated inversion recovery images, whereas arachnoid cysts have similar signal to cerebrospinal fluid.

The correct answer is (**d**). The other statements are false. Similar to arachnoid cysts, epidermoid cysts have low T1 signal, high T2 signal, and do not enhance.

2. Of the following statements comparing the differences between epidermoid and dermoid inclusion cysts, which one is true?
   a) Unlike dermoid cysts, epidermoid cysts have skin appendages that form cholesterol.
   b) Epidermoid cysts tend to have a midline location, whereas dermoid cysts are more frequently lateral.
   c) Dermoid cysts have high signal in T1 secondary to fatty content.
   d) Epidermoid cysts do not show signal on diffusion-weighted imaging (DWI), whereas dermoid cysts demonstrate high DWI signal.

The correct answer is (**c**). Dermoids have high signal in T1 secondary to fatty content. All other statements are false.

■ Case 58
....

1. Which is the most common mass in the cerebellopontine angle (CPA)?
   a) Meningioma
   b) Arachnoid cyst
   c) Acoustic schwannoma
   d) Aneurysm
   e) Metastasis

The correct answer is (**c**). Acoustic schwannomas make up 70 to 80% of the CPA masses, followed by meningiomas and epidermoid inclusion cysts.

2. Which of the following characteristics is *not* typical of a CPA schwannoma?
   a) Microhemorrhage
   b) Dural tail
   c) Avid enhancement
   d) Increased T2 signal
   e) Arise in the internal auditory canal (IAC)

The correct answer is (**b**). Schwannomas can exhibit microhemorrhage, avid enhancement, increased T2 signal, and arise in the IAC. The presence of a dural tail favors meningioma.

■ Case 59
....

1. Which of the following is characteristic of plasmacytomas?
   a) Sclerotic margins
   b) Osteoblastic appearance on CT images
   c) Involvement of appendicular bones
   d) Variable patterns of enhancement

The correct answer is (**d**). Plasmacytomas have nonsclerotic margins, occur more commonly in flat bones, and are lytic on CT image.

2. After age 50, which is the most common malignant bone tumor in adults?
   a) Multiple myeloma
   b) Plasmacytoma
   c) Metastasis
   d) Sarcoma

The correct answer is (**c**). After age 50, bone metastases are the most common malignant bone tumor encountered.

■ Case 60
....

1. Which of the following is not a feature of adhesive arachnoiditis?
   a) Enlargement of the nerve root sleeve and neural foramen
   b) Thickening and clumping of nerve roots
   c) Adhesion of nerve roots to peripheral dura ("empty sac" sign)
   d) Soft tissue mass (pseudomass)
   e) History of lumbar surgery, trauma, spinal meningitis, spinal anesthesia

The correct answer is (**a**). Adhesive arachnoiditis does not cause neural foraminal enlargement. All of the others are features of adhesive arachnoiditis.

2. Causes of thickening of the nerve roots include all of the following except...
   a) Carcinomatous meningitis
   b) Intradural metastases
   c) Chronic polyneuropathies
   d) Viral myelitis
   e) Lymphoma

The correct answer is (**d**). Viral myelitis is an acute inflammatory insult of the spinal cord due to direct viral infection or postviral immunologic attack. It does not cause thickening of the nerve roots.

■ Case 61
....

1. What is the most frequent cause of spinal epidural abscess?
   a) Bacterial spondylodiskitis
   b) Mycobacterial spondylodiskitis
   c) Postsurgical complication
   d) Hematogenous spread of infection
   e) Indwelling catheters

The correct answer is (**a**). Epidural abscesses are most frequently associated with spondylodiskitis.

2. Which intervention is indicated in patients with extensive epidural abscess?
   a) Percutaneous fluoroscopy-guided aspiration
   b) Percutaneous insertion of an epidural drain
   c) Intravenous antibiotics with no intervention
   d) Open spine surgical drainage

The correct answer is (**d**). Open surgical drainage is the treatment of choice in cases of extensive epidural abscesses.

■ Case 62
....

1. Which is a characteristic of pyogenic spondylodiskitis?
   a) Sparing of the intervertebral disk
   b) Prevertebral soft tissue edema
   c) Involvement of the posterior elements
   d) Noncontiguous spread of infection

The correct answer is (**b**). Prevertebral edema is a common feature of pyogenic spondylodiskitis and aids in differentiating it from degenerative spondylosis. Sparing of the disk, involvement of the posterior elements, and noncontiguous spread of infection are more common in tuberculous spondylitis.

2. Which is a sign of resolution of infection in pyogenic spondylodiskitis?
   a) Restoration of normal fat signal in the bone marrow
   b) Paravertebral enhancement
   c) End plate sclerosis
   d) Phlegmon formation

The correct answer is (**a**). Restoration of normal fat signal in the bone marrow and reduction in the degree and extension of paravertebral enhancement are sensitive signs of treatment response.

■ Case 63
....

1. In immunosuppressed patients, which of the following entities tend to develop hemorrhage?
   a) Cryptococcal infection
   b) Progressive multifocal leukoencephalopathy (PML)
   c) HIV encephalopathy
   d) Septic emboli
   e) Toxoplasmosis

The correct answer is (**d**). Septic emboli have a high rate of hemorrhage. *Cryptococcus*, PML, HIV encephalopathy, and toxoplasmosis do not typically present with hemorrhage. This feature can help focus the differential diagnosis.

2. Which of the following lesions *do not* show enhancement in immunosuppressed patients?
   a) Toxoplasmosis
   b) Lymphoma
   c) Septic emboli
   d) HIV encephalitis
   e) PML immune reconstitution inflammatory syndrome (IRIS)

The correct answer is (**d**). HIV encephalitis does not enhance. Lymphoma, septic emboli, PML-IRIS, and toxoplasmosis will demonstrate enhancement as an imaging feature.

■ Case 64
....

1. Which is true regarding fungal central nervous system (CNS) infections?
   a) The primary site of infection is the CNS.
   b) Meningitis is a rare manifestation.
   c) They may occur in immunocompetent hosts.
   d) All pathogens have identical imaging features.

The correct answer is (**c**). Although more common in the immunosuppressed host, fungal infections may occur in healthy individuals.

2. Which is not a typical route of access of fungal infections to the brain?
   a) Hematogenous
   b) Direct invasion from the sinonasal cavity
   c) Incidentally following trauma
   d) Spread from a pulmonary focus

The correct answer is (**c**). It is uncommon that a previously healthy individual develops a fungal CNS infection following a traumatic event.

■ Case 65
....

1. The following entities are complications of facial soft tissue infections except...
   a) Bezold abscess
   b) Pott's puffy tumor
   c) Ludwig angina
   d) Orbital pseudotumor

The correct answer is (**d**). Orbital pseudotumor refers to a nonspecific orbital inflammation not due to any known etiology or systemic illness. It is not an infectious process. Bezold abscess (acute otomastoiditis eroding through the cortex medial to the attachment of sternocleidomastoid), Pott's puffy tumor, and Ludwig angina (rapidly progressive cellulitis of the floor of the mouth causing risk of rapid airway compromise) are all complications of facial infections.

2. Which of the following is true regarding sinus conditions?
   a) Tolosa–Hunt syndrome is a painful ophthalmoplegia caused by nonspecific inflammation of the cavernous sinus or superior orbital fissure.
   b) Rosai–Dorfman disease is secondary to spread of ethmoid cellulitis.
   c) Subperiosteal orbital abscess is a histiocytic proliferative disorder that affects the sinuses, skin, and upper respiratory tract.
   d) Ramsay Hunt syndrome is a granulomatous vasculitis that may involve the sinuses.

The correct answer is (**a**). Tolosa–Hunt syndrome is a painful ophthalmoplegia caused by nonspecific inflammation of the cavernous sinus or superior orbital fissure. All of the other statements are false. Ramsay Hunt syndrome refers to varicella zoster virus infection involving sensory fibers of cranial nerves VII and VIII, and portions of the external ear supplied by the auriculotemporal nerve. Subperiosteal orbital abscess is a secondary to the spread of ethmoid cellulitis. Rosai–Dorfman disease is a histiocytic proliferative disorder that affects the sinuses, skin, and upper respiratory tract. Granulomatosis with polyangiitis (Wegener granulomatosis) is a granulomatous vasculitis that may involve the sinuses.

■ Case 66

1. Apical pseudotumor of the orbit extending to the cavernous sinus associated with painful ophthalmoplegia is known as which one of the following?
   a) Ramsay Hunt syndrome
   b) Tolosa–Hunt syndrome
   c) Horner syndrome
   d) Gradenigo syndrome
   e) Bell's palsy

The correct answer is (**b**). This is the definition of Tolosa–Hunt syndrome. Ramsay Hunt syndrome is varicella zoster virus infection affecting the sensory fibers of cranial nerves VII and VIII. Horner syndrome is an interruption of the cervical sympathetic pathway. Gradenigo syndrome is petrous apicitis that presents with retro-orbital pain and cranial nerve palsies. Bell's palsy is facial nerve paralysis secondary to herpes simplex infection.

2. In a patient with pseudotumor, which of the following is the best imaging characteristic that suggests the cause is immunoglobulin-4 (IgG4) related?
   a) Patchy enhancement
   b) Low T1 signal
   c) Low T2 signal
   d) High T1 signal
   e) High T2 signal

The correct answer is (**c**). IgG4 pseudotumor presents on imaging as low signal on a T2-weighted image; this helps differentiate them from lymphomas that tend to show increased signal on T2-weighted images relative to muscle.

■ Case 67

1. Which condition typically courses with thick, nodular leptomeningeal enhancement?
   a) Fungal meningitis
   b) Viral meningitis
   c) Bacterial meningitis
   d) Intracranial hypotension

The correct answer is (**a**). Fungal meningitis generally presents with thick, nodular leptomeningeal enhancement. Viral and bacterial meningitis shows thinner, linear enhancement. Intracranial hypotension shows pachymeningeal enhancement.

2. Which is true regarding pyogenic meningitis?
   a) Exclusive to the immunocompromised host
   b) Generally self-limiting course
   c) Increased T2/fluid-attenuated inversion recovery (FLAIR) signal within the cerebral sulci
   d) Easily distinguished from viral meningitis

The correct answer is (**c**). Increased T2/FLAIR signal within the cerebral sulci. Increased T2/FLAIR signal within the cerebral sulci is a common imaging feature in pyogenic meningitis. This condition is not exclusive to the immunocompromised host, can be identical to viral meningitis on imaging, and requires antibiotic treatment.

■ Case 68

1. The reason for restricted diffusion in cerebral abscess is which of the following?
   a) High cellularity in the capsule
   b) Proteinaceous content of the purulent material
   c) Subacute blood products in the necrotic debris
   d) Manganese in the necrotic debris

The correct answer is (**b**), proteinaceous content of the purulent material and increased viscosity of the fluid. High cellularity in neoplastic lesions causes restricted diffusion. Extracellular methemoglobin causes restricted diffusion un subacute hematomas. Manganese is present in fungal infections and contributes to their low T2 signal.

2. Which of the following lesions shows a center of restricted diffusion on diffusion-weighted imaging (DWI)?
   a) Abscess
   b) Progressive multifocal leukoencephalopathy
   c) Primary CNS lymphoma
   d) Cerebral toxoplasmosis
   e) Demyelinating lesions

The correct answer is (**a**). DWI restriction in an abscess is located predominantly within the purulent debris in center of the lesion. All the other entities may feature DWI restriction at the periphery of the lesion.

■ Case 69
....

1. Which imaging finding suggests immune inflammatory reconstitution syndrome (IRIS) in a patient with progressive multifocal leukoencephalopathy (PML)?
   a) New enhancement in the lesions
   b) Hemorrhagic transformation of the lesions
   c) Cortical involvement of previously seen lesions
   d) Development of symmetric periventricular hyperintensities
   e) Cystic degeneration of the lesions

The correct answer is (**a**). New area of enhancement and edema of a lesion are indicators of IRIS.

2. Which of the following entities in patients with HIV does not enhance?
   a) HIV encephalopathy
   b) PML-IRIS
   c) Toxoplasmosis
   d) Lymphoma
   e) Septic emboli

The correct answer is (**a**). HIV encephalopathy does not show enhancement. PML-IRIS, toxoplasmosis, lymphoma, and septic emboli typically show enhancement.

■ Case 70
....

1. Which is not considered a risk factor for AIDS dementia complex?
   a) Young age at infection
   b) Prolonged HIV infection
   c) Low CD4 counts
   d) Older age at seroconversion

The correct answer is (**a**). Young age at the time of infection is not a risk factor for developing AIDS dementia complex. Low CD4 counts, older age at seroconversion, and prolonged HIV infection are.

2. Which is a typical feature of AIDS dementia complex?
   a) Restricted diffusion involving deep white matter
   b) White matter signal abnormality in the posterior fossa
   c) Parietal lobe predominance
   d) Lack of mass effect

The correct answer is (**d**). AIDS dementia complex does not course with mass effect or enhancement.

■ Case 71
....

1. Which of the following is *not* associated with dilatation of the perivascular spaces?
   a) Mucopolysaccharidosis
   b) Hydrocephalus
   c) Cryptococcosis

The correct answer is (**b**). Hydrocephalus is not a cause of dilated perivascular spaces. Mucopolysaccharidosis and cryptococcosis are known causes of prominence of the perivascular spaces.

2. Conditions that mimic subarachnoid hemorrhage on CT scans include all of the following except...
   a) Diffuse cerebral edema
   b) Leptomeningeal cryptococcosis
   c) Racemose neurocysticercosis
   d) Hyperoxygenation artifact from mechanical ventilation

The correct answer is (**d**). Hyperoxygenation artifact from mechanical ventilation will cause abnormal signal in the subarachnoid space in T2/FLAIR sequences. However, this entity will not cause abnormal density on CT. Diffuse cerebral edema may give the appearance of "pseudosubarachnoid hemorrhage." Leptomeningeal cryptococcosis and racemose neurocysticercosis can have abnormal density of the subarachnoid space on CT.

■ Case 72
....

1. Which of the following characteristics favor toxoplasmosis over lymphoma?
   a) The presence of ring enhancing lesions affecting the basal ganglia
   b) Hemorrhagic transformation and gliosis in lesions after treatment
   c) Ventricular subependymal enhancement
   d) The presence of vasogenic edema around ring enhancing lesions

The correct answer is (**b**). Hemorrhagic transformation and gliosis in lesions after treatment is typically seen only in toxoplasmosis. The presence of ring enhancing lesions affecting the basal ganglia and vasogenic edema around ring enhancing lesions is seen in both diseases. Ventricular subependymal enhancement is only seen in lymphoma.

2. The "eccentric target sign" is described in patients with HIV who have which of the following conditions?
   a) Progressive multifocal leukoencephalopathy
   b) Toxoplasmosis
   c) Cryptococcosis
   d) Primary central nervous system lymphoma
   e) HIV encephalitis

The correct answer is (**b**). The "eccentric target sign" has been described in toxoplasmosis.

■ Case 73
· ·

1. Central restricted diffusion is present in which of the following conditions?
   a) Metastasis
   b) Abscess
   c) Cyst
   d) Primary brain neoplasm

The correct answer is (**b**). High diffusion-weighted imaging signal with low apparent diffusion coefficient values are typically present centrally within cerebral abscesses, representing true restricted diffusion.

2. Low internal T2 signal within a cerebral lesion may indicate which of the following?
   a) Proteinaceous fluid
   b) Melanin
   c) High cellularity
   d) Hemoglobin degradation products
   e) All of the above

The correct answer is (**e**). Any of the aforementioned substances can result in low T2 signal within intracranial lesions.

■ Case 74
· ·

1. In the assessment of opportunistic infection, which is correct?
   a) HIV encephalitis causes mass effect and asymmetric periventricular or subcortical white matter disease.
   b) Progressive multifocal leukoencephalopathy (PML) white matter lesions tend to be symmetric.
   c) Toxoplasma, lymphoma, and tuberculosis may present as ring enhancing lesions.
   d) PML tends to spare the subcortical U-fibers.

The correct answer is (**c**). Toxoplasma, lymphoma, and tuberculosis may present as ring enhancing lesions. HIV encephalitis causes atrophy and symmetric periventricular or unilateral white matter disease. PML white matter lesions tend to be asymmetric. PML tends to affect the subcortical U-fibers.

2. Regarding PML, which statement is true?
   a) In PML-IRIS, there is a relapse or recurrence of preexisting infectious disease.
   b) In PML-IRIS, the reconstitution of the immune system causes an abnormal immune response to infectious/noninfectious antigens.
   c) In PML–non-IRIS the lesions tend to be symmetric, whereas in PML-IRIS they are asymmetric.
   d) PML–non-IRIS is characterized by ring enhancing lesions, whereas PML-IRIS shows asymmetric white matter lesions without mass effect.

The correct answer is (**b**). In PML-IRIS, the reconstitution of the immune system causes an abnormal immune response to infectious/noninfectious antigens. In PML–non-IRIS, there is a reactivation of a preexisting infection by the JC virus. In both PML–non-IRIS and PML-IRIS, the lesions tend to be asymmetric. PML–non-IRIS is not characterized by ring enhancing lesions.

■ Case 75
· ·

1. Which of the following is a characteristic of the typical presentation of epidural hematomas?
   a) Will not cross the sutures
   b) Crescent in shape
   c) Content is venous blood
   d) Will not cross the dural folds
   e) 50% are infratentorial secondary to skull base fractures

The correct answer is (**a**). Epidural hematomas typically will not cross the sutures and they have a biconvex shape, the content is arterial blood, they will cross the dural folds, and > 90% are supratentorial in location.

2. Which of the following is an MR characteristic of hyperacute epidural hematomas?
   a) Typically present as a crescent-shaped lesion
   b) Core shows hyperintensity on diffusion-weighted imaging (DWI)
   c) Diffusely enhance with gadolinium
   d) Associated with underlying sinus disease
   e) Are seen within the cerebral sulci with minimal mass effect

The correct answer is (**b**). The core of hyperacute epidural hematomas shows hyperintensity on DWI due to the presence of oxygenated hemoglobin. They should not enhance with gadolinium and are not typically associated with underlying sinus disease as empyemas do. Subarachnoid hemorrhage is the one that is seen within the cerebral sulci with minimal mass effect.

■ Case 76

1. Which of the following is true with respect to alar ligament rupture?
   a) Associated with occipital condyle avulsion fractures
   b) Associated with hyperextension
   c) Presents with posterior displacement of the dens
   d) Usually secondary to C1 burst and lateral mass fractures.

The correct answer is (**a**). Alar ligament rupture is associated to type III occipital condyle avulsion fractures. Alar ligament rupture is more common in children, is caused by flexion and rotation and does not generally present with posterior displacement of the dens. Transverse ligament rupture is usually secondary to C1 burst and lateral mass fractures.

2. Which of the following structures is a continuation of the posterior longitudinal ligament?
   a) Apical ligament
   b) Cruciate ligament
   c) Alar ligament
   d) Tectorial membrane

The correct answer is (**d**). Tectorial membrane. The tectorial membrane is the rostral continuation of the posterior longitudinal ligament.

■ Case 77

1. Regarding spinal cord injury, which statement is true?
   a) Fractures with bony retropulsion, disk extrusions, and epidural hematomas do not frequently cause spinal cord compression.
   b) In spinal cord injury without radiographic abnormality (SCIWORA), there are no fractures on x-ray or CT images but there may be cord signal abnormalities on MRI.
   c) In SCIWORA, the patients present clinically with myelopathy but demonstrate normal findings on x-ray, CT, and MRI images.
   d) Patients with cord swelling tend to have a worse prognosis than patients with cord hemorrhage.

The correct answer is (**b**). In SCIWORA, there are no fractures on x-ray or CT images but there may be cord signal abnormalities on MRI. Fractures with bony retropulsion, disk extrusions, and epidural hematomas frequently cause spinal cord compression, playing a significant role in patients with clinical signs of myelopathy. In SCIWORA, the patients present clinically with myelopathy but demonstrate normal findings on x-ray and CT images, with or without MRI abnormalities. Patients with cord hemorrhage tend to have a worse prognosis than patients with only cord swelling.

2. Regarding spinal cord injuries the following are true except...
   a) Patients with incomplete neurologic deficit and spinal instability need to be treated emergently due to the risk of progression of the neurologic deficit.
   b) Patients with complete neurologic deficit have a higher chance of recovery than patients with incomplete cord or nerve root injury.
   c) Patients with injuries around the L1 level are at risk of conus medullaris syndrome, with paralysis of the sacrally innervated bowel and bladder but possible preservation of lower limb motor function.
   d) Patients with incomplete neurologic deficit and extrinsic cord compression need to be treated emergently due to the risk of progression of the neurologic deficit.

The correct answer is (**b**). Patients with complete neurologic deficit have a higher chance of recovery than patients with incomplete cord or nerve root injury. Patients with incomplete neurologic deficit presenting with spinal instability or with extrinsic compression need to be treated emergently to avoid the risk of progression of the neurologic deficit. Patients with injuries around the L1 level are at risk of conus medullaris syndrome, with paralysis of the sacrally innervated bowel and bladder. The motor function of the lower limbs may be preserved.

■ Case 78

1. Which is true regarding Duret hemorrhages?
   a) Occur secondary to upward transtentorial herniation
   b) Result in tonsillar herniation
   c) Are more common in the medulla
   d) Are generally centrally located

The correct answer is (**d**). Duret hemorrhages are typically centrally located. They are caused by downward transtentorial herniation, they do not necessarily result in tonsillar herniation and are more common in the midbrain and pons.

2. Which is *not* a sign of cerebral edema?
   a) Enlargement of the ventricles
   b) Effacement of the cerebral sulci
   c) Loss of gray–white matter differentiation
   d) Diffuse cerebral hypoattenuation

The correct answer is (**a**). Enlargement of the ventricles. Cerebral edema generally causes slitlike ventricles unless there is an added component of hydrocephalus.

■ Case 79

1. Which MRI feature favors pathologic fracture over traumatic compression fracture?
   a) Bone marrow edema
   b) Convex posterior border of the vertebral body
   c) Biconcave morphology of the end plates
   d) Wedge deformity of the vertebral body

The correct answer is (**b**). Convex posterior border of the vertebral body is secondary to expansion of the vertebral body in the setting of an underlying tumor, and it is not seen in fractures due to trauma on normal bone. Bone marrow edema, biconcave morphology of the end plates, and wedge deformity of the vertebral body are nonspecific features of fractures that do not help to determine the etiology.

2. Which of the following MRI features is seen in both osteoporotic compression fracture and pathologic fracture?
   a) Associated soft tissue mass
   b) Restricted diffusion
   c) No signal dropout in T1-weighted out-of-phase imaging
   d) Bone marrow edema

The correct answer is (**c**). Bone marrow edema has an appearance similar to osteoporotic compression fractures and pathologic fractures. Associated soft tissue mass, restricted diffusion, and lack of signal dropout on T1-weighted out-of-phase imaging are features of pathologic fractures that help to differentiate them from osteoporotic compression fractures.

■ Case 80

1. Which of the following is true in relation to diffuse axonal injury (DAI)?
   a) T2* gradient echo is better than susceptibility-weighted imaging (SWI) in detection of microhemorrhages.
   b) Diffusion tensor image shows increased fractional anisotropy in regions of the brain with DAI.
   c) The genu is the most frequent site of shear injuries in the corpus callosum.
   d) Diffusion-weighted image (DWI) will show increased signal in the areas of injury.
   e) CT is better in the detection of microbleed as compared to MR.

The correct answer is (**d**). Diffusion weighted images will demonstrate areas of increased signal at the site of DAI. MR is superior to CT in the detection of microbleeds, and the most sensitive sequence is SWI.

2. An MR image of the brain of a 58-year-old patient shows multiple subcortical microbleeds on SWI in the brain with no involvement of the basal ganglia, normal fluid-attenuated inversion recovery (FLAIR) and DWI in a patient with no history of recent trauma, the most likely diagnosis would be:
   a) DAI
   b) Type IV cavernous angiomas
   c) Amyloid angiopathy
   d) Hypertensive angiopathy
   e) Cardiac emboli

The correct answer is (**c**). Amyloid angiopathy tends to be seen mostly in the subcortical white matter in patients with no evidence of chronic microvascular disease; in this case, with normal FLAIR. DAI favors the subcortical white matter, corpus callosum, and brainstem; the lesions tend to be positive on DWI; and a history of trauma should be present. Type IV cavernous angiomas present with diffuse scattered microhemorrhage with no predilection for the subcortical white matter. Cardiac emboli should show restricted diffusion.

■ Case 81

1. Regarding Chance fracture, which statement is true?
   a) There is no distraction of the posterior elements.
   b) There is fracture of the pedicles and variable involvement of the posterior elements.
   c) It is more frequently centered in the craniocervical junction.
   d) The anterior ligamentous complex is frequently involved.

The correct answer is (**b**). There is fracture of the pedicles and variable involvement of the posterior elements. Chance fractures are more frequently centered at the thoracolumbar (not craniocervical) junction. Distraction of the posterior elements and involvement of the posterior (not anterior) ligamentous complex are common.

2. Which statement regarding distraction injuries is false?
   a) In distraction injuries, one part of the spinal column is separated from the other, leaving a space in between.
   b) They can be secondary to soft tissue injury, bone fracture, or both.
   c) Extension injuries are not included in the category of distraction injuries.
   d) Distraction injuries are often very unstable.
   e) Distraction extension injuries are usually seen in patients with diffuse idiopathic skeletal hyperostosis or ankylosing spondylitis.

The correct answer is (**c**). Extension injuries are indeed included in the category of distraction injuries (B3 injury in the AOSpine Thoracolumbar Spine Injury Classification system). Distraction extension injuries are usually seen in patients with diffuse idiopathic skeletal hyperostosis or ankylosing spondylitis. In distraction injuries, one part of the spinal column is separated from the other, leaving a space in between. Distraction injuries can be secondary to soft tissue injury, bone fracture, or both, and they often are very unstable.

■ Case 82

1. What is the main role of MR in the setting of cervical trauma?
   a) Detect the extent of spinal cord injury
   b) Evaluate for the prevertebral soft tissues
   c) Identify the fracture tracts
   d) Evaluate for bone marrow edema
   e) Identify the presence of enhancement

The correct answer is (**a**). The main role of MR is detection of the type and extent of spinal cord injury, which affects patient management. MR is better suited for exclusion of spinal cord lesions than detection of ligamentous or other soft tissue injuries.

2. Which of the following is a characteristic commonly shared by translational and distraction injuries of the cervical spine?
   a) Lesion to the spinal cord
   b) Involvement of the discoligamentous complex (DLC)
   c) Sparing of the ligaments
   d) Compression deformity of the vertebral bodies

The correct answer is (**b**). Both distraction and translational injuries of the subaxial cervical spine typically course with DLC involvement.

■ Case 83

1. With respect to avulsion fractures in hyperextension dislocation, which is correct?
   a) They are more common in the upper cervical spine.
   b) They are pathognomonic of hyperextension injuries.
   c) They tend to be more horizontally oriented.
   d) They occur at the posteroinferior aspect of the vertebral body.

The correct answer is (**c**). They tend to be more horizontally oriented. Hyperextension dislocation may be associated with avulsion fractures of the anteroinferior vertebral body. They are more horizontally oriented and occur in the inferior cervical spine.

2. Which is *not* a component of the posterior ligament complex?
   a) Posterior longitudinal ligament
   b) Interspinous ligament
   c) Ligamentum flavum
   d) Supraspinous ligament

The correct answer is (**a**). The posterior longitudinal ligament is not part of the posterior ligament complex.

■ Case 84

1. Regarding parenchymal contusions, which statement is false?
   a) Are a cause of bilateral frontal atrophy
   b) May present with or without hemorrhage
   c) Are secondary to shear forces in the axons
   d) Are secondary to direct impact of the cortex against the calvarium
   e) Are more frequent in the anterior and middle cranial fossa

The correct answer is (**c**). Diffuse axonal injuries, not parenchymal contusions, are secondary to shear forces in the axons. Parenchymal contusions are a cause of bilateral frontal atrophy, may present with or without hemorrhage, are secondary to direct impact of the cortex against the calvarium, and are more common in the anterior and middle cranial fossa.

2. Regarding the assessment of traumatic brain injury, which is correct?
   a) MRI of the brain is used to rule out subarachnoid hemorrhage in patients with persistent headache and normal brain CT images.
   b) Fluid-attenuated inversion recovery (FLAIR) sequences are the most sensitive to detect acute, subacute, and chronic blood products.
   c) Diffusion-weighted imaging (DWI), FLAIR, and gradient echo (GRE) are helpful in the evaluation of diffuse axonal injury.
   d) MR angiography is the modality of choice to assess traumatic vascular injury.

The correct answer is (**c**). DWI, FLAIR, and GRE are helpful in the evaluation of diffuse axonal injury. $T2^*$ and susceptibility-weighted imaging MRI sequences (not FLAIR) are most sensitive to detect acute, early subacute, and chronic stages of diffuse axonal injury.

■ **Case 85**

1. Regarding the McDonald criteria for multiple sclerosis (MS), which statement is true?
   a) Spinal cord and optic nerve lesions are not included in the determination of dissemination in space.
   b) Dissemination in space can be shown by involvement of at least three of five areas of the central nervous system (three or more periventricular lesions, one or more infratentorial lesion, one or more spinal cord lesion, one or more optic nerve lesion, one or more cortical or juxtacortical lesion).
   c) Dissemination in time cannot be established in the absence of a prior comparison MRI exam.
   d) Dissemination in time can be established by the presence of at least one new T2 or gadolinium enhancing lesion on follow-up MRI scan, with reference to a baseline scan, irrespective of the timing of the baseline MRI scan.

The correct answer is (**d**). Dissemination in time can be established by the following: presence of at least one new T2 or gadolinium enhancing lesion on follow-up MRI scan, with reference to a baseline scan, irrespective of the timing of the baseline MRI scan; or the simultaneous presence of asymptomatic gadolinium enhancing and nonenhancing lesions at any time.

2. Which feature is more commonly seen in white matter hyperintensities from demyelinating disease as compared to leukoaraiosis?
   a) Heterogeneous T2 signal intensity
   b) Indistinct borders
   c) Ovoid shape
   d) Punctate in size

The correct answer is (**c**). White matter T2 hyperintensities related to demyelination are more likely to be ovoid, > 3 mm (as opposed to being punctate), well circumscribed, homogenous in signal intensity, and located in periventricular or juxtacortical locations.

■ **Case 86**

1. The following features favor the diagnosis of chronic lymphocytic inflammation with pontine perivascular enhancement responsive to steroids (CLIPPERS) except…
   a) Subacute progressive ataxia, diplopia, and other clinical features of brainstem dysfunction
   b) Significant clinical and radiologic response to glucocorticosteroids
   c) Mass effect and necrosis on MRI scans
   d) Linear and punctate contrast enhancement
   e) Minimal or absent findings in T2 and fluid-attenuated inversion recovery (FLAIR) sequences

The correct answer is (**c**). Mass effect and necrosis on MRI scans are not characteristic features of CLIPPERS and should prompt an investigation of alternative etiologies. Subacute progressive ataxia, diplopia, and other clinical features of brainstem dysfunction, significant clinical and radiologic response to glucocorticosteroids, linear and punctate contrast enhancement, and minimal or absent findings in T2 and FLAIR sequences are all features of CLIPPERS.

2. Regarding the diagnosis of CLIPPERS, which is true?
   a) It demonstrates a ring enhancement pattern, with or without areas of central necrosis.
   b) It is confined to the pons, and extrapontine involvement should prompt an investigation of other etiologies.
   c) It typically demonstrates restricted diffusion.
   d) FLAIR and T2-weighted images tend to show minimal or absent signal abnormalities.
   e) Cerebral angiography demonstrates a beaded appearance of the posterior circulation vessels.

The correct answer is (**d**). All other statements are false. CLIPPERS usually demonstrates linear and punctate areas of enhancement, possibly with a radiating pattern. It is not always confined to the pons; it may involve the other areas of the brainstem, cerebellum, spinal cord, basal ganglia, or cerebral white matter. CLIPPERS does not demonstrate restricted diffusion or abnormalities on cerebral angiography.

■ **Case 87**

1. Which of the following conditions presents with lesions that are cigar-shaped on sagittal imaging, wedge-shaped on axial imaging, are eccentrically located, and are less than or equal to two vertebral bodies in length?
   a) Multiple sclerosis
   b) Neuromyelitis optica (NMO)
   c) Transverse myelitis
   d) Spinal cord infarction
   e) Subacute combined degeneration

The correct answer is (**a**). MS lesions in the spinal cord typically have these features on MR imaging.

2. Which of the following is a characteristic of spinal involvement of NMO?
   a) Cystic lesions
   b) Hemosiderin cap
   c) Lesions involving < 50% of the cross-sectional area of the cord
   d) Patchy enhancement in areas of relapse
   e) Lesions less than three vertebral bodies in length

The correct answer is (**d**). NMO presents as patchy enhancement in areas of relapse, the lesions cover more than half of the area of the spinal cord in cross section, and they are not associated with cysts or hemorrhage.

■ Case 88

1. Which is true regarding spinal cord infarcts?
   a) They more commonly involve the posterior half of the cord.
   b) They generally have an insidious course.
   c) Anterior cord infarcts are more commonly bilateral.
   d) Clinical presentation is generally painless flaccid paralysis.

The correct answer is (**c**). Anterior cord infarcts are generally bilateral because of the single sulcal artery giving rise to the blood supply of the bilateral ventral horns. Presentation is typically acute back pain and more commonly affects the anterior cord.

2. Which is true regarding the spinal cord vascular supply?
   a) The majority of blood supply is provided by medullary branches of the radicular arteries.
   b) The anterior spinal artery is formed by the confluence of the radicular arteries.
   c) A single posterior spinal artery courses along the medial dorsal cord.
   d) Pial circumferential plexus branches supply the majority of blood to the gray matter.

The correct answer is (**a**). The majority of the blood supply is provided by the medullary branches of the radicular arteries. The anterior spinal artery is formed by the confluence of the intracranial vertebral arteries. The pial plexus supplies the peripheral white matter, and the posterior spinal arteries are paired structures that course along the bilateral posterolateral aspect of the spinal cord.

■ Case 89

1. Regarding ossification of the posterior longitudinal ligament (PLL), which of the following is true?
   a) It typically presents with syndesmophytes, with paraspinous ligamentous or disk ossification bridging two adjacent vertebral bodies.
   b) It tends to be an incidental finding in asymptomatic patients.
   c) It may coexist with diffuse idiopathic skeletal hyperostosis (DISH) or ossification of the ligamentum flavum.
   d) It predisposes patients to atypical fractures and pseudoarthrosis.

The correct answer is (**c**). It may coexist with DISH or ossification of the ligamentum flavum. Ankylosing spondylitis typically presents with syndesmophytes, with paraspinous ligamentous or disk ossification bridging two adjacent vertebral bodies. Ankylosing spondylitis also predisposes patients to atypical fractures and pseudoarthrosis. DISH tends to be an incidental finding in asymptomatic patients. Although ossification of the posterior longitudinal ligament (OPLL) may be asymptomatic, it causes spinal canal stenosis and frequently leads to myelopathy or myeloradiculopathy.

2. Regarding the diagnosis of OPLL, which of the following is false?
   a) MRI is used to evaluate cord abutment and myelopathy.
   b) It is defined as flowing ossification of the PLL spanning at least four contiguous vertebral bodies.
   c) DISH can coexist with OPLL in ~25% of cases.
   d) Bridge-type OPLL causes loss of segmental motion and may lead to segmental instability.

The correct answer is (**b**). DISH is defined as flowing ossification of the anterior (not posterior) longitudinal ligament spanning at least four contiguous vertebral bodies. All other statements are true: MRI is used to evaluate cord abutment and myelopathy, DISH can coexist with OPLL in ~25% of cases, and bridge-type OPLL causes loss of segmental motion and may lead to segmental instability.

■ Case 90

1. Which of the following is a characteristic of posterior reversible encephalopathy syndrome (PRES)?
   a) Half of the cases show lesions with restricted diffusion.
   b) Lesions are typically asymmetric.
   c) It is caused by severe vasoconstriction.
   d) Lesions favor the brainstem.
   e) Lesions typically reverse completely.

The correct answer is (**e**). Lesions in PRES typically reverse completely. Approximately 10% of the cases show lesions with restricted diffusion. The lesions are typically symmetric. It is secondary to a disorder in vascular autoregulation. Lesions favor the occipital and parietal lobes.

2. Which of the following can be seen as a complication of PRES?
   a) Hemorrhage
   b) Deep vein thrombosis
   c) Cortical thrombosis
   d) Basilar artery occlusion
   e) Hydrocephalus

The correct answer is (**a**), hemorrhage. Deep vein thrombosis, cortical thrombosis, basilar artery occlusion, and hydrocephalus are not associated with PRES.

■ **Case 91**

1. Which of the following is a characteristic imaging feature of hypertrophic olivary degeneration (HOD)?
   a) Postcontrast enhancement
   b) Unilateral or bilateral involvement
   c) Early onset of hypertrophy following the insult
   d) Decreased T2 signal

The correct answer is (**b**). HOD may demonstrate unilateral or bilateral involvement. On the other hand, T2 signal is usually high, there is no enhancement, and there is late onset of hypertrophy following the insult.

2. Which is true regarding HOD?
   a) It is caused by damage to the corticospinal tract.
   b) T2 hyperintensity may persist indefinitely.
   c) Typically, it first appears as atrophy of the nucleus followed by hypertrophy.
   d) Hypertrophy occurs before T2 signal change.

The correct answer is (**b**). Although hypertrophy may subside, T2 hyperintensity may persist indefinitely. HOD occurs secondary to injury of the dentato-rubro-olivary pathway, and increased T2 signal precedes hypertrophy.

■ **Case 92**

1. Which of the following statements is true?
   a) Chiasmatic herniation is more common in primary empty sella configuration.
   b) Most patients with chiasmatic herniation present with visual field disturbances.
   c) Downward angulation and tilting of the optic chiasm is characteristic of chiasmatic herniation.
   d) Herniation of the anterior and inferior third ventricle into the sella is more common than herniation of the chiasm.
   e) Chiasmatic herniation normally presents with absence of the septum pellucidum.

The correct answer is (**c**). Downward angulation and tilting of the optic chiasm is characteristic of chiasmatic herniation. Chiasmatic herniation is more common in secondary not primary empty sella configuration. Most patients with chiasmatic herniation are asymptomatic. Herniation of the anterior and inferior third ventricle into the sella is less frequent that herniation of the chiasm. Chiasmatic herniation has not been described in correlation with absence of the septum pellucidum.

2. Which of the following entities courses with chiasmatic hypoplasia?
   a) Chiasmatic herniation secondary to a primary empty sella
   b) Septo-optic dysplasia
   c) Lobar holoprosencephaly
   d) Rathke cleft cyst
   e) Pituitary hamartoma

The correct answer is (**b**), septo-optic dysplasia. Chiasmatic herniation secondary to a primary empty sella, lobar holoprosencephaly, Rathke cleft cyst and pituitary hamartoma are not associated with chiasmatic hypoplasia.

■ **Case 93**

1. Which areas of the brain are generally spared of cortical involvement in hepatic encephalopathy?
   a) Frontal lobes
   b) Temporal lobes
   c) Insulae
   d) Occipital lobes

The correct answer is (**d**), occipital lobes. Cortical/subcortical involvement tends to be more variable and asymmetric. Generally, there is relative sparing of the occipital and perirolandic regions.

2. Which is true regarding MR spectroscopy (MRS) in hepatic encephalopathy?
   a) Metabolic abnormalities are irreversible in hepatic encephalopathy.
   b) Changes on MRS do not correlate to severity of hepatic encephalopathy.
   c) MRS can show elevation of glutamine/glutamate.
   d) MRS can show elevation of myoinositol.

The correct answer is (**c**). MRS shows an elevation of glutamine/glutamate with a decrease of myoinositol and choline. The degree of metabolic abnormalities is usually proportional to the severity of the hepatic encephalopathy and can be reversible with treatment.

■ **Case 94**

1. Imaging findings of mesial temporal sclerosis (MTS) include which of the following?
   a) Small or atrophic hippocampus ipsilateral to the seizure focus with increased T1 signal
   b) Loss of internal architecture and loss of hippocampal head digitations
   c) Dilatation of the contralateral temporal horn
   d) Decreased T2 signal intensity of the ipsilateral amygdala
   e) Atrophy of contralateral mammillary body and fornix

The correct answer is (**b**). Findings of MTS include loss of internal architecture and loss of hippocampal head digitations. Findings also include small or atrophic hippocampus ipsilateral to the seizure focus with increased T2 (not T1) signal, dilatation of the ipsilateral temporal horn, increased (not decreased) T2 signal intensity of the ipsilateral amygdala, and atrophy of ipsilateral (not contralateral) mammillary body and fornix.

2. Regarding the differential diagnosis of MTS, which is true?
   a) In limbic encephalitis, signal changes are confined to the limbic system.
   b) Dual pathology implies the presence of MTS and another potentially epileptogenic extrahippocampal anomaly.
   c) Bilateral MTS is easier to recognize than unilateral MTS.
   d) Cortical dysplasia and gliotic lesions are not recognized causes of dual pathology.

The correct answer is (**b**). Dual pathology implies the presence of MTS and another potentially epileptogenic extrahippocampal anomaly. In limbic encephalitis, signal changes are *not always* confined to the limbic system. Bilateral MTS may be difficult to recognize. Cortical dysplasia and gliotic lesions are *common* causes of dual pathology.

■ Case 95

1. Which of the following is considered a variant of multiple sclerosis (MS)?
   a) Baló disease
   b) Acute disseminated encephalomyelitis (ADEM)
   c) Neuromyelitis optica (NMO)
   d) Central pontine myelinolysis
   e) Susac syndrome

The correct answer is (**a**). Baló concentric sclerosis is considered an atypical variant of MS along with tumefactive MS, Schilder disease, and Marburg disease.

2. The presence of aquaporin-4 (AQP4) in cerebrospinal fluid is related to which of the following entities?
   a) Baló disease
   b) ADEM
   c) NMO
   d) Central pontine myelinolysis
   e) Susac syndrome

The correct answer is (**c**). NMO lesions express AQP4.

■ Case 96

1. Which is true regarding multiple myeloma (MM)?
   a) Spinal compression fractures are a common occurrence.
   b) Active myeloma lesions do not tend to enhance.
   c) MM is most commonly seen in females.
   d) MM is the second most common primary osseous malignancy.

The correct answer is (**a**). Spinal compression fractures may occur in up to 70% of cases. Active myeloma lesions tend to enhance, MM is more common in males, and MM is the most common primary osseous malignancy in adults.

2. Which is true with respect to imaging in MM?
   a) Imaging is unreliable for assessing treatment response.
   b) CT imaging shows blastic lesions.
   c) There is a high predilection for bones with low red marrow concentration.
   d) Fat suppression techniques allow for greater conspicuity of lesions.

The correct answer is (**d**). MRI with fat saturation provides better contrast and conspicuity of lesions.

■ Case 97

1. Which is a characteristic feature of radiation necrosis?
   a) Well-defined margins
   b) Solid enhancement
   c) Decreased lesion size
   d) Increased surrounding T2 fluid-attenuated inversion recovery (FLAIR) changes

The correct answer is (**d**). Increased surrounding T2 FLAIR changes. Initially, there is an increase in surrounding edema followed by volume loss. The margins are ill-defined or feathery, the lesion tends to increase in size, and the enhancement is similar to soap bubbles or Swiss cheese.

2. Which is true regarding advanced imaging in radiation necrosis?
   a) Increased *N*-acetylaspartate (NAA) on MR spectroscopy (MRS) images
   b) Hypometabolism on fluorodeoxyglucose–positron emission tomography (FDG-PET) scan
   c) Increased relative cerebral blood volume (rCBV) on MR perfusion images
   d) Myoinositol peak on MRS images

The correct answer is (**b**). Radiation necrosis is generally hypometabolic on FDG-PET. NAA decreases, rCBV is low or normal, and there is no myoinositol peak on MRS images.

■ Case 98

1. Which of the following is the most common location of synovial cysts in the spine?
   a) Craniocervical junction
   b) Subaxial cervical spine
   c) Thoracic spine
   d) Lumbar spine
   e) Sacrum

The correct answer is (**d**). The lumbar spine is the most frequent location of synovial cysts.

2. Which of the following is a characteristic of a synovial cyst of the spine?
   a) Has no synovial lining
   b) Connected to the facet joint
   c) Secondary to a disruption of a disk fragment from a disk extrusion
   d) Meningothelial origin with avid enhancement
   e) Always shows increased signal on T1-weighted image

The correct answer is (**b**). Synovial cysts are always connected to the facet joint, they have a synovial lining, and although they can show increased signal on T1-weighted images, typically they show low intensity on these sequences. Secondary to a disruption of a disk fragment from a disk extrusion is consistent with a disk sequestration. Meningothelial origin with avid enhancement is consistent with a meningioma.

■ Case 99

1. Which of the following characteristics is seen in a sequestered disk?
   a) Peripheral enhancement
   b) Continuity with a disk extrusion
   c) Posterior location in the spinal canal
   d) Hemorrhage
   e) Foraminal location

The correct answer is (**a**). Sequestered disks show peripheral enhancement in the inflammatory phase.

2. A focal disk defect where in at least one plane, the diameter of the base of the herniated material is narrower than the diameter of the herniated material is the definition of which of the following?
   a) An annular bulge
   b) A sequestered disk
   c) A disk protrusion
   d) A disk extrusion
   e) An annular fissure

The correct answer (**d**). This is the definition of a disk extrusion.

■ Case 100

1. Which is true regarding basal encephaloceles?
   a) They are generally clinically evident as a nasal mass.
   b) No clear connection is seen with the subarachnoid space.
   c) A tract is generally present with the foramen cecum.
   d) Transethmoidal and transsphenoidal are its most common variants.

The correct answer is (**d**). Transethmoidal and transsphenoidal are its most common variants. They are generally not seen externally. A connection is present with the subarachnoid space, and they occur posterior to the foramen cecum at the cribriform plate and through the floor of the sella.

2. Which of the encephalocele categories is the most common?
   a) Occipital
   b) Sincipital
   c) Basal
   d) All are equally prevalent.

The correct answer is (**a**). Encephaloceles are classified into three categories: occipital (75%), sincipital (15%), and basal (10%).

Further Readings

■ Case 1

Bosemani T, Orman G, Boltshauser E, Tekes A, Huisman TA, Poretti A. Congenital abnormalities of the posterior fossa. RadioGraphics 2015;35(1):200–220

Osborn AG. Posterior fossa malformations. Osborn's Brain: Imaging, Pathology, and Anatomy. Philadelphia, PA: Lippincott Williams & Wilkins; 2012:1055–1083

Yousem DM, Grossman RI. Neuroradiology: The Requisites. 3rd ed. Philadelphia, PA: Mosby Elsevier; 2010:773–809

■ Case 2

Geerdink N, van der Vliet T, Rotteveel JJ, Feuth T, Roeleveld N, Mullaart RA. Essential features of Chiari II malformation in MR imaging: an interobserver reliability study—part 1. Childs Nerv Syst 2012;28(7):977–985

Stevenson KL. Chiari type II malformation: past, present, and future. Neurosurg Focus 2004;16(2):E5

■ Case 3

Poretti A, Boltshauser E, Huisman TA. Cerebellar and brainstem malformations. Neuroimaging Clin N Am 2016; 26(3):341–357

■ Case 4

Barkovich AJ, Raybaud C. Pediatric Neuroimaging. 5th ed. Philadelphia, PA: Lippincott Williams & Wilkins; 2012

Hetts SW, Sherr EH, Chao S, et al. Anomalies of the corpus callosum: an MR analysis of the phenotypic spectrum of associated malformations. AJR 2016;187(5):1343–1348

Osborn AG. Nonneoplastic cysts. Osborn's Brain: Imaging, Pathology, and Anatomy. Philadelphia, PA: Lippincott Williams & Wilkins; 2012

Stroustrup Smith A, Levine D. Appearance of an interhemispheric cyst associated with agenesis of the corpus callosum. AJNR Am J Neuroradiol 2004;25(6):1037–1040

■ Case 5

Cotes C, Bonfante E, Lazor J, et al. Congenital basis of posterior fossa anomalies. Neuroradiol J 2015;28(3):238–253

Doherty D. Joubert syndrome: insights into brain development, cilium biology, and complex disease. Semin Pediatr Neurol 2009;16(3):143–154

Merritt L. Recognition of the clinical signs and symptoms of Joubert syndrome. Adv Neonatal Care 2003;3(4): 178–186, quiz 187–188

■ Case 6

McKinney AM, Nascene D, Miller WP, et al. Childhood cerebral X-linked adrenoleukodystrophy: diffusion tensor imaging measurements for prediction of clinical outcome after hematopoietic stem cell transplantation. AJNR Am J Neuroradiol 2013;34(3):641–649

■ Case 7

Osborn AG. Nonneoplastic cysts. Osborn's Brain: Imaging, Pathology, and Anatomy. Philadelphia, PA: Lippincott Williams & Wilkins; 2012:773–809

Osborn AG, Preece MT. Intracranial cysts: radiologic-pathologic correlation and imaging approach. Radiology 2006;239(3):650–664

Yousem DM, Grossman RI. Neuroradiology: The Requisites. 3rd ed. Philadelphia, PA: Mosby Elsevier; 2010

■ Case 8

Dubourg C, Bendavid C, Pasquier L, Henry C, Odent S, David V. Holoprosencephaly. Orphanet J Rare Dis 2007; 2(8):8

Hahn JS, Pinter JD. Holoprosencephaly: genetic, neuroradiological, and clinical advances. Semin Pediatr Neurol 2002;9(4):309–319

Winter TC, Kennedy AM, Woodward PJ. Holoprosencephaly: a survey of the entity, with embryology and fetal imaging. RadioGraphics 2015;35(1):275–290

■ Case 9

Rossi A, Cama A, Piatelli G, Ravegnani M, Biancheri R, Tortori-Donati P. Spinal dysraphism: MR imaging rationale. J Neuroradiol 2004;31(1):3–24

■ Case 10

Barkovich AJ, Guerrini R, Kuzniecky RI, Jackson GD, Dobyns WB. A developmental and genetic classification for malformations of cortical development: update 2012. Brain 2012;135(Pt 5):1348–1369

Prayson RA. Classification and pathological characteristics of the cortical dysplasias. Childs Nerv Syst 2014;30(11): 1805–1812

Raybaud C, Widjaja E. Development and dysgenesis of the cerebral cortex: malformations of cortical development. Neuroimaging Clin N Am 2011;21(3):483–543, vii

■ Case 11

Severino M, Allegri AE, Pistorio A, et al. Midbrain-hindbrain involvement in septo-optic dysplasia. AJNR Am J Neuroradiol 2014;35(8):1586–1592

Winter TC, Kennedy AM, Woodward PJ. Holoprosencephaly: a survey of the entity, with embryology and fetal imaging. RadioGraphics 2015;35(1):275–290

■ Case 12

Arii J, Tanabe Y. Leigh syndrome: serial MR imaging and clinical follow-up. AJNR Am J Neuroradiol 2000;21(8): 1502–1509

Barkovich AJ, Good WV, Koch TK, Berg BO. Mitochondrial disorders: analysis of their clinical and imaging characteristics. AJNR Am J Neuroradiol 1993;14(5):1119–1137

Bonfante E, Koenig MK, Adejumo RB, Perinjelil V, Riascos RF. The neuroimaging of Leigh syndrome: case series and review of the literature. Pediatr Radiol 2016;46(4):443–451

Osborn AG. Inherited metabolic disorders. Osborn's Brain: Imaging, Pathology, and Anatomy. Philadelphia, PA: Lippincott Williams & Wilkins; 2012:853–907

Saneto RP, Friedman SD, Shaw DWW. Neuroimaging of mitochondrial disease. Mitochondrion 2008;8(5-6): 396–413

Yousem DM, Grossman RI. Neuroradiology: The Requisites. 3rd ed. Philadelphia, PA: Mosby Elsevier; 2010

■ Case 13

Chao CP, Zaleski CG, Patton AC. Neonatal hypoxic-ischemic encephalopathy: multimodality imaging findings. RadioGraphics 2006;26(Suppl 1):S159–S172

Liauw L, Palm-Meinders IH, van der Grond J, et al. Differentiating normal myelination from hypoxic-ischemic encephalopathy on T1-weighted MR Images: a new approach. AJNR Am J Neuroradiol 2007;28(4): 660–665

Wong DS, Poskitt KJ, Chau V, et al. Brain injury patterns in hypoglycemia in neonatal encephalopathy. AJNR Am J Neuroradiol 2013;34(7):1456–1461

■ Case 14

Reichert R, Campos LG, Vairo F, et al. Neuroimaging findings in patients with mucopolysaccharidosis: what you really need to know. RadioGraphics 2016;36(5): 1448–1462

Palmucci S, Attinà G, Lanza ML, et al. Imaging findings of mucopolysaccharidoses: a pictorial review. Insights Imaging 2013;4(4):443–459

Zafeiriou DI, Batzios SP. Brain and spinal MR imaging findings in mucopolysaccharidoses: a review. AJNR Am J Neuroradiol 2013;34(1):5–13

■ Case 15

Barkovich AJ, Raybaud C. Pediatric Neuroimaging. 5th ed. Philadelphia, PA: Lippincott Williams & Wilkins; 2012

Raghavan N, Barkovich AJ, Edwards M, Norman D. MR imaging in the tethered spinal cord syndrome. AJR 1989;152(4):843–852

Yousem DM, Grossman RI. Neuroradiology: The Requisites. 3rd ed. Philadelphia, PA: Mosby Elsevier; 2010

Zaleska-Dorobisz U, Bladowska J, Biel A, Pałka LW, Hołownia D. MRI diagnosis of diastematomyelia in a 78-year-old woman: case report and literature review. Pol J Radiol 2010;75(2):82–87

■ Case 16

Cecchetto G, Milanese L, Giordano R, Viero A, Suma V, Manara R. Looking at the missing brain: hydranencephaly case series and literature review. Pediatr Neurol 2013;48(2):152–158

RadCases.thieme.com   RadCases Plus Q&A Neuro Imaging   **233**

Naidich TP, Griffiths PD, Rosenbloom L. Central nervous system injury in utero: selected entities. Pediatr Radiol 2015;45(Suppl 3):S454–S462

Sepulveda W, Cortes-Yepes H, Wong AE, Dezerega V, Corral E, Malinger G. Prenatal sonography in hydranencephaly: findings during the early stages of disease. J Ultrasound Med 2012;31(5):799–804

Winter TC, Kennedy AM, Byrne J, Woodward PJ. The cavum septi pellucidi: why is it important? J Ultrasound Med 2010;29(3):427–444

■ Case 17

Barkovich AJ, Raybaud C. Pediatric Neuroimaging. 5th ed. Philadelphia, PA: Lippincott Williams & Wilkins; 2012.

Blümcke I, Thom M, Aronica E, et al. The clinicopathologic spectrum of focal cortical dysplasias: a consensus classification proposed by an ad hoc Task Force of the ILAE Diagnostic Methods Commission. Epilepsia 2011;52(1):158–174

Colombo N, Tassi L, Galli C, et al. Focal cortical dysplasias: MR imaging, histopathologic, and clinical correlations in surgically treated patients with epilepsy. AJNR Am J Neuroradiol 2003;24(4):724–733

Kabat J, Król P. Focal cortical dysplasia—review. Pol J Radiol 2012;77(2):35–43

■ Case 18

Saleem SN, Said AH, Lee DH. Lesions of the hypothalamus: MR imaging diagnostic features. RadioGraphics 2007; 27(4):1087–1108

Vézina G. Neuroimaging of phakomatoses: overview and advances. Pediatr Radiol 2015;45(Suppl 3):S433–S442

■ Case 19

Cai W, Kassarjian A, Bredella MA, et al. Tumor burden in patients with neurofibromatosis types 1 and 2 and schwannomatosis: determination on whole-body MR images. Radiology 2009;250(3):665–673

Kissil JL, Blakeley JO, Ferner RE, et al. What's new in neurofibromatosis? Proceedings from the 2009 NF Conference: new frontiers. Am J Med Genet A 2010;152A(2):269–283

■ Case 20

Baron Y, Barkovich AJ. MR imaging of tuberous sclerosis in neonates and young infants. AJNR Am J Neuroradiol 1999;20(5):907–916

Osborn AG. Neurocutaneous syndromes. Osborn's Brain: Imaging, Pathology, and Anatomy. Philadelphia, PA: Lippincott Williams & Wilkins; 2012:1131–1171

Umeoka S, Koyama T, Miki Y, Akai M, Tsutsui K, Togashi K. Pictorial review of tuberous sclerosis in various organs. RadioGraphics 2008;28(7):e32

■ Case 21

Shanbhogue KP, Hoch M, Fatterpaker G, Chandarana H. von Hippel-Lindau disease: review of genetics and imaging. Radiol Clin North Am 2016;54(3):409–422

■ Case 22

Al-Shahi Salman R, Berg MJ, Morrison L, Awad IA; Angioma Alliance Scientific Advisory Board. Hemorrhage from cavernous malformations of the brain: definition and reporting standards. Stroke 2008;39(12):3222–3230

Jeon JS, Kim JE, Chung YS, et al. A risk factor analysis of prospective symptomatic haemorrhage in adult patients with cerebral cavernous malformation. J Neurol Neurosurg Psychiatry 2014;85(12):1366–1370

Nikoubashman O, Di Rocco F, Davagnanam I, Mankad K, Zerah M, Wiesmann M. Prospective hemorrhage rates of cerebral cavernous malformations in children and adolescents based on MRI appearance. AJNR Am J Neuroradiol 2015;36(11):2177–2183

Yun TJ, Na DG, Kwon BJ, et al. A T1 hyperintense perilesional signal aids in the differentiation of a cavernous angioma from other hemorrhagic masses. AJNR Am J Neuroradiol 2008;29(3):494–500

■ Case 23

Abdel Razek AA, Alvarez H, Bagg S, Refaat S, Castillo M. Imaging spectrum of CNS vasculitis. RadioGraphics 2014;34(4):873–894

Marder CP, Donohue MM, Weinstein JR, Fink KR. Multimodal imaging of reversible cerebral vasoconstriction syndrome: a series of 6 cases. AJNR Am J Neuroradiol 2012;33(7):1403–1410

Miller TR, Shivashankar R, Mossa-Basha M, Gandhi D. Reversible cerebral vasoconstriction syndrome, part 2: diagnostic work-up, imaging evaluation, and differential diagnosis. AJNR Am J Neuroradiol 2015;36(9): 1580–1588

Patsalides AD, Atac G, Hedge U, et al. Lymphomatoid granulomatosis: abnormalities of the brain at MR imaging. Radiology 2005;237(1):265–273

■ Case 24
....

Biondi A. Truncal intracranial aneurysms: dissecting and fusiform aneurysms. Neuroimaging Clin N Am 2006;16(3):453–465, viii

Krings T, Choi IS. The many faces of intracranial arterial dissections. Interv Neuroradiol 2010;16(2):151–160

■ Case 25
....

Esnault P, Cardinale M, et al. Blunt cerebrovascular injuries in severe traumatic brain injury: incidence, risk factors, and evolution. J Neurosurg 2016;29:1–7

Flis CM, Jäger HR, Sidhu PS. Carotid and vertebral artery dissections: clinical aspects, imaging features and endovascular treatment. Eur Radiol 2007;17(3):820–834

Galyfos G, Filis K, Sigala F, Sianou A. Traumatic carotid artery dissection: a different entity without specific guidelines. Vasc Spec Int 2016;32(1):1–5

■ Case 26
....

Leach JL, Fortuna RB, Jones BV, Gaskill-Shipley MF. Imaging of cerebral venous thrombosis: current techniques, spectrum of findings, and diagnostic pitfalls. RadioGraphics 2006;26(Suppl 1):S19–S41, discussion S42–S43

Osborn AG. Osborn's Brain: Imaging, Pathology, and Anatomy. Philadelphia, PA: Lippincott Williams & Wilkins; 2012:215–243

■ Case 27
....

Guey S, Tournier-Lasserve E, Hervé D, Kossorotoff M. Moyamoya disease and syndromes: from genetics to clinical management. Appl Clin Genet 2015;8:49–68

Liu W, Xu G, Liu X. Neuroimaging diagnosis and the collateral circulation in moyamoya disease. Interv Neurol 2013;1(2):77–86

■ Case 28
....

Feng C, Xu Y, Bai X, et al. Basilar artery atherosclerosis and hypertensive small vessel disease in isolated pontine infarctions: a study based on high-resolution MRI. Eur Neurol 2013;70(1-2):16–21

Kwon HM, Kim JH, Lim JS, Park JH, Lee SH, Lee YS. Basilar artery dolichoectasia is associated with paramedian pontine infarction. Cerebrovasc Dis 2009;27(2):114–118

■ Case 29
....

Geibprasert S, Pongpech S, Jiarakongmun P, Shroff MM, Armstrong DC, Krings T. Radiologic assessment of brain arteriovenous malformations: what clinicians need to know. RadioGraphics 2010;30(2):483–501

Kumar S, Patel AM, Vaghela DU, Singh K, Solanki RN, Shah HR. The brain arteriovenous malformations (BAVMs): a pictorial essay with emphasis on role of imaging in management. Indian J Radiol Imaging 2006;16:757–764

Osborn AG. Vascular malformations. Osborn's Brain: Imaging, Pathology, and Anatomy. Philadelphia, PA: Lippincott Williams & Wilkins; 2012:135–169

Yousem DM, Grossman RI. Vascular diseases of the brain. Neuroradiology: The Requisites. 3rd ed. Philadelphia, PA: Mosby Elsevier; 2010

■ Case 30
....

Kim LJ, Spetzler RF. Classification and surgical management of spinal arteriovenous lesions: arteriovenous fistulae and arteriovenous malformations. Neurosurgery 2006; 59(5, Suppl 3)S195–S201, discussion S3–S13

Mull M, Nijenhuis RJ, Backes WH, Krings T, Wilmink JT, Thron A. Value and limitations of contrast-enhanced MR angiography in spinal arteriovenous malformations and dural arteriovenous fistulas. AJNR Am J Neuroradiol 2007;28(7):1249–1258

Yang HK, Lee JW, Jo SE, et al. MRI findings of spinal arteriovenous fistulas: focusing on localisation of fistulas and differentiation between spinal dural and perimedullary arteriovenous fistulas. Clin Radiol 2016;71(4):381–388

■ Case 31
....

Briet C, Salenave S, Bonneville JF, Laws ER, Chanson P. Pituitary apoplexy. Endocr Rev 2015;36(6):622–645

Semple PL, Jane JA, Lopes MB, Laws ER. Pituitary apoplexy: correlation between magnetic resonance imaging and histopathological results. J Neurosurg 2008;108(5):909–915

Case 32

Arbelaez A, Castillo M, Mukherji SK. Diffusion-weighted MR imaging of global cerebral anoxia. AJNR Am J Neuroradiol 1999;20(6):999–1007

Huang BY, Castillo M. Hypoxic-ischemic brain injury: imaging findings from birth to adulthood. RadioGraphics 2008;28(2):417–439, quiz 617

Muttikkal TJ, Wintermark M. MRI patterns of global hypoxic-ischemic injury in adults. J Neuroradiol 2013; 40(3):164–171

Case 33

Cianfoni A, Caulo M, Cerase A, et al. Seizure-induced brain lesions: a wide spectrum of variably reversible MRI abnormalities. Eur J Radiol 2013;82(11):1964–1972

Masterson K, Vargas MI, Delavelle J. Postictal deficit mimicking stroke: role of perfusion CT. J Neuroradiol 2009;36(1):48–51

Rupprecht S, Schwab M, Fitzek C, Witte OW, Terborg C, Hagemann G. Hemispheric hypoperfusion in postictal paresis mimics early brain ischemia. Epilepsy Res 2010; 89(2-3):355–359

Case 34

Auriel E, Charidimou A, Gurol ME, et al. Validation of clinicoradiological criteria for the diagnosis of cerebral amyloid angiopathy-related inflammation. JAMA Neurol 2016;73(2):197–202

Yamada M. Cerebral amyloid angiopathy: emerging concepts. J Stroke 2015;17(1):17–30

Case 35

Kumar N. Neuroimaging in superficial siderosis: an in-depth look. AJNR Am J Neuroradiol 2010;31(1):5–14

Osborn AG. Subarachnoid hemorrhage and aneurysms. Osborn's Brain: Imaging, Pathology, and Anatomy. Philadelphia, PA: Lippincott Williams & Wilkins; 2012: 105–135

Rodriguez FR, Srinivasan A. Superficial siderosis of the CNS. AJR Am J Roentgenol 2011;197(1):W149–152

Case 36

Bang OY, Goyal M, Liebeskind DS. Collateral circulation in ischemic stroke: assessment tools and therapeutic strategies. Stroke 2015;46(11):3302–3309

Miller TR, Shivashankar R, Mossa-Basha M, Gandhi D. Reversible cerebral vasoconstriction syndrome, part 2: diagnostic work-up, imaging evaluation, and differential diagnosis. AJNR Am J Neuroradiol 2015;36(9): 1580–1588

Nambiar V, Sohn SI, Almekhlafi MA, et al. CTA collateral status and response to recanalization in patients with acute ischemic stroke. AJNR Am J Neuroradiol 2014; 35(5):884–890

Case 37

Feng C, Xu Y, Bai X, et al. Basilar artery atherosclerosis and hypertensive small vessel disease in isolated pontine infarctions: a study based on high-resolution MRI. Eur Neurol 2013;70(1-2):16–21

Kwon HM, Kim JH, Lim JS, Park JH, Lee SH, Lee YS. Basilar artery dolichoectasia is associated with paramedian pontine infarction. Cerebrovasc Dis 2009;27(2): 114–118

Case 38

Akgun V, Battal B, Bozkurt Y, et al. Normal anatomical features and variations of the vertebrobasilar circulation and its branches: an analysis with 64-detector row CT and 3T MR angiographies. Sci World J 2013;2013: 620162

Dimmick SJ, Faulder KC. Normal variants of the cerebral circulation at multidetector CT angiography. RadioGraphics 2009;29(4):1027–1043

Osborn AG. Arterial anatomy and strokes. Osborn's Brain: Imaging, Pathology, and Anatomy. Philadelphia, PA: Lippincott Williams & Wilkins; 2012:169–215

Yousem DM, Grossman RI. Neuroradiology: The Requisites. 3rd ed. Philadelphia, PA: Mosby Elsevier; 2010

Case 39

Delgado Almandoz JE, Yoo AJ, Stone MJ, et al. The spot sign score in primary intracerebral hemorrhage identifies patients at highest risk of in-hospital mortality and poor outcome among survivors. Stroke 2010; 41(1):54–60

Wada R, Aviv RI, Fox AJ, et al. CT angiography "spot sign" predicts hematoma expansion in acute intracerebral hemorrhage. Stroke 2007;38(4):1257–1262

■ Case 40

Dalesandro MF, Andre JB. Posttreatment evaluation of brain gliomas. Neuroimaging Clin N Am 2016;26(4):581–599

■ Case 41

Kim DH, Kim JH, Choi SH, et al. Differentiation between intramedullary spinal ependymoma and astrocytoma: comparative MRI analysis. Clin Radiol 2014;69(1):29–35

Koeller KK, Rosenblum RS, Morrison AL. Neoplasms of the spinal cord and filum terminale: radiologic-pathologic correlation. RadioGraphics 2000;20(6):1721–1749

Yuh EL, Barkovich AJ, Gupta N. Imaging of ependymomas: MRI and CT. Childs Nerv Syst 2009;25(10):1203–1213

■ Case 42

Poretti A, Meoded A, Huisman TA. Neuroimaging of pediatric posterior fossa tumors including review of the literature. J Magn Reson Imaging 2012;35(1):32–47

Rasalkar DD, Chu WC, Paunipagar BK, Cheng FW, Li CK. Paediatric intra-axial posterior fossa tumours: pictorial review. Postgrad Med J 2013;89(1047):39–46

Zamora C, Huisman TA, Izbudak I. Supratentorial tumors in pediatric patients. Neuroimaging Clin N Am 2017;27(1):39–67

■ Case 43

Castillo M, Davis PC, Takei Y, Hoffman JC Jr. Intracranial ganglioglioma: MR, CT, and clinical findings in 18 patients. AJR Am J Roentgenol 1990;154(3):607–612

Koeller KK, Henry JM; Armed Forces Institute of Pathology. From the archives of the AFIP: superficial gliomas: radiologic-pathologic correlation. RadioGraphics 2001;21(6):1533–1556

Provenzale JM, Ali U, Barboriak DP, Kallmes DF, Delong DM, McLendon RE. Comparison of patient age with MR imaging features of gangliogliomas. AJR Am J Roentgenol 2000;174(3):859–862

■ Case 44

Osborn AG. Pineal and germ cell tumors. Osborn's Brain: Imaging, Pathology, and Anatomy. Philadelphia, PA: Lippincott Williams & Wilkins; 2012:539–561

Smirniotopoulos JG, Rushing EJ, Mena H. Pineal region masses: differential diagnosis. RadioGraphics 1992;12(3):577–596

Smith AB, Rushing EJ, Smirniotopoulos JG. From the archives of the AFIP: lesions of the pineal region: radiologic-pathologic correlation. RadioGraphics 2010;30(7):2001–2020

Yousem DM, Grossman RI. Neuroradiology: The Requisites. 3rd ed. Philadelphia, PA: Mosby Elsevier; 2010

■ Case 45

Agarwal A, Kanekar S. Intraventricular tumors. Semin Ultrasound CT MR 2016;37(2):150–158

Vandesteen L, Drier A, Galanaud D, et al. Imaging findings of intraventricular and ependymal lesions. J Neuroradiol 2013;40(4):229–244

■ Case 46

Choi SH, Kwon BJ, Na DG, Kim JH, Han MH, Chang KH. Pituitary adenoma, craniopharyngioma, and Rathke cleft cyst involving both intrasellar and suprasellar regions: differentiation using MRI. Clin Radiol 2007;62(5):453–462

Garnett MR, Puget S, Grill J, Sainte-Rose C. Craniopharyngioma. Orphanet J Rare Dis 2007;2:18

Lubuulwa J, Lei T. Pathological and topographical classification of craniopharyngiomas: a literature review. J Neurol Surg Rep 2016;77(3):e121–e127

■ Case 47

Griessenauer CJ, Rizk E, Miller JH, et al. Pediatric tectal plate gliomas: clinical and radiological progression, MR imaging characteristics, and management of hydrocephalus. J Neurosurg Pediatr 2014;13(1):13–20

Osborn AG. Astrocytomas. Osborn's Brain: Imaging, Pathology, and Anatomy. Philadelphia, PA: Lippincott Williams & Wilkins; 2012:453–493

Poussaint TY, Kowal JR, Barnes PD, et al. Tectal tumors of childhood: clinical and imaging follow-up. AJNR Am J Neuroradiol 1998;19(5):977–983

Smith AB, Rushing EJ, Smirniotopoulos JG. From the archives of the AFIP: lesions of the pineal region: radiologic-pathologic correlation. RadioGraphics 2010; 30(7):2001–2020

Yousem DM, Grossman RI. Neuroradiology: The Requisites. 3rd ed. Philadelphia, PA: Mosby Elsevier; 2010

■ Case 48

Gonçalves VT, Reis F, Queiroz LdeS, França M Jr. Pleomorphic xanthoastrocytoma: magnetic resonance imaging findings in a series of cases with histopathological confirmation. Arq Neuropsiquiatr 2013;71(1):35–39

Moore W, Mathis D, Gargan L, et al. Pleomorphic xanthoastrocytoma of childhood: MR imaging and diffusion MR imaging features. AJNR Am J Neuroradiol 2014;35(11):2192–2196

Raz E, Zagzag D, Saba L, et al. Cyst with a mural nodule tumor of the brain. Cancer Imaging 2012;12:237–244

■ Case 49

Johnson DR, Diehn FE, Giannini C, et al. Genetically defined oligodendroglioma is characterized by indistinct tumor borders at MRI. AJNR Am J Neuroradiol 2017;38(4): 678–684

■ Case 50

Altman DA, Atkinson DS Jr, Brat DJ. Best cases from the AFIP: glioblastoma multiforme. RadioGraphics 2007;27(3):883–888

Louis DN, Perry A, Reifenberger G, et al. The 2016 World Health Organization Classification of tumors of the central nervous system: a summary. Acta Neuropathol 2016;131(6):803–820

Osborn AG. Nonneoplastic cysts. Osborn's Brain: Imaging, Pathology, and Anatomy. Philadelphia, PA: Lippincott Williams & Wilkins; 2012

Yousem DM, Grossman RI. Neuroradiology: The Requisites. 3rd ed. Philadelphia, PA: Mosby Elsevier; 2010

■ Case 51

Macellari F, Paciaroni M, Agnelli G, Caso V. Neuroimaging in intracerebral hemorrhage. Stroke 2014;45(3):903–908

Patnana M, Bronstein Y, Szklaruk J, et al. Multimethod imaging, staging, and spectrum of manifestations of metastatic melanoma. Clin Radiol 2011;66(3):224–236

■ Case 52

Park MS, Suh DC, Choi WS, Lee SY, Kang GH. Multifocal meningioangiomatosis: a report of two cases. AJNR Am J Neuroradiol 1999;20(4):677–680

Strojan P, Popović M, Jereb B. Secondary intracranial meningiomas after high-dose cranial irradiation: report of five cases and review of the literature. Int J Radiat Oncol Biol Phys 2000;48(1):65–73

■ Case 53

Chung EM, Specht CS, Schroeder JW. From the archives of the AFIP: pediatric orbit tumors and tumorlike lesions: neuroepithelial lesions of the ocular globe and optic nerve. RadioGraphics 2007;27(4):1159–1186

Kornreich L, Blaser S, Schwarz M, et al. Optic pathway glioma: correlation of imaging findings with the presence of neurofibromatosis. AJNR Am J Neuroradiol 2001;22(10):1963–1969

Yousem DM, Grossman RI. Neuroradiology: The Requisites. 3rd ed. Philadelphia, PA: Mosby Elsevier; 2010

■ Case 54

Vandesteen L, Drier A, Galanaud D, et al. Imaging findings of intraventricular and ependymal lesions. J Neuroradiol 2013;40(4):229–244

■ Case 55

Fukui MB, Meltzer CC, Kanal E, Smirniotopoulos JG. MR imaging of the meninges. Part II. Neoplastic disease. Radiology 1996;201(3):605–612

Fukuoka H, Hirai T, Okuda T, et al. Comparison of the added value of contrast-enhanced 3D fluid-attenuated inversion recovery and magnetization-prepared rapid acquisition of gradient echo sequences in relation to conventional postcontrast T1-weighted images for the evaluation of leptomeningeal diseases at 3T. AJNR Am J Neuroradiol 2010;31(5):868–873

◼ Case 56

Erdem E, Angtuaco EC, Van Hemert R, Park JS, Al-Mefty O. Comprehensive review of intracranial chordoma. RadioGraphics 2003;23(4):995–1009

Oot RF, Melville GE, New PFJ, et al. The role of MR and CT in evaluating clival chordomas and chondrosarcomas. AJR Am J Roentgenol 1988;151(3):567–575

Osborn AG. Miscellaneous tumors and tumor-like conditions. Osborn's Brain: Imaging, Pathology, and Anatomy. Philadelphia, PA: Lippincott Williams & Wilkins; 2012:727–745

Yeom KW, Lober RM, Mobley BC, et al. Diffusion-weighted MRI: distinction of skull base chordoma from chondrosarcoma. AJNR Am J Neuroradiol 2013;34(5): 1056–1061, S1

◼ Case 57

Bonneville F, Savatovsky J, Chiras J. Imaging of cerebello-pontine angle lesions: an update. Part 2: intra-axial lesions, skull base lesions that may invade the CPA region, and non-enhancing extra-axial lesions. Eur Radiol 2007; 17(11):2908–2920

Demir MK, Yapıcıer O, Onat E, et al. Rare and challenging extra-axial brain lesions: CT and MRI findings with clinico-radiological differential diagnosis and pathological correlation. Diagn Interv Radiol 2014;20(5):448–452

◼ Case 58

Kim DY, Lee JH, Goh MJ, et al. Clinical significance of an increased cochlear 3D fluid-attenuated inversion recovery signal intensity on an MR imaging examination in patients with acoustic neuroma. AJNR Am J Neuroradiol 2014;35(9):1825–1829

Lakshmi M, Glastonbury CM. Imaging of the cerebellopontine angle. Neuroimaging Clin N Am 2009;19(3):393–406

◼ Case 59

Angtuaco EJC, Fassas ABT, Walker R, Sethi R, Barlogie B. Multiple myeloma: clinical review and diagnostic imaging. Radiology 2004;231(1):11–23

Lloret I, Server A, Taksdal I. Calvarial lesions: a radiological approach to diagnosis. Acta Radiol 2009;50(5):531–542

Major NM, Helms CA, Richardson WJ. The "mini brain": plasmacytoma in a vertebral body on MR imaging. AJR Am J Roentgenol 2000;175(1):261–263

◼ Case 60

Maulucci CM, Ghobrial GM, Oppenlander ME, Flanders AE, Vaccaro AR, Harrop JS. Arachnoiditis ossificans: clinical series and review of the literature. Clin Neurol Neurosurg 2014;124:16–20

Petty PG, Hudgson P, Hare WS. Symptomatic lumbar spinal arachnoiditis: fact or fallacy? J Clin Neurosci 2000;7(5): 395–399

◼ Case 61

Cugati G, Singh M, Pande A, et al. Primary spinal epidural lymphomas. J Craniovertebr Junction Spine 2011;2(1): 3–11

Gala FB, Aswani Y. Imaging in spinal posterior epidural space lesions: a pictorial essay. Indian J Radiol Imaging 2016;26(3):299–315

Gold M. Magnetic resonance imaging of spinal emergencies. Top Magn Reson Imaging 2015;24(6):325–330

◼ Case 62

Gouliouris T, Aliyu SH, Brown NM. Spondylodiscitis: update on diagnosis and management. J Antimicrob Chemother 2010;65(Suppl 3):iii11–iii24

Hong SH, Choi JY, Lee JW, Kim NR, Choi JA, Kang HS. MR imaging assessment of the spine: infection or an imitation? RadioGraphics 2009;29(2):599–612

Yousem DM, Grossman RI. Neuroradiology: The Requisites. 3rd ed. Philadelphia, PA: Mosby Elsevier; 2010

◼ Case 63

Smirniotopoulos JG, Murphy FM, Rushing EJ, Rees JH, Schroeder JW. From the archives of the AFIP: patterns of contrast enhancement in the brain and meninges RadioGraphics 2007;27:525–551

◼ Case 64

Jain KK, Mittal SK, Kumar S, Gupta RK. Imaging features of central nervous system fungal infections. Neurol India 2007;55(3):241–250

Shih RY, Koeller KK. Bacterial, fungal, and parasitic infections of the central nervous system: radiologic-pathologic correlation and historical perspectives. RadioGraphics 2015;35(4):1141–1169

Starkey J, Moritani T, Kirby P. MRI of CNS fungal infections: review of aspergillosis to histoplasmosis and everything in between. Clin Neuroradiol 2014;24(3):217–230

■ Case 65

Suwan PT, Mogal S, Chaudhary S. Pott's puffy tumor: an uncommon clinical entity. Case Rep Pediatr 2012;2012: 386104

■ Case 66

Kline LB, Hoyt WF. The Tolosa-Hunt syndrome. J Neurol Neurosurg Psychiatry 2001;71(5):577–582

Wasmeier C, Pfadenhauer K, Rösler A. Idiopathic inflammatory pseudotumor of the orbit and Tolosa-Hunt syndrome—are they the same disease? J Neurol 2002;249(9):1237–1241

■ Case 67

Kastrup O, Wanke I, Maschke M. Neuroimaging of infections. NeuroRx 2005;2(2):324–332

Osborn AG. Congenital, acquired pyogenic, and acquired viral infections Osborn's Brain: Imaging, Pathology, and Anatomy. Philadelphia, PA: Lippincott Williams & Wilkins; 2012:297–337

Smirniotopoulos JG, Murphy FM, Rushing EJ, Rees JH, Schroeder JW. Patterns of contrast enhancement in the brain and meninges. RadioGraphics 2007;27(2):525–551

Yousem DM, Grossman RI. Neuroradiology: The Requisites. 3rd ed. Philadelphia, PA: Mosby Elsevier; 2010

■ Case 68

Finelli PF, Foxman EB. The etiology of ring lesions on diffusion-weighted imaging. Neuroradiol J 2014;27(3): 280–287

Kapsalaki EZ, Gotsis ED, Fountas KN. The role of proton magnetic resonance spectroscopy in the diagnosis and categorization of cerebral abscesses. Neurosurg Focus 2008;24(6):E7

Lai PH, Weng HH, Chen CY, et al. In vivo differentiation of aerobic brain abscesses and necrotic glioblastomas multiforme using proton MR spectroscopic imaging. AJNR Am J Neuroradiol 2008;29(8):1511–1518

Whang JS, Kolber M, Powell DK, Libfeld E. Diffusion-weighted signal patterns of intracranial haemorrhage. Clin Radiol 2015;70(8):909–916

■ Case 69

Gottumukkala RV, Romero JM, Riascos RF, Rojas R, Glikstein RS. Imaging of the brain in patients with human immunodeficiency virus infection. Top Magn Reson Imaging 2014;23(5):275–291

Smith AB, Smirniotopoulos JG, Rushing EJ. From the archives of the AFIP: central nervous system infections associated with human immunodeficiency virus infection: radiologic-pathologic correlation. RadioGraphics 2008;28:2033–2058

■ Case 70

Osborn AG. HIV/AIDS. Osborn's Brain: Imaging, Pathology, and Anatomy. Philadelphia, PA: Lippincott Williams & Wilkins; 2012:375–405

Smith AB, Smirniotopoulos JG, Rushing EJ. From the archives of the AFIP: central nervous system infections associated with human immunodeficiency virus infection: radiologic-pathologic correlation. RadioGraphics 2008;28(7):2033–2058

Yousem DM, Grossman RI. Neuroradiology: The Requisites. 3rd ed. Philadelphia, PA: Mosby Elsevier; 2010

■ Case 71

Bowen LN, Smith B, Reich D, Quezado M, Nath A. HIV-associated opportunistic CNS infections: pathophysiology, diagnosis and treatment. Nat Rev Neurol 2016;12(11):662–674

Nakae Y, Kudo Y, Yamamoto R, Johkura K. Pseudo-subarachnoid hemorrhage in cryptococcal meningitis: MRI findings and pathological study. Neurol Sci 2013; 34(12):2227–2229

■ Case 72

Gottumukkala RV, Romero JM, Riascos RF, Rojas R, Glikstein RS. Imaging of the brain in patients with human immunodeficiency virus infection. Top Magn Reson Imaging 2014;23(5):275–291

Smith AB, Smirniotopoulos JG, Rushing EJ. From the archives of the AFIP: central nervous system infections associated with human immunodeficiency virus infection: radiologic-pathologic correlation. RadioGraphics 2008;28(7):2033–2058

■ Case 73

Kimura-Hayama ET, Higuera JA, Corona-Cedillo R, et al. Neurocysticercosis: radiologic-pathologic correlation. RadioGraphics 2010;30(6):1705–1719

Shih RY, Koeller KK. Bacterial, fungal, and parasitic infections of the central nervous system: radiologic-pathologic correlation and historical perspectives. RadioGraphics 2015;35(4):1141–1169

■ Case 74

Berger JR, Aksamit AJ, Clifford DB, et al. PML diagnostic criteria: consensus statement from the AAN Neuroinfectious Disease Section. Neurology 2013;80(15): 1430–1438

Sahraian MA, Radue EW, Eshaghi A, Besliu S, Minagar A. Progressive multifocal leukoencephalopathy: a review of the neuroimaging features and differential diagnosis. Eur J Neurol 2012;19(8):1060–1069

■ Case 75

Silvera S, Oppenheim C, Touzé E, et al. Spontaneous intracerebral hematoma on diffusion-weighted images: influence of T2-shine-through and T2-blackout effects. AJNR Am J Neuroradiol 2005;26(2):236–241

Young RJ, Destian S. Imaging of traumatic intracranial hemorrhage. Neuroimaging Clin N Am 2002;12(2):189–204

■ Case 76

Riascos R, Bonfante E, Cotes C, Guirguis M, Hakimelahi R, West C. Imaging of atlanto-occipital and atlantoaxial traumatic injuries: what the radiologist needs to know. RadioGraphics 2015;35(7):2121–2134

■ Case 77

Leypold BG, Flanders AE, Burns AS. The early evolution of spinal cord lesions on MR imaging following traumatic spinal cord injury. AJNR Am J Neuroradiol 2008;29(5): 1012–1016

Mahajan P, Jaffe DM, Olsen CS, et al. Spinal cord injury without radiologic abnormality in children imaged with magnetic resonance imaging. J Trauma Acute Care Surg 2013;75(5):843–847

Miyanji F, Furlan JC, Aarabi B, Arnold PM, Fehlings MG. Acute cervical traumatic spinal cord injury: MR imaging findings correlated with neurologic outcome—prospective study with 100 consecutive patients. Radiology 2007;243(3):820–827

Potter K, Saifuddin A. Pictorial review: MRI of chronic spinal cord injury. Br J Radiol 2003;76(905):347–352

■ Case 78

Osborn AG. Secondary effects and sequelae of CNS trauma. Osborn's Brain: Imaging, Pathology, and Anatomy. Philadelphia, PA: Lippincott Williams & Wilkins; 2012:51–73

Yousem DM, Grossman RI. Neuroradiology: The Requisites. 3rd ed. Philadelphia, PA: Mosby Elsevier; 2010

■ Case 79

Cicala D, Briganti F, Casale L, et al. Atraumatic vertebral compression fractures: differential diagnosis between benign osteoporotic and malignant fractures by MRI. Musculoskelet Surg 2013;97(Suppl 2):S169–S179

Jung HS, Jee WH, McCauley TR, Ha KY, Choi KH. Discrimination of metastatic from acute osteoporotic compression spinal fractures with MR imaging. RadioGraphics 2003;23(1):179–187

■ Case 80

Currie S, Saleem N, Straiton JA, Macmullen-Price J, Warren DJ, Craven IJ. Imaging assessment of traumatic brain injury. Postgrad Med J 2016;92(1083):41–50

Kuo KH, Pan YJ, Lai YJ, Cheung WK, Chang FC, Jarosz J. Dynamic MR imaging patterns of cerebral fat embolism: a systematic review with illustrative cases. AJNR Am J Neuroradiol 2014;35(6):1052–1057

Liu J, Kou Z, Tian Y. Diffuse axonal injury after traumatic cerebral microbleeds: an evaluation of imaging techniques. Neural Regen Res 2014;9(12):1222–1230

Mechtler LL, Shastri KK, Crutchfield KE. Advanced neuroimaging of mild traumatic brain injury. Neurol Clin 2014;32(1):31–58

■ Case 81

Lopez AJ, Scheer JK, Smith ZA, Dahdaleh NS. Management of flexion distraction injuries to the thoracolumbar spine. J Clin Neurosci 2015;22(12):1853–1856

Swischuk LE, Jadhav SP, Chung DH. Aortic injury with Chance fracture in a child. Emerg Radiol 2008;15(5):285–287

Vaccaro AR, Oner C, Kepler CK, et al; AOSpine Spinal Cord Injury & Trauma Knowledge Forum. AOSpine thoracolumbar spine injury classification system: fracture description, neurological status, and key modifiers. Spine 2013;38(23):2028–2037

■ Case 82

Vaccaro AR, Hulbert RJ, Patel AA, et al; Spine Trauma Study Group. The subaxial cervical spine injury classification system: a novel approach to recognize the importance of morphology, neurology, and integrity of the disco-ligamentous complex. Spine 2007;32(21):2365–2374

■ Case 83

Bernstein MP, Baxter AB. Cervical spine trauma: pearls and pitfalls. ARRS Categorical Course 2012:21–25

Rao SK, Wasyliw C, Nunez DB Jr. Spectrum of imaging findings in hyperextension injuries of the neck. RadioGraphics 2005;25(5):1239–1254

■ Case 84

Bodanapally UK, Sours C, Zhuo J, Shanmuganathan K. Imaging of traumatic brain injury. Radiol Clin North Am 2015;53(4):695–715, viii

Wintermark M, Sanelli PC, Anzai Y, Tsiouris AJ, Whitlow CT; ACR Head Injury Institute; ACR Head Injury Institute. Imaging evidence and recommendations for traumatic brain injury: conventional neuroimaging techniques. J Am Coll Radiol 2015;12(2):e1–e14

■ Case 85

Filippi M, Rocca MA, Ciccarelli O, et al; MAGNIMS Study Group. MRI criteria for the diagnosis of multiple sclerosis: MAGNIMS consensus guidelines. Lancet Neurol 2016;15(3):292–303

Grueter BE, Schulz UG. Age-related cerebral white matter disease (leukoaraiosis): a review. Postgrad Med J 2012; 88(1036):79–87

Miller TR, Mohan S, Choudhri AF, Gandhi D, Jindal G. Advances in multiple sclerosis and its variants: conventional and newer imaging techniques. Radiol Clin North Am 2014;52(2):321–336

Okuda DT. Incidental lesions suggesting multiple sclerosis. Continuum (Minneap Minn) 2016;22(3):730–743

■ Case 86

Dudesek A, Rimmele F, Tesar S, et al. CLIPPERS: chronic lymphocytic inflammation with pontine perivascular enhancement responsive to steroids. Review of an increasingly recognized entity within the spectrum of inflammatory central nervous system disorders. Clin Exp Immunol 2014;175(3):385–396

Hou X, Wang X, Xie B, et al. Horizontal eyeball akinesia as an initial manifestation of CLIPPERS: case report and review of literature. Medicine (Baltimore) 2016;95(34): e4640

Simon NG, Parratt JD, Barnett MH, et al. Expanding the clinical, radiological and neuropathological phenotype of chronic lymphocytic inflammation with pontine perivascular enhancement responsive to steroids (CLIPPERS). J Neurol Neurosurg Psychiatry 2012;83(1):15–22

■ Case 87

Wan H, He H, Zhang F, Sha Y, Tian G. Diffusion-weighted imaging helps differentiate multiple sclerosis and neuromyelitis optica-related acute optic neuritis. J Magn Reson Imaging 2017;45(6):1780–1785

■ Case 88

Alblas CL, Bouvy WH, Lycklama À Nijeholt GJ, Boiten J. Acute spinal-cord ischemia: evolution of MRI findings. J Clin Neurol 2012;8(3):218–223

Masson C, Pruvo JP, Meder JF, et al; Study Group on Spinal Cord Infarction of the French Neurovascular Society. Spinal cord infarction: clinical and magnetic resonance imaging findings and short term outcome. J Neurol Neurosurg Psychiatry 2004;75(10):1431–1435

Poe LB. The owl's eyes sign. Radsource, March 2015. http://radsource.us/the-owls-eyes-sign/

■ Case 89

Abiola R, Rubery P, Mesfin A. Ossification of the posterior longitudinal ligament: etiology, diagnosis, and outcomes of nonoperative and operative management. Global Spine J 2016;6(2):195–204

Saetia K, Cho D, Lee S, Kim DH, Kim SD. Ossification of the posterior longitudinal ligament: a review. Neurosurg Focus 2011;30(3):E1

Sartip KA, Dong T, Ndukwe M, et al. Ossification of the posterior longitudinal ligament: imaging findings in the era of cross-sectional imaging. J Comput Assist Tomogr 2015;39(6):835–841

■ Case 90

Bartynski WS. Posterior reversible encephalopathy syndrome, part 1: fundamental imaging and clinical features. AJNR Am J Neuroradiol 2008;29(6):1036–1042

Schweitzer AD, Parikh NS, Askin G, et al. Imaging characteristics associated with clinical outcomes in posterior reversible encephalopathy syndrome. Neuroradiology 2017;59(4):379–386

■ Case 91

Goyal M, Versnick E, Tuite P, et al. Hypertrophic olivary degeneration: metaanalysis of the temporal evolution of MR findings. AJNR Am J Neuroradiol 2000;21(6): 1073–1077

Yousem DM, Grossman RI. Neuroradiology: The Requisites. 3rd ed. Philadelphia, PA: Mosby Elsevier; 2010

■ Case 92

Dhanwal DK, Sharma AK. Brain and optic chiasmal herniations into sella after cabergoline therapy of giant prolactinoma. Pituitary 2011;14(4):384–387

Kaufman B, Tomsak RL, Kaufman BA, et al. Herniation of the suprasellar visual system and third ventricle into empty sellae: morphologic and clinical considerations. AJR Am J Roentgenol 1989;152(3):597–608

Saindane AM, Lim PP, Aiken A, Chen Z, Hudgins PA. Factors determining the clinical significance of an "empty" sella turcica. AJR Am J Roentgenol 2013;200:1125–1131

■ Case 93

Rovira A, Alonso J, Córdoba J. MR imaging findings in hepatic encephalopathy. AJNR Am J Neuroradiol 2008;29(9):1612–1621

Sharma P, Eesa M, Scott JN. Toxic and acquired metabolic encephalopathies: MRI appearance. AJR Am J Roentgenol 2009;193(3):879–886

U-King-Im JM, Yu E, Bartlett E, Soobrah R, Kucharczyk W. Acute hyperammonemic encephalopathy in adults: imaging findings. AJNR Am J Neuroradiol 2011;32(2): 413–418

Willson KJ, Nott LM, Broadbridge VT, Price T. Hepatic encephalopathy associated with cancer or anticancer therapy. Gastrointest Cancer Res 2013;6(1):11–16

■ Case 94

Bote RP, Blázquez-Llorca L, Fernández-Gil MA, Alonso-Nanclares L, Muñoz A, De Felipe J. Hippocampal sclerosis: histopathology substrate and magnetic resonance imaging. Semin Ultrasound CT MR 2008;29(1):2–14

da Rocha AJ, Nunes RH, Maia ACM Jr, do Amaral LLF. Recognizing autoimmune-mediated encephalitis in the differential diagnosis of limbic disorders. AJNR Am J Neuroradiol 2015;36(12):2196–2205

Van Paesschen W. Qualitative and quantitative imaging of the hippocampus in mesial temporal lobe epilepsy with hippocampal sclerosis. Neuroimaging Clin N Am 2004;14(3):373–400, vii

■ Case 95

Hardy TA, Tobin WO, Lucchinetti CF. Exploring the overlap between multiple sclerosis, tumefactive demyelination and Baló's concentric sclerosis. Mult Scler 2016;22(8):986–992

Karaarslan E, Altintas A, Senol U, et al. Baló's concentric sclerosis: clinical and radiologic features of five cases. AJNR Am J Neuroradiol 2001;22(7):1362–1367

Pietroboni AM, Arighi A, De Riz MA, et al. Baló's concentric sclerosis: still to be considered as a variant of multiple sclerosis? Neurol Sci 2015;36(12):2277–2280

■ Case 96

Angtuaco EJC, Fassas ABT, Walker R, Sethi R, Barlogie B. Multiple myeloma: clinical review and diagnostic imaging. Radiology 2004;231(1):11–23

Hanrahan CJ, Christensen CR, Crim JR. Current concepts in the evaluation of multiple myeloma with MR imaging and FDG PET/CT. RadioGraphics 2010;30(1):127–142

Healy CF, Murray JG, Eustace SJ, Madewell J, O'Gorman PJ, O'Sullivan P. Multiple myeloma: a review of imaging features and radiological techniques. Bone Marrow Res 2011;2011:583439

Yousem DM, Grossman RI. Neuroradiology: The Requisites. 3rd ed. Philadelphia, PA: Mosby Elsevier; 2010

■ Case 97

Ruzevick J, Kleinberg L, Rigamonti D. Imaging changes following stereotactic radiosurgery for metastatic intracranial tumors: differentiating pseudoprogression from tumor progression and its effect on clinical practice. Neurosurg Rev 2014;37(2):193–201, discussion 201

Shah R, Vattoth S, Jacob R, et al. Radiation necrosis in the brain: imaging features and differentiation from tumor recurrence. RadioGraphics 2012;32(5):1343–1359

Sundgren PC. MR spectroscopy in radiation injury. AJNR Am J Neuroradiol 2009;30(8):1469–1476

■ Case 98

Apostolaki E, Davies AM, Evans N, Cassar-Pullicino VN. MR imaging of lumbar facet joint synovial cysts. Eur Radiol 2000;10(4):615–623

Cambron SC, McIntyre JJ, Guerin SJ, Li Z, Pastel DA. Lumbar facet joint synovial cysts: does T2 signal intensity predict outcomes after percutaneous rupture? AJNR Am J Neuroradiol 2013;34(8):1661–1664

■ Case 99

Fardon DF, Williams AL, Dohring EJ, Murtagh FR, Gabriel Rothman SL, Sze GK. Lumbar disc nomenclature: version 2.0: recommendations of the combined task forces of the North American Spine Society, the American Society of Spine Radiology, and the American Society of Neuroradiology. Spine 2014;39(24): E1448–E1465

Williams AL, Murtagh FR, Rothman SL, Sze GK. Lumbar disc nomenclature: version 2.0. AJNR Am J Neuroradiol 2014;35(11):2029

■ Case 100

Lowe LH, Booth TN, Joglar JM, Rollins NK. Midface anomalies in children. RadioGraphics 2000;20(4):907–922, quiz 1106–1107, 1112

Morón FE, Morriss MC, Jones JJ, Hunter JV. Lumps and bumps on the head in children: use of CT and MR imaging in solving the clinical diagnostic dilemma. RadioGraphics 2004;24(6):1655–1674

Index

Locators refer to case number. Locators in boldface indicate primary diagnosis.